Revision Total Knee Arthroplasty

Hosam E. Matar • Benjamin V. Bloch •
Hugh U. Cameron • Peter J. James

Revision Total Knee Arthroplasty

A Practical Guide

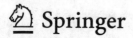

Hosam E. Matar
Nottingham Elective Orthopaedic Services
Nottingham University Hospitals NHS Trust
Nottingham, UK

Benjamin V. Bloch
Nottingham Elective Orthopaedic Services
Nottingham University Hospitals NHS Trust
Nottingham, UK

Hugh U. Cameron
Sunnybrook Health Sciences Centre
University of Toronto
Toronto, Canada

Peter J. James
Nottingham Elective Orthopaedic Services
Nottingham University Hospitals NHS Trust
Nottingham, UK

ISBN 978-3-030-81287-4   ISBN 978-3-030-81285-0   (eBook)
https://doi.org/10.1007/978-3-030-81285-0

This Springer imprint is published by the registered company Springer Nature Switzerland AG
The registered company address is: Gewerbestrasse 11, 6330 Cham, Switzerland

Foreword I

In the lower extremity arthroplasty arena, I have seen no greater advancement in my 35 years of practice than in the field of revision total knee arthroplasty. "Revision Total knee Arthroplasty: A Practical Guide" is published at an opportune time where the present state of many advances in revision knee arthroplasty technique has matured to the point where expert surgeons and clinical investigators have optimized these newly developed techniques and even more importantly, in this "evidence based" era of medicine, accumulated carefully defined outcomes of these techniques to help the surgeon and patient understand the results of treatment that can be expected. The worldly recognized surgeons in the field of revision knee arthroplasty who have edited this book, Matar, Bloch, Cameron and James, have drawn on decades of their own experience to provide an international perspective on this subject.

There is no greater challenge than in revision knee surgery where a toolbox of options is needed to obtain a successful outcome. "Revision Total Knee Arthroplasty: A Practical Guide" has outlined, in a novel and organized way, the preoperative considerations, intraoperative assessment, preparation of the bony and ligamentous anatomy, and the decision-making process and execution of the reconstruction needed for a surgeon to obtain a successful and durable revision arthroplasty outcome. The novelty of the editors' approach is in the uniform structure of the chapters. Each chapter begins with a thought-provoking quote. This is followed by a brief summary of the chapter objectives. They go on to combine surgical, pre- and intraoperative planning and thought processes, detailed intraoperative execution and postoperative considerations needed to for the success of the subject matter they outline. Data available in the literature and the authors' own data, from their experience with the content presented, is dispersed throughout the chapters. Techniques are demonstrated with detailed illustrations and high-quality intraoperative photos. Each chapter has voluminous case examples with high-resolution preoperative, intraoperative, postoperative and follow-up radiographs. Finally, Top Tips are outlined in bold throughout the text. Compliments also go to the Springer Nature production team for these detailed and organized layouts.

Reviewing the table of contents, the reader observes a thorough outline of the essentials, including principles learned from routine and complex primary arthroplasty surgery, to plan, perform and rehabilitate revision arthroplasty cases. The chapter on historical challenges of these procedures in the beginning demonstrates how far we have come in this discipline of revision surgery. Detailed aspects of indications, preoperative planning, pain management, removal of components, soft tissue and component reconstruction (including all of the various successfully proven options available today), and rehabilitation are described and illustrated along with the up-to-date results of the various procedures. Salvage procedures, including cases with large defects, as well as options for infected cases and treatment of periprosthetic fractures are described and illustrated (both with high-resolution serial radiographs and intraoperative photos of illustrative cases). Reflection on the advancements made over the last three to four decades through the eyes of two experienced senior surgeons is a fitting epilogue to the book.

"Revision Total Knee Arthroplasty: A Practical Guide" should provide practical solutions for arthroplasty surgeons (whether they be in high- or low-volume revision practices) and their patients in need of revision knee arthroplasty through this global perspective.

John J. Callaghan M.D.
The Lawrence and Marilyn Dorr
Emeritus Chair, Immediate Past
President, US Knee Society
University of Iowa
Iowa City, US

Foreword II

Revision knee arthroplasty is one of the technically and surgically most demanding techniques in musculoskeletal surgery. The challenge starts with surgical planning, e.g. cementless or cemented stems, the need for additional metaphyseal fixation with sleeves, bone reconstruction with cement or allograft or wedges, the amount of constraint and much more. Hence, there is a tremendous need for a comprehensive guide covering all aspects of revision total knee arthroplasty (rTKA).

Theoretical knowledge and clinical experience are the most important factors of success today. The combination of lessons learned over the past decades and the latest scientific findings offered by four of the most experienced revision knee surgeons is an exceptional strength of this book. The reasons for failure of TKA have changed over the past few years, with wear and implant fractures disappearing almost completely. Better imaging modalities and increasing knowledge of serologic markers to identify not only infection but also metal wear and corrosion have changed surgical strategies. The need for an enhanced implant design to reach a virtually natural behaviour is much better understood today. Furthermore, revision knees like primary knees need a radius of curvature that allows a more physiological roll-back. Better ingrowth surfaces by 3D printing, new concepts for implant fixation together with a longer follow-up of the established techniques will allow us to better predict clinical results and achieve longer survival rates if our technologies are used in a proper manner.

The authors of *Revision Total Knee Arthroplasty: A Practical Guide* have done a remarkable job of compiling the most up-to-date knowledge of surgical techniques and underlying theoretical knowledge for successful revision knee arthroplasty.

The book includes their clinical experience as well as the results of their scientific work, which is why it is a perfect source for every revision knee arthroplasty surgeon today. Every aspect of revision total knee arthroplasty has been addressed and detailed practical insights into all aspects of this field will help solve different challenges of every individual case. Tips and tricks for surgery, intraoperative photos and X-rays are included in well-organized and well-structured chapters.

In conclusion, I would therefore like to congratulate the authors on a remarkably well-done guide and recommend it to all general orthopaedic surgeons as well as specialist knee arthroplasty surgeons. This book serves as an excellent source for advice in practical work and for continuous improvement of clinical results.

Carsten Perka
Chair, Orthopaedic Department
Director, Center for Musculoskeletal Surgery
Charité - Universitätsmedizin Berlin
Berlin, Germany

Foreword III

Revision Total Knee Arthroplasty: A Practical Guide

The continued growth of knee arthroplasty surgery around the world has been driven by successful clinical outcomes. Despite the excellent survivorship of knee replacements, primary surgery inevitably leads to revision surgery in a proportion of cases. The management of these unfortunate patients presents a significant challenge both with the surgical decision-making, as well as the complexity of operative intervention, and specifically the variety of skills, techniques and implants that surgeons need to be familiar with.

Therefore, this new book—Revision total knee arthroplasty: A Practical Guide —is a welcome addition for knee surgeons around the world. Importantly it focuses on practical issues that arise from managing the many different reasons why revision surgery may be required. Safe decision-making is a cornerstone to delivering safe revision surgery and this book is a key resource for revision knee surgeons of all grades and experience.

Andrew Price
Nuffield Orthopaedic Centre
Oxford, UK

Andrew Toms
Exeter Knee Reconstruction Unit
Exeter, UK

Preface

Total knee arthroplasty is a successful, cost-effective and durable operation that has helped millions of patients, offering them pain relief and improvements in function and quality of life. The demand for total knee arthroplasty is increasing worldwide with younger and higher demand patients having new knees every year with higher functional expectations than ever. This will inevitably lead to increased demand for revision knee surgery, which carries a significant burden on healthcare systems and surgeons worldwide. Historically, the outcomes of revision knee surgery have not been as good as those of primary knees. This is an area of subspecialization that requires training in advanced revision techniques and a multi-disciplinary team approach with significant resources to achieve satisfactory outcomes.

Revision Total Knee Arthroplasty: A Practical Guide is a unique book that provides arthroplasty surgeons with a framework and set of principles, philosophies and advanced surgical techniques that are the cumulative experience of renowned experts with decades of practice in this field. Our approach has been to always revert back to the first principles of a primary knee arthroplasty and to apply those principles to revision surgery. The success of this approach is reflected by the excellent outcomes we have achieved over the years. During years of practice, we have made mistakes, learnt lessons, honed our skills and developed new techniques which we are proud to share in this book.

The book is structured in a logical way to follow the patients' journey from the time of a primary knee, through indications and techniques for revision surgery to limb salvage options. Reading through the chapters, you will find *top tips* that we hope would be of use in moments of doubt, for example, when deciding whether to offer a patient with a unhappy knee a revision, when planning for a complex re-revision case or when faced with a challenging situation in the operating theatre.

We hope that this book will be a useful aid and a practical guide to arthroplasty surgeons worldwide as they strive to relieve patients' pain and offer them a new lease of life; a noble effort in which spirit this book has been written.

Nottingham, UK   Hosam E. Matar
Nottingham, UK   Benjamin V. Bloch
Toronto, Canada   Hugh U. Cameron
Nottingham, UK   ·   Peter J. James

Contents

1   Philosophy of Primary Total Knee Arthroplasty: Back to the
Beginning 1

2   Complex Primary Total Knee Arthroplasty 17

3   Assessment of Painful Total Knee Arthroplasty 59

4   Indications for Revision Total Knee Arthroplasty 67

5   Challenges of Surgical Exposure 93

6   Removal of Well-Fixed Components 107

7   Principles of Surgical Reconstruction: Back to the Beginning...
Again 123

8   Fixation in Revision Total Knee Arthroplasty 139

9   Kinematics of Constrained Condylar Revision Implants: A
Practical Perspective 163

10   Rotating-Hinge Implants 169

11   Salvage Revision Total Knee Arthroplasty 195

12   Managing Infection in Revision Total Knee Arthroplasty: A
Practical Perspective 223

13   Orthoplastics and Revision Knee Arthroplasty 245

14   Managing Chronic Patella Dislocations in Revision Knee
Arthroplasty: Surgical Technique 251

15   Extensor Mechanism Failure and Allograft Reconstruction 269

16   Periprosthetic Knee Fractures: An Arthroplasty Perspective 287

17   Mortality in Revision Knee Arthroplasty 305

18   Starting Out in Revision Knee Arthroplasty   315

19   A Lifetime of Revision Knee Arthroplasty   319

20   A Lifetime of Revision Knee Arthroplasty   331

Index   339

About the Authors

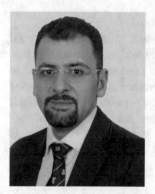

Hosam E. Matar is a fellowship trained consultant arthroplasty surgeon with special interest in revision surgery. He is well-published and has a vast experience in clinical research with particular interest in improving outcomes of arthroplasty patients and evidence-based orthopaedics.

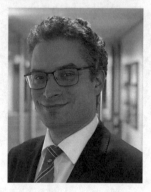

Benjamin V. Bloch is a fellowship trained consultant arthroplasty surgeon with special interest in revision knee surgery. He has an extensive background in teaching and training with numerous peer-reviewed publications.

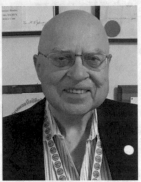

Hugh U. Cameron is a world-renowned arthroplasty surgeon, and internationally recognized for his expertise in total joint replacement and revision surgery for arthritis of the hip and knee. He lectures extensively throughout the world and has published widely. He is currently an Associate Professor in the Department of Surgery and Bioengineering at Sunnybrook Health Sciences Centre, Toronto, Canada.

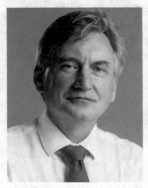

Peter J. James is a renowned arthroplasty surgeon, who has developed a national and international reputation for revision and complex knee replacement. He has particular expertise and experience in high-performance knee replacements for active patients and difficult revision knee surgery. He has been involved in both design and evaluation of revision knee prostheses/systems and lectures widely on all aspects of primary and revision knee surgery.

Philosophy of Primary Total Knee Arthroplasty: Back to the Beginning

1

Progress is man's ability to complicate simplicity.

Thor Heyerdahl

1.1 Introduction

The modern era of total knee arthroplasty (TKA) arguably began in 1973 with the introduction of the Total Condylar prosthesis designed by *Insall* and colleagues [1]. Although influenced by previous designs, this cemented prosthesis in which both cruciate ligaments were sacrificed and with sagittal plane stability provided by the articular surface geometry has set the standard for survivorship of TKA. Modern designs have retained most of the original features. Recent pooled registry data (14 registries) revealed excellent 25-year survivorship of TKAs at 82.3% (95% CI 81·3–83·2) [2].

The demand for TKA is ever increasing. An estimated 700,000 TKAs are performed each year in the USA alone with a projected increase in demand to over 3.48 million procedures by 2030 [3, 4]. However, despite the successes and rapid adoption of TKA, several studies have found that about 1 in 5 patients undergoing TKA are dissatisfied with the results of their surgery [5]. Over the years, and in an attempt to improve patients' outcomes and satisfaction, surgeons and manufacturers have introduced a number of modifications to TKA from surgical approach to patient specific instrumentation (PSI) and navigation techniques. Some of these techniques have seen a cycle of gaining initial popularity before falling out of favour, only to surface again a decade or so later such as early unicondylar and bicompartmental designs [6, 7]. Whilst novel techniques aim to achieve better clinical outcomes, it is important to consider there may be added costs, particularly with the inflationary costs of healthcare and the potential complications associated

© The Author(s), under exclusive license to Springer Nature Switzerland AG 2021
H. E. Matar et al., *Revision Total Knee Arthroplasty*,
https://doi.org/10.1007/978-3-030-81285-0_1

Table 1.1 Summary of randomised controlled trials in primary TKA (from Matar et al. [8])

Category	No. RCTs	Sample size	No. RCTs (%) with significant findings
Surgical approach	34	2459	3
Tourniquet	31	2560	4
MIS	13	1036	1
PSI	30	2517	2
Knee design	37	3702	2
Component Fixation	27	2956	0
Mobile bearing	47	5488	1
Navigation	50	5936	10
Polyethylene	19	2600	0
Technique	27	2387	4
Cement	6	3495	3
Robotics	3	150	0
Kinematic alignment	4	454	0
Patella resurfacing	26	6766	2
Patella management	14	1588	1
Drain	19	1801	0
Closure	16	1780	0
Total	**403**	**47,675**	**33 (8.2%)**

with adopting new technologies and their learning curve. In a unique overview of all randomised controlled trials (RCTs; 403 RCTs, n = 47,675 patients) published on primary TKA, we found that only 8.2% of trials reported significant differences between interventions [8]. Interestingly, 20% of navigation trials reported significant differences in radiological outcomes but no differences in clinical or patients' reported outcomes (Table 1.1).

Over recent decades and with improved polyethylene manufacturing and production processes, modes of TKA failure have changed with far fewer failures due to osteolysis and polyethylene related issues and with infection, loosening and instability now the main causes of revision TKA worldwide [9–13].

1.2   Stability in TKA

Leaving the argument of cruciate-retaining versus sacrificing aside, the first step during TKA is a soft tissue clearance of the knee including the menisci, which are important stabilisers of the native knee, the anterior cruciate ligament (ACL) in every case, and often the posterior cruciate ligament (PCL) as well. So, as part of our surgical approach to get to the knee and prepare the joint before making any bone cuts, we create instability. We should therefore aim to limit the amount of instability that we create. The medial collateral ligament (MCL) and lateral collateral ligament (LCL) are in this context sacrosanct. Our clinical experience suggests that those ligaments do not contract or shorten, although they may stretch or attenuate in gross neglected deformity, particularly in elderly patients. In the majority of cases they remain largely intact and surgical release is to be avoided.

The second premise is to recognise the native knee joint's stabilisers on the medial, lateral, posterior and anterior aspects with a deep understanding of what structures provide the stability in flexion and extension to work out where the problem lies when assessing deformity. If we take a knee with a fixed deformity in extension and we put that knee into flexion, the deformity will almost certainly correct. We seldom see people sitting with the knee at 90° on a chair with a massive deformity. Usually when they sit down the deformity corrects as they are predominantly weight-bearing deformities and they become fixed as the knee approaches extension from flexion. Here, we try to work out the deforming forces and stabilising structures in both flexion and extension to understand what structures are tight and how to correct the soft tissue deformity.

Top Tip: Most fixed knee deformities are extension deformities and correct in flexion.

In a valgus knee, for example, the only stabilisers on the lateral side of the knee, if you take PCL (which we do routinely as it makes gap balancing easier) out of the equation, are the LCL, popliteus and posterolateral capsule. Popliteus is often injured during surgery, either during tibial resection or more commonly at the posterolateral aspect during posterior femoral condyle preparation where it is most at risk. This leaves the LCL as the only reliable stabiliser of the knee in flexion, and as there is no residual deformity with the knee in a flexed position; it is clear that the LCL is not tight and therefore should not be released. The structures that are tight and can be released are the posterolateral capsule and potentially the iliotibial band, as an extra-capsular stabiliser, but not much else.

Top Tip: In most valgus knees, extension deformity can be corrected by a posterolateral capsular release.

On the other hand, in a varus deformity, the deep MCL is tight in extension but has very little effect on flexion as it blends into the posteromedial capsule. So, in flexion it is the superficial MCL that keeps the knee stable. If one over-releases the MCL to correct a varus deformity you will achieve correction in extension but instability in flexion. Here, we have to recognise that the native knee joint is generally slacker on the lateral side in flexion than medial side, so if we try to get absolute equal tension on both medial and lateral sides, we are then changing the alignment and kinematics of the knee. Interestingly, many unhappy knees in clinical practice are as a result of this chase of a zero-degree mechanical alignment which may be good for longevity of the implant, and we understand the mechanical principles and why engineers might want us to achieve this; but this may not be necessarily a comfortable position for patients to be in particularly having had, for example, a lifelong varus deformity. With continuous improvement and advancement of modern technology and more accuracy in positioning components, it is quite likely that we will be heading towards more kinematically aligned knee replacements, in a widespread fashion within certain parameters, as there are limits to what can be achieved.

Top Tip: In most varus knees, extension deformity can be corrected by a posteromedial capsular release.

It is a common experience in revision knee clinics to see unhappy knees with reasonable X-rays, but the chief complaint of instability which has been surgically created rather than due to a patient's or implant's factors. A happy TKA must be put within a *balanced soft tissue envelope*.

1.3 Balanced Soft Tissue Envelope

Early pioneers of TKA all recognised that a successful TKA depends on a surgeons' ability to position the implant within a stable collateral ligament frame *(The Frame Principle)* (Fig. 1.1).

We believe that adhering to the frame principle is fundamental to the success of knee arthroplasty both in primary and revision cases. If we strip back to this basic principle it starts to make sense and it follows that wherever we put one component

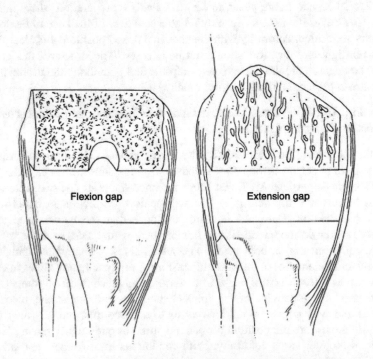

Fig. 1.1 Flexion and Extension gap (with permission from Insall's Philosophy of TKA)

should dictate where we put the other within this 'ligament frame'. If we accept that the ligaments are not contracted and remain intact then correct and linked component placement to respect and equalise soft tissue tension throughout the range of motion is a logical surgical goal which can be achieved by a gap balanced approach building the knee from the tibial cut. If we place the two components completely independently, we have no control over the relationship between those components and the collateral ligaments with increased risk of subtle instability in mid-flexion and flexion.

In practice, there is a measured resection approach which is still probably the most commonly performed around the world. Often the femur is prepared first and it relies on certain anatomical landmarks to position the components, which works in extension because it is a valgus cut on the femur and a perpendicular cut on the tibia. However, it is in flexion and mid-flexion where we potentially run into problems. The landmarks used are the trans-epicondylar axis, which is sometimes quite difficult to find reliably and reproducibly, and Whiteside's line. Most surgeons, however, rely on posterior referencing using the posterior condyles of the femur to dial in a fixed amount of 3°–5° of external rotation depending on the system used. However, in almost every knee with advanced OA there is a degree of posterior condylar wear. In varus knees, for example, there is posterior medial condylar wear and if we are measuring 3° of external rotation it is quite likely that we are achieving more than 3°, and vice versa in valgus knees which have the added complexity of not only wear but also possible lateral condylar hypoplasia. So, there are many potential variations in how we position the femoral component based on a measured resection technique. Femoral component rotation, in turn, affects the flexion gap.

Within this technique, the tibial component is also positioned independently trying to get it roughly at 90° to the mechanical axis of the tibia. So, if we inadvertently increase external rotation of the femoral component then we will run the risk of medial laxity and flexion instability, because it is not linked to the tibial component within the collateral frame. Similarly, if we do not externally rotate enough, it may have an impact on patella tracking and more importantly MCL tension. If it is too tight on the medial side, patients get medial pain and stiffness.

Therefore, what makes more sense is to build the knee in a stepwise fashion which the vast majority of revision knee surgeons would agree is the only way for a successful operation in revision TKA. So why not apply those same principles in primary TKA?

Top Tip: A successful TKA depends on a surgeons' ability to position the implant within a stable collateral ligament frame *(The Frame Principle).*

1.4   Gap Balanced Approach (Figs. 1.2, 1.3, 1.4, 1.5, 1.6 and 1.7)

This simply means having a stable tibial platform, and intact medial and lateral collateral ligaments, which allows us to then position the femoral component within this frame. Although you can choose whether to take off the PCL or not, in our experience it is easier and more reproducible if you do take it out, and then build the knee on a gap balanced technique. This means the tibial cut is performed first, or straight after the distal femoral cut, as the idea is to assess the extension gap first and balance the knee in extension, clearing the posterior osteophytes off the femur, the posteromedial osteophyte off the tibia (which is often missed), releasing the tight posteromedial capsule off the tibia to correct any varus deformity and to elevate the tight posterior capsule in advanced disease (Figs. 1.2, 1.3, 1.4, 1.5, 1.6 and 1.7).

Remember, if you think about a varus knee that is fixed in flexion, the soft tissue tightness will be in the posteromedial capsule as it is always the fixed flexion deformity which predominates as a varus knee that comes fully straight to full extension is always correctable. Every varus knee that has a fixed deformity, will have a degree of associated fixed flexion deformity which implies that the tight soft tissue structure is the posteromedial capsule rather than the MCL. This is usually caused by medial tibial osteophytes, femoral osteophytes and some scarring and tightness from the posteromedial capsule, and once we address them early it usually corrects.

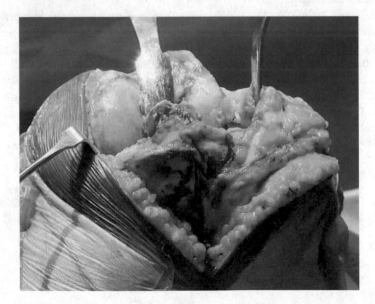

Fig. 1.2 Tibial cut first and clearing osteophytes

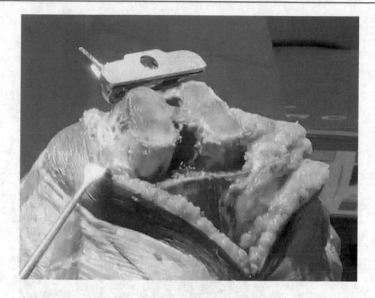

Fig. 1.3 Distal femoral cut and clearing posterior osteophytes

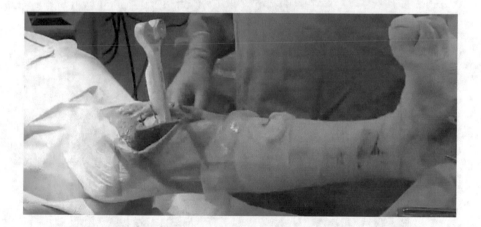

Fig. 1.4 Balancing in extension

What if it doesn't? In this case you should not take the superficial MCL, but re-examine the knee making sure the posteromedial capsule is released, all osteophytes removed, ensure that enough bone has been resected, check the angle of the tibial cut, and finally lift off the deep MCL/deep oblique ligament; all of which should be done in a stepwise fashion. If the knee is still tight the options here are to

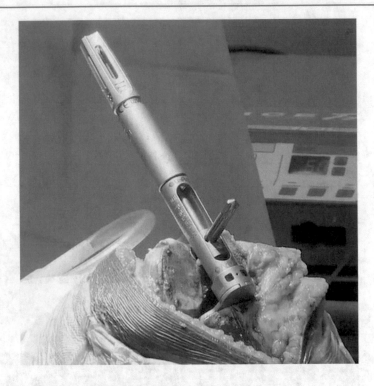

Fig. 1.5 Positioning a gap balancer in 90° flexion

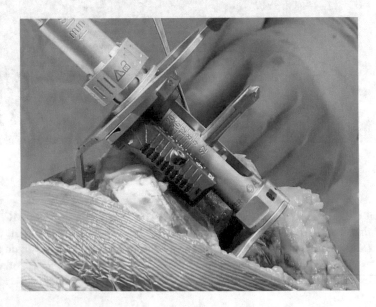

Fig. 1.6 Creating flexion gap equal to the extension gap linking the femoral component positioning to a stable tibial platform within a balanced collaterals frame

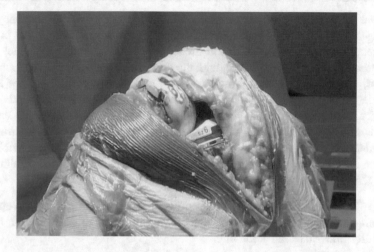

Fig. 1.7 Well-balanced knee with trials in flexion, no lift-off, patella tracking well with adequate height and tension

do a transverse capsular release or more of a kinematic alignment by adjusting the bone cuts; that is our preference as we do not want to destabilise the joint, so we accept some residual varus to allow the joint to be balanced in extension.

To Tip: Do not destabilise the joint in pursuit of mechanical alignment.

1.5   What About Tibial Slope?

The philosophy of PCL retention or resection affects how we think about the tibial slope.

If you keep the PCL, then you need to match the patient's native tibial slope as the PCL is naturally tensioned on the slope that they had throughout their lives. So, having a single arbitrary slope setting in the jig is not accurate for all CR knees. If you are a CR user, then it is our opinion that you should match the patient's native slope.

If, on the other hand, you sacrifice the PCL then the flexion gap will open up, and you will need less slope but should still take into consideration the requirements of the implant design to be used, to avoid either laxity or tightness in flexion.

The issue with tibial slope is that as surgeons we are not necessarily accurate in restoring the native tibial slope; rather than cutting the slope in a true anteroposterior (AP) direction, it is unfortunately commonly cut in anteromedial to posterolateral direction as it is easier to apply the tibial jig to the exposed anteromedial tibial surface. This leads us to build in a compound slope which will then affect both flexion and extension gaps. Knee designs which require a zero-degree slope are therefore more forgiving from this point of view. However, if the implant design requires 5° or 7° AP slope it is imperative that all efforts are made to cut in a true AP direction to avoid issues with soft tissue balancing and instability issues which are difficult to resolve without re-cutting the tibia which causes iatrogenic bone loss.

Also, in patients who are morbidly obese, the thick soft tissue envelope around the tibia pushes the tibial cutting guide away from the tibia which adds to the difficulty in getting the desired slope angle. The use of intra-medullary jigs can help as in revision cases. If you are more used to extra-medullary jigs, then ensure you have adequate exposure and a good view of the tibia. The patella in combination with the deep fat layer can make this difficult so consider sliding the patella rather than everting and creating a little pocket laterally to park the patella.

Top Tip: Know the thickness of your implant and make sure you have resected enough tibia. Don't over-resect the femur as this will create flexion instability and raise the joint line.

1.6   Balancing the Knee in Extension

Having cut the tibia, the femur is cut at an appropriate valgus angle. The extension gap is then created, sized and balanced. If you are still struggling to balance the extension gap at this stage we advise re-visiting the steps described above, concentrating on osteophyte removal from both femur and posteromedial tibia to ensure the posteromedial capsule is not tethered or tight. It may be the case that the medial side remains tighter even after these manoeuvres. It is imperative that the MCL is not released to gain correction. We believe it is better advised to adjust the angle of the bone cuts, either on the tibial side by cutting in slight varus (no more than 3° is advised) to match the anatomic alignment of the tibia or to decrease the valgus angle cut on the femur to offload the medial side. Our preferred option is to alter the valgus cut on the femur by reducing down to 3° or 4° rather than the more usual 5–6°. Either way we are aiming to achieve a more kinematically aligned knee within the frame of that individual's collateral ligaments rather than chasing a neutral mechanical axis which would need ligament release; hence creating potential instability.

In doing so, in achieving kinematic alignment, one might argue that we are not loading the poly insert equally on medial and lateral sides, but it is our view that it is more important that we balance the knee to equalise tension and load across the tibiofemoral joint. By creating a 'balanced' knee we believe it is more protective of fixation and implant wear than chasing mechanical alignment. The Oxford experience in unicompartmental knees supports this view.

Top Tip: a *'balanced'* knee is more protective of fixation and implant wear than *'unbalanced'* mechanically aligned knee.

1.7 Balancing the Knee in Flexion

On the *flexion balanced workflow*, the femoral rotation is based on your medial and lateral collateral ligaments balance (the top side of the frame in flexion). The posterior femoral cuts should be parallel to the tibial cut when the collateral ligaments are appropriately tensioned. The flexion gap size is controlled by the femoral component size relative to the AP size of the native femur and the size of the posterior femoral bone cuts made. This gap can therefore be manipulated by upsizing and downsizing the femoral component to help achieve flexion/extension balance. The AP placement of the femoral component can also be manipulated to balance the flexion space by anteriorising or posteriorising the component. Lastly gap size is altered by femoral component flexion. Slight femoral flexion has the effect of tightening up the flexion space. All of these options should be remembered when addressing the femoral gap in surgery.

Femoral gap balance with respect to medial and lateral sided tension is controlled by femoral component rotation. By tensioning the knee in flexion, the femoral component can be positioned so the posterior femoral bone cuts are parallel to the cut tibia; thus, ensuring a rectangular flexion gap. Balancing devices, computer assisted surgical workflows and even simple laminar spreaders can be used to achieve this goal.

When following a gap balanced approach, it is important that we respect the joint line by not over-resecting the distal femur [a common mistake in TKA performed for patients with fixed flexion deformity (FFD)]. In most cases the FFD is produced by a combination of osteophytes and tight posterior capsule, and not any changes of the native femur itself. Therefore, we should not take more bone off the distal femur because as soon as we do so to combat that FFD, we have inadvertently raised the joint line instead of addressing the tightness in the capsule which is mostly osteophytic in nature.

Whilst this approach may allow the extension gap to be created and balanced it will impact on flexion stability in a significant way. The problem in these knees sits in the posterior space which tightens the posterior capsule. In this plane, bony resection to balance the soft tissues will address the extension gap only. As soon as the knee is flexed the tight posterior capsule is lost and stability is then increasingly driven by the collateral ligaments. Joint line elevation to address a tight posterior capsule will not reliably tension the collaterals throughout the range of motion. Understanding the relationship between joint line, component sizing and component orientation including rotation are the fundamentals which underpin TKA surgery.

Top Tip: In FFD deformity, femurs don't grow in size and over-resection will not solve the problem. Clear any posterior osteophytes and release the tight capsule.

1.8 A Word of Caution

If you use a measured resection technique and you want to cut your tibia in few degrees of varus having first externally rotated the femur, then you will have medial instability which is very difficult to fix. The patella will track in these scenarios but you will have medial instability in flexion.

Maltracking patellae are more often seen in valgus knees, and it is in these cases where measured resection has a higher risk of leading to a malrotated femoral component due to the bony anatomy often present in this scenario. We believe that in these cases it is imperative to consider a balanced workflow.

1.9 Mobile Versus Fixed Bearings

The literature suggests that there is no difference in clinical outcomes [8, 14]. There are theoretical advantages to each. The ability to de-couple motion and protect polyethylene and tibial fixation is often quoted in support of mobile-bearing knees, although poly wear is less of an issue with modern polyethylene.

The other advantage is being able to use the implant to give better stability, for example the longest published track record is on Low Contact Stress (LCS) rotating platform (RP) knees with 98% 20-year survivorship using revision for any cause as an endpoint and with an excellent mean Knee Society Score of 87.3 [15]. Here, the principle of having a very conforming polyethylene geometry that closely matches the femur enhances AP stability and will help with all surgical aspects building some stability in the implant while losing the torsional torque (which is the downside of conformity) by having a rotating-platform.

We would also argue that using an RP-design would enhance a surgeon's skills as surgeons would have to balance the knee throughout ROM, otherwise they risk insert spin-out which is classically due to over release. This is particularly seen in valgus knees, usually in a figure-of-four position, where the medial side remains engaged in flexion. If the lateral side had been over-released and not balanced against a tight medial side, then the insert could spin-out. So, knowing and understanding that you cannot leave the knee unbalanced, makes you a better knee replacement surgeon. This is not saying that that the implant is better but rather you are having to address stability and flexion balance better which a lot of fixed-bearing surgeons may not necessarily worry about as much [16].

It is important here not to mix this surgical philosophy with the principle of rotating-platform and measured resection surgical technique. A high rate of spinout was seen in some systems using CR-RP implants performed with a measured resection technique as the flexion space was not well-balanced [17–19].

Top Tip: We would caution surgeons against using an RP device with a measured resection technique. An RP device is best used with a balanced approach.

Getting the knee balanced using a gap balancing approach works equally well with fixed bearings although it is not quite as forgiving on tibial component rotation. Here, it is worth mentioning that you can get better bone coverage of the tibia with an RP implant which will accept a few degrees of malrotation as the RP insert usually self-aligns.

Another related concept is tibial rotation; as the knee goes from flexion to extension it rotates. Here, two philosophies apply; either you can compromise with a lack of conformity and stability in a fixed bearing to allow the rotation to occur between the femoral component and the top surface of the poly insert, or allow that rotation to occur on the under-surface of the more conforming poly insert against the tibial tray. The latter has the dual advantage of stability with conformity of the femur-poly interface and disperses the torsional torque in the under-surface-poly-tibia-interface.

We have to also acknowledge that a number of registries have shown that RP do less well. We feel this may be because they are used by measured resection surgeons so it is a technique related rather than implant or philosophy related issue [20, 21].

1.10   PCL-Retention and Gap Balancing

The question is what are we balancing against with an intact PCL? A tight PCL in the context of OA or the collateral ligaments?

In flexion, with the posterior capsule slack and redundant, we usually take the PCL out in order to balance against the intact collaterals with some feedback from the extensor mechanism on the lateral side. We know that the lateral side in varus knees is always a bit slacker than the medial side, so on the whole this does not really have any significant influence on rotation. In fact, it has a protective effect against excessive external rotation of the femoral component.

On the other hand, if we keep the PCL and start to distract the flexion space then how do we know which of the three structures we are trying to balance against tightens first? The PCL is already tight and will therefore be tensioned first giving erroneous rotation not dictated by the collaterals but rather by a tight PCL. If we are then faced with lift-off and we then recess the PCL to improve flexion, that tension and balance is then lost.

Top Tip: A balanced approach is more reproducible using either a cruciate-substituting (CS)/ or posterior-stabilised (PS) implant.

In a related topic, there is some evidence to suggest that patients with high BMI have higher rate of tibial failure and therefore stemmed implants are a good way to improve fixation and reduce early aseptic failure of tibial trays [22–24]. In those circumstances, we will often need a 0° slope to get stems into the tibia safely and for that PS knees are better than CR designs which usually require increased tibial slope.

1.11　Patella Resurfacing

Interestingly, this continues to be a divisive topic with some surgeons always resurfacing and others who never do. The truth may well be somewhere in between. There are many arguments for and against with no real long-term advantage from high quality trials [8]. If the patella is healthy and tracks well, removing the osteophytes is all that is needed and there is very little benefit in resurfacing. For PS knees however, due to issues related to the box, there is an argument to resurface those routinely not only medicolegally, but to genuinely reduce the risk of crepitus and anterior knee pain accepting that there is the potential for patella-resurfacing related complications which can be very challenging to manage. Another indication for routine resurfacing is in cases where the patella component can be medialised to help subtle patella maltracking without any other gross abnormalities with component positioning and knee kinematics. Our philosophy is to routinely resurface in cases of primary patellofemoral OA, inflammatory arthropathy and when a PS femur is used; otherwise a selective approach to resurfacing is taken.

In conclusion, a successful TKA depends on positioning the implant within a stable collateral ligament frame. Adhering to the frame principle is fundamental to the success of knee arthroplasty both in primary and revision cases.

References

1. Insall J, et al. Total condylar knee replacment: preliminary report. Clin Orthop Relat Res. 1976;120:149–54.
2. Evans JT, et al. How long does a knee replacement last? A systematic review and meta-analysis of case series and national registry reports with more than 15 years of follow-up. Lancet. 2019;393(10172):655–63.
3. Nguyen LC, Lehil MS, Bozic KJ. Trends in total knee arthroplasty implant utilization. J Arthroplasty. 2015;30(5):739–42.
4. Kurtz S, et al. Projections of primary and revision hip and knee arthroplasty in the United States from 2005 to 2030. J Bone Joint Surg Am. 2007;89(4):780–5.
5. Bourne RB, et al. Patient satisfaction after total knee arthroplasty: who is satisfied and who is not? Clin Orthop Relat Res. 2010;468(1):57–63.
6. Insall JN, et al. A comparison of four models of total knee-replacement prostheses. J Bone Joint Surg Am. 1976;58(6):754–65.
7. Ranawat CS. History of total knee replacement. J South Orthop Assoc. 2002;11(4):218–26.
8. Matar HE, et al. Overview of Randomized Controlled Trials in Total Knee Arthroplasty (47,675 Patients): What Have We Learnt? J Arthroplasty. 2020;35(6):1729–1736.e1.
9. Lum ZC, Shieh AK, Dorr LD. Why total knees fail-A modern perspective review. World J Orthop. 2018;9(4):60–4.
10. Sadoghi P, et al. Revision surgery after total joint arthroplasty: a complication-based analysis using worldwide arthroplasty registers. J Arthroplasty. 2013;28(8):1329–32.
11. Sharkey PF, et al. Why are total knee arthroplasties failing today–has anything changed after 10 years? J Arthroplasty. 2014;29(9):1774–8.
12. Fehring TK, et al. Early failures in total knee arthroplasty. Clin Orthop Relat Res. 2001;392:315–8.
13. Cameron HU, Hunter GA. Failure in total knee arthroplasty: mechanisms, revisions, and results. Clin Orthop Relat Res. 1982;170:141–6.

14. Fransen BL, et al. No differences between fixed- and mobile-bearing total knee arthroplasty. Knee Surg Sports Traumatol Arthrosc. 2017;25(6):1757–77.
15. Milligan DJ, et al. Twenty-year survivorship of a cemented mobile bearing Total Knee Arthroplasty. Knee. 2019;26(4):933–40.
16. Geary MB, et al. Why Do Revision Total Knee Arthroplasties Fail? A Single-Center Review of 1632 Revision Total Knees Comparing Historic and Modern Cohorts. J Arthroplasty. 2020.
17. Callaghan JJ, et al. Cemented rotating-platform total knee replacement a concise follow-up, at a minimum of fifteen years, of a previous report. J Bone Joint Surg Am. 2005;87(9):1995–8.
18. Gupta SK, et al. The P.F.C. sigma RP-F TKA designed for improved performance: a matched-pair study. Orthopedics. 2006;29(9 Suppl):S49–52.
19. Callaghan JJ. Mobile-bearing knee replacement: clinical results: a review of the literature. Clin Orthop Relat Res. 2001;392:221–5.
20. Gothesen O, et al. Increased risk of aseptic loosening for 43,525 rotating-platform vs. fixed-bearing total knee replacements. Acta Orthop. 2017;88(6):649–656.
21. Namba RS, et al. Risk of revision for fixed versus mobile-bearing primary total knee replacements. J Bone Joint Surg Am. 2012;94(21):1929–35.
22. Garceau SP, et al. Reduced Aseptic Loosening With Fully Cemented Short-Stemmed Tibial Components in Primary Cemented Total Knee Arthroplasty. J Arthroplasty. 2020;35(6):1591-1594.e3.
23. Fournier G, et al. Increased survival rate in extension stemmed TKA in obese patients at minimum 2 years follow-up. Knee Surg Sports Traumatol Arthrosc. 2020;28(12):3919–25.
24. Schultz BJ, DeBaun MR, Huddleston JI 3rd. The use of stems for morbid obesity in total knee arthroplasty. J Knee Surg. 2019;32(7):607–10.

Complex Primary Total Knee Arthroplasty

2

All animals are equal, but some animals are more equal than others!

George Orwell

2.1 Introduction

The term "complex primary TKA" is an umbrella term that describes a variety of conditions and scenarios of difficult cases that require extra planning and contingencies with revision systems available in the operating room. On the whole, it is a subjective term with no agreed definition in the literature. What is agreed, however, is that these cases carry higher risk of complications both in the short- and long-term. In their long-term outcome study of complex primaries from the Mayo clinic, Martin et al. reported outcomes of 427 knees that had a varus-valgus constrained (VVC) design and 246 knees that had rotating-hinge arthroplasties. They found that the rate of component revision for any reason at 10 years was over 2 times higher, and over 3 times higher at 20 years, compared to a large group of complex primaries with unconstrained implants [1]. In their study from the Norwegian registry of 401 condylar-constrained knee (CCK) or hinged implants, Badawy et al. reported 2 years survivorship of 94.8% (95% CI 91.4–98.2) and 93.5% after 5 years for the primary CCK and 91.0% (CI 86.6–95.4) after 2 years and 85.5% after 5 years for the primary hinged TKA [2]. Mancino et al., in their study of CCK implants used in primary TKA with severe coronal deformity and/or intraoperative instability (54 knees; mean 9 years follow up), overall survivorship was 93.6% [3]. This variation in the literature reflects this heterogenous group of patients with different conditions and degrees of complexities (deformity, bone defects, ligamentous instability, surgeon's experience, patients' factors) where each case is different which makes any generalisation less accurate.

© The Author(s), under exclusive license to Springer Nature Switzerland AG 2021
H. E. Matar et al., *Revision Total Knee Arthroplasty*,
https://doi.org/10.1007/978-3-030-81285-0_2

In this chapter, we will provide some tips and lessons that we have learnt over years of practice dealing with complex and unusual cases with some common themes and basic principles that would apply to most complex cases.

2.2 So, What Makes a Complex TKA?

The three main aspects are the status of the surrounding soft tissues, deformity, and lack of suitable bone for fixation.

Previous surgery or trauma can compromise the soft tissue envelope leaving multiple scars which may interfere with the standard surgical approaches to the knee. Severe varus or valgus deformities, or the more challenging large fixed flexion deformity (FFD) are commonly encountered examples. Less frequently, we may see patients with skeletal dysplasia, short stature, or even rickets. In everyday practice, previous fractures either in the distal femur or proximal tibia with a degree or malunion or retained metalwork are commonly seen. Lack of suitable bone for fixation can be seen in isolation or as a result of previous trauma or bone loss due to severe deformity (Fig. 2.1). Morbid obesity and high BMI are also considered a complex procedure due to the difficulty in exposure and particular consideration should be given to using stemmed implants with the aim of spreading the load and protecting fixation (Fig. 2.2) [4, 5].

Top Tip: **The three main aspects that make a knee complex are the status of the surrounding soft tissues, deformity, and lack of suitable bone for fixation.**

2.3 Surgical Approach

Getting adequate exposure is one of the main challenges in complex cases, particularly in the presence of multiple scars from previous surgeries (Fig. 2.3), previous fracture, high BMI, or deformity. For example, in a previous high tibial osteotomy (HTO) which alters the relationship between alignment and ligamentous position, there is often associated patella baja, making exposure more challenging. Multiplanar osteotomies have increased in recent years and add another layer of complexity with the translation that they produce, resulting in significant alterations to the anatomy which can make knee balancing incredibly difficult [6–10].

Top Tip: **Involve a plastic surgeon early on, plan your way in and ensure getting adequate soft tissue cover before undertaking any reconstruction.**

In stiff knees, getting a safe access to the joint is all about protecting the extensors and the collateral ligaments. We have a low threshold for using extended exposures early on which not only saves valuable surgical time but also gives the best protection to these vital structures. The posterolateral corner of the tibia is by far the most difficult area to get to in difficult exposures. Therefore, attempting to

(i)

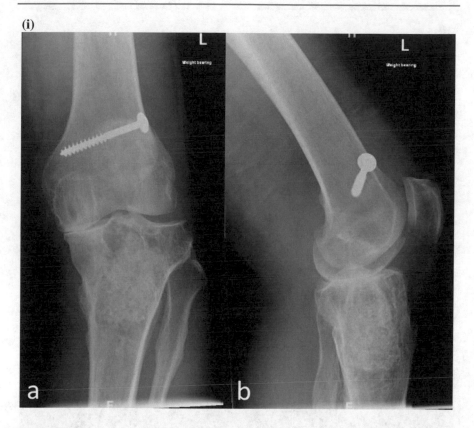

Fig. 2.1 i Radiographs of a 54 years old man with advanced varus OA and previous Gore-tex ACL reconstruction and a large lytic lesion in the proximal tibia which had been bone grafted 8 years earlier. **ii** Follow up radiographs following reconstruction using metaphyseal sleeve on the tibial side to address the issue of fixation in this case

improve the exposure by working proximally on the quads offers very little help; as does anything above the patella. Surgeons are generally less worried about performing a quadriceps snip or a turndown because they can repair it at the end with sutures. However, logically, you will need to sever the quads tendon completely to get any meaningful exposure. Further, the long-term outcomes of such proximal soft tissue work are fraught with potential complications, weakness and extensor lag. Tibial crest osteotomy, on the other hand, with a long bone-bed, protects the extensor apparatus and allows excellent exposure to the tibia. It is a safe and reliable option particularly for cases with patella baja and is used routinely in rTKA for stiff knees and when explanting stemmed components (see Chap. 5 on surgical exposure in rTKA for more details) (Fig. 2.4).

Top Tip: Tibial crest osteotomy is safe and reliable with excellent functional outcomes protecting the extensor mechanism and allowing excellent exposure.

(ii)

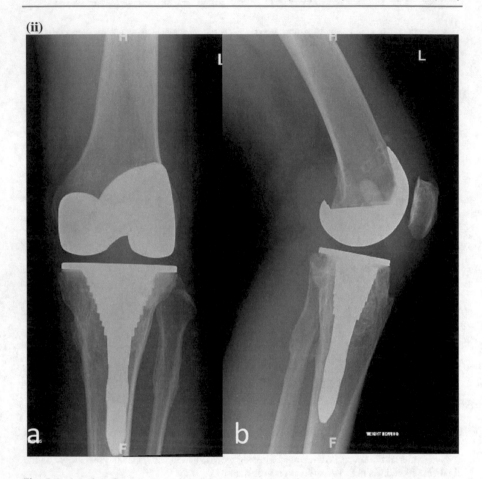

Fig. 2.1 (continued)

(i)

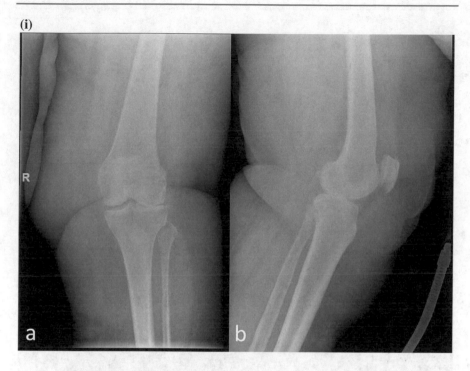

Fig. 2.2 i Preoperative radiographs of 78 years old lady with mild valgus knee but complicated by a high BMI of 49 kg/m². **ii** Postoperative radiographs following reconstruction with a stemmed cemented tibia, CS knee with a fixed bearing and a drain in situ (left for 24 hours). The morphology of her tibial canal allowed for a stemmed tibia on a CS articulation. However, in other cases, PS design may be more appropriate with a zero slope on the tibia to ensure central position of the stem and avoid perforation or fractures

(ii)

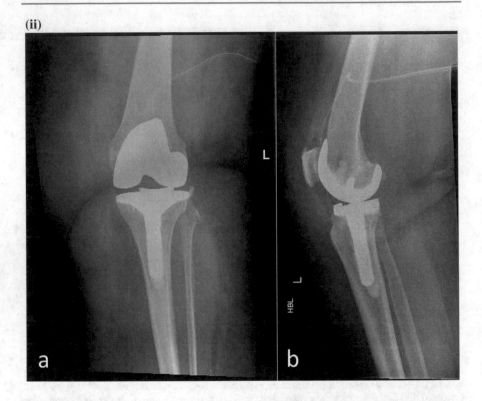

Fig. 2.2 (continued)

Fig. 2.3 Example of a
patient with symptomatic
advanced OA being
considered for TKA. He has
had multiple surgeries in the
past following a road traffic
accident years ago. This
would be a complex primary
that requires input from a
plastic surgeon to plan the
most appropriate surgical
approach and ensure adequate
soft tissue cover

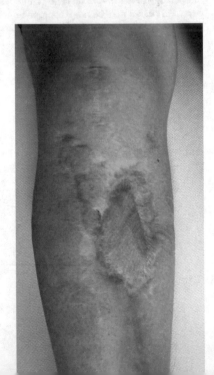

(i)

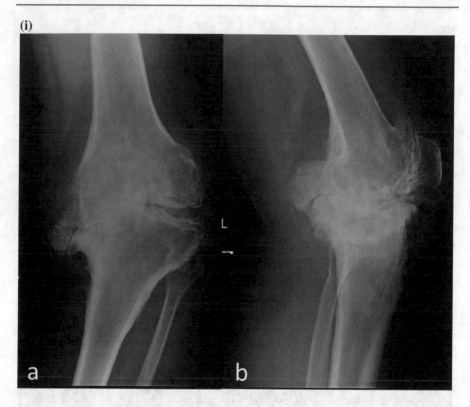

Fig. 2.4 i Weight-bearing anteroposterior and lateral radiographs of left knee in a 76-year old farmer with bilateral severe OA and significant deformity with ROM 30–45. **ii** Postoperative radiographs following a complex primary reconstruction with crest osteotomy for adequate exposure and rotating-hinge implant (SMILES system). **iii** Subsequent follow up radiographs with a healed osteotomy and good clinical function of the same patient

(ii)

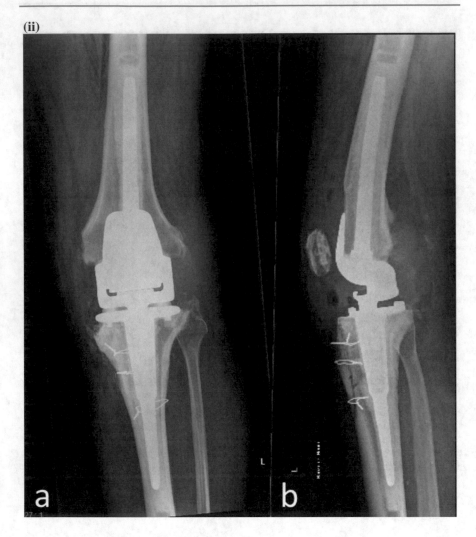

Fig. 2.4 (continued)

(iii)

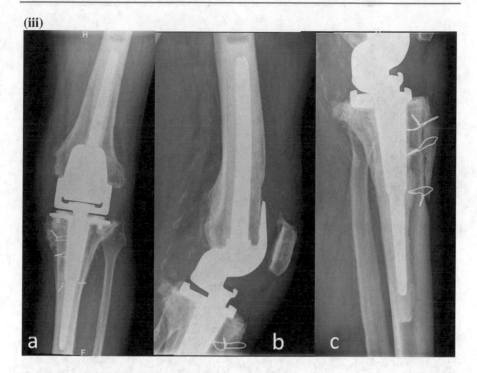

Fig. 2.4 (continued)

2.4 Chronic Fixed Flexion Deformity

The dilemma here is what are we trying to achieve when faced with elderly, chair-shaped patients with agonising arthritic pain which usually is bilateral. This is quite different form younger active patients with post-traumatic FFD. Postoperative mobilisation is very difficult, so consider a simultaneous procedure, if medically appropriate, or staged within short period of time.

Operatively, all the posterior structures are shortened and tight and lengthening procedures put the neurovascular structures at risk. So, logically, the principle here is getting enough space in extension for the implant and being able to get to the posterior aspect of the knee. Therefore, adequate bony cuts are needed with significant soft tissue releases which may necessitate the use of a hinged implant. It is usually the case that once a significant posterior capsular release is done, stability can only be achieved with a hinged implant (Fig. 2.4).

Similarly, in historic polio patients or more commonly neuromuscular patients or those with spinal stenosis who tend to have weak quadriceps and acquired back-knee gait and recurvatum with posterior capsular failure. Again, those would require a hinge design.

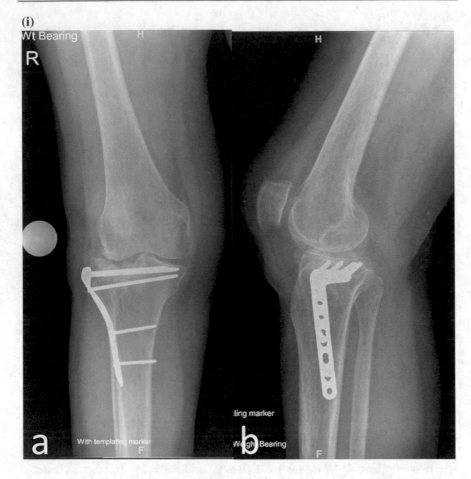

Fig. 2.5 i Anteroposterior and lateral radiographs of a 58 years old female with post-traumatic osteoarthritis with previous tibial plateau fracture which was fixed with a lateral locking plate. **ii** Postoperative radiographs following removal of metal work and primary TKA

2.5 Previous Periarticular Fractures

The issue here is not about limb alignment as much as implant fixation. Leaving plates or screws in situ from previous fixation brings no harm, as long as they do not get in the way, keeping the long bones protected allowing the option of simply resurfacing with conventional implants. If, on the other hand, the periarticular region and the metaphyseal bone is sufficiently disrupted that adequate fixation is compromised, then intramedullary fixation with stems or sleeves is mandatory in order to get a platform to stabilise and build the knee. The frame principle would apply with intact collaterals akin to a primary balanced approach even though we

(ii)

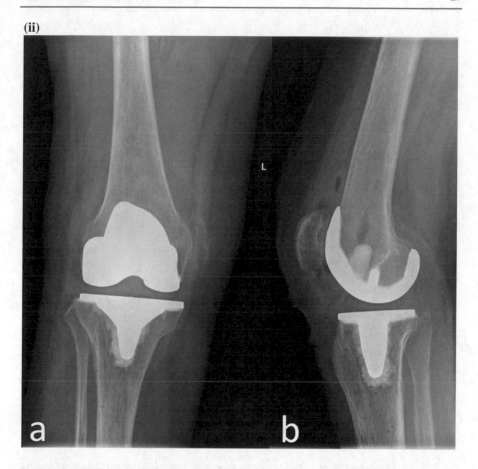

Fig. 2.5 (continued)

are using revision components to ensure adequate fixation. When metalwork is to be removed, a single- or two-stage approach is acceptable as is a single- or two-incision technique. Tissue sampling to rule out deep infection is to be encouraged particularly in a staged approach of removing the metalwork before any major reconstruction is undertaking (Figs. 2.5, 2.6, 2.7 and 2.8).

(i)

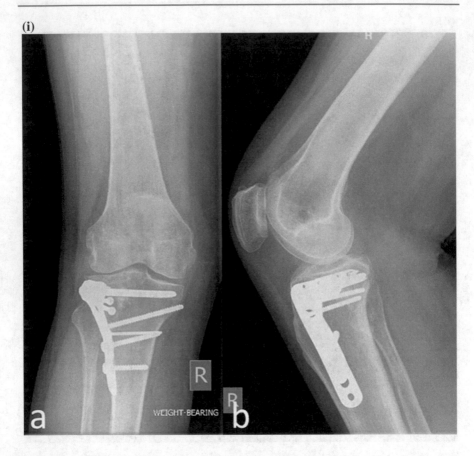

Fig. 2.6 i Another example of a periarticular fracture with anteroposterior and lateral radiographs of a 70 years old woman with plate fixation for tibial plateau fracture. ii Postoperative radiographs at 3 years follow up following partial removal of metalwork and a primary TKA

(ii)

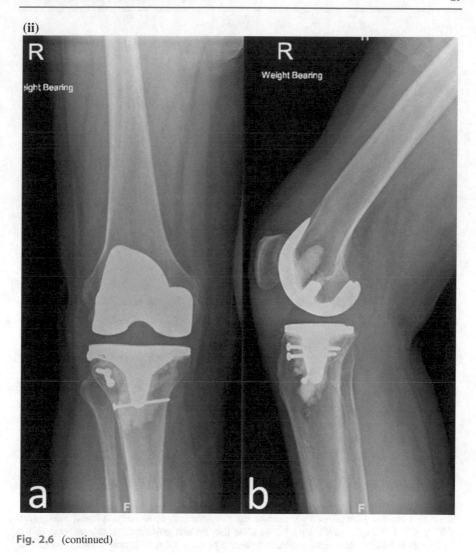

Fig. 2.6 (continued)

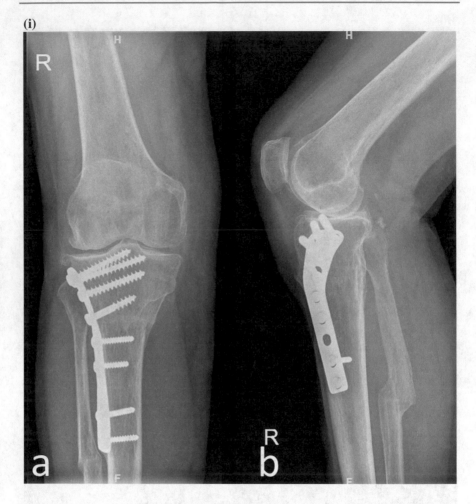

Fig. 2.7 i Another example of a periarticular fracture with anteroposterior and lateral radiographs of 75 years old woman with a long lateral plate fixation and posttraumatic osteoarthritis of her right knee. **ii** Postoperative radiographs following a primary TKA with retained lateral plate and only removing the proximal screws

(ii)

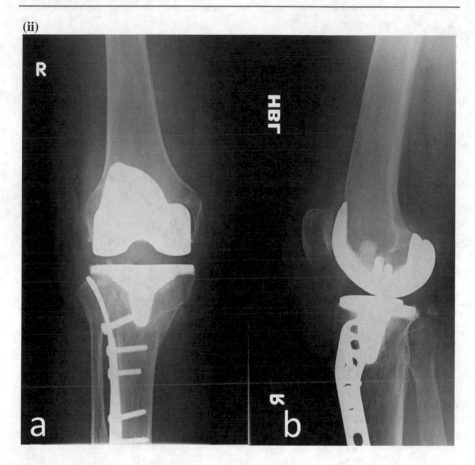

Fig. 2.7 (continued)

(i)

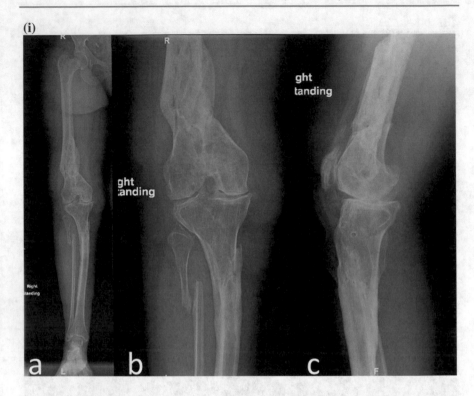

Fig. 2.8 i An example of a complex primary case in 47 years old man with previous multiple malunited femoral and tibial fractures. ii Postoperative radiographs at 5 years follow up following primary TKA demonstrating the principle that *'sometimes less is more'* accepting that resorting neutral mechanical alignment would have required multiple complex osteotomies

(ii)

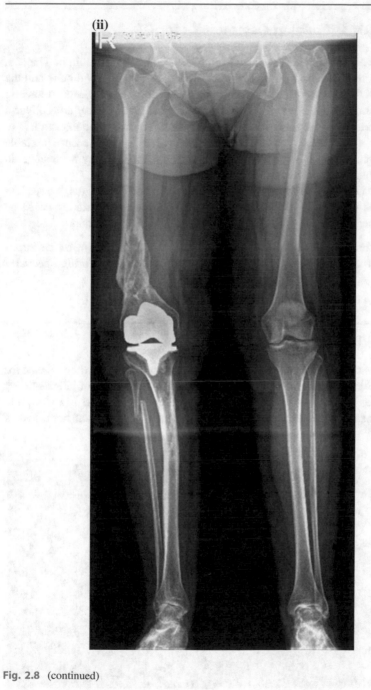

Fig. 2.8 (continued)

2.6   Previous Offloading Osteotomies for OA

With HTO we are sometimes faced with a varus OA and a valgus limb. This can
lead to alterations in the usual relationship between the ligaments and bone and the
usual approach for a primary may not be sufficient to achieved a balanced knee in
the usual fashion. The issue is primarily in the tibial cut which may not deliver a
stable platform to build from, so you have to be wary of these variations and it is in
those patients where extra constraint may be required to help ensure a stable
construct. As previously discussed, the presence of patella baja may necessitate an
extensile approach early on.

In the less commonly performed distal femoral osteotomy for valgus, we see less
of a problem as we can adjust the distal femoral cut and femoral rotation based on
the gap balanced approach without significant problems in this group.

**Top Tip: In complex cases with altered anatomy, a balanced approach and a
more constrained implant is often necessary to provide extra added security
and stability.**

2.7   Revising Partial Knees

Unicompartmental (Figs. 2.9 and 2.10): in most cases, particularly when revised for
polyethylene wear, there is little bone loss and the tibial cut at time of index surgery
is conservative. We tend to cut at the level of the tibial plate and use a slightly
thicker poly insert with standard primary components. If significant bone loss is

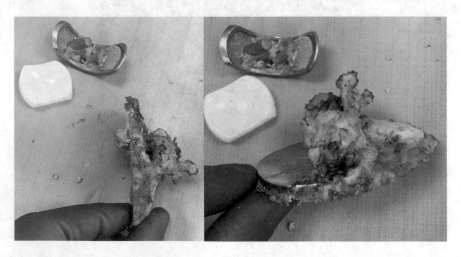

Fig. 2.9 Example of removing a medial unicompartmental implant with minimal bone loss by
cutting the tibia at the level of the implant

(i)

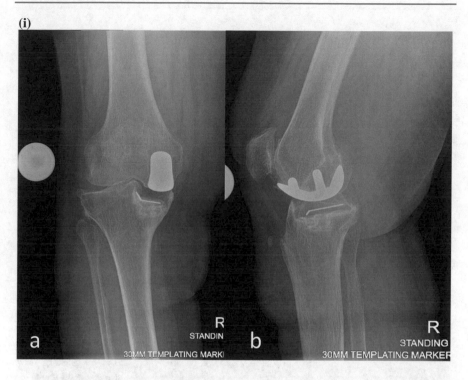

Fig. 2.10 i Preoperative radiographs of right knee in a 79 years old lady with a failed medial unicompartmental knee replacement and proximal tibial bone loss. **ii** Postoperative radiographs at 3 years following revision using metaphyseal sleeve on the tibia and primary PS component on the femur with satisfactory outcomes

encountered, then stems, sleeves or augments might be needed. On the femoral side, we often find that it has been over-resected posteriorly. Again, augments might be needed and we use revision implants in those circumstances which in turns mandates the use of a stem to ensure adequate implant fixation; either a short cemented or cementless stem.

Patellofemoral Joint Arthroplasty (PJFA) (Figs. 2.11 and 2.12): Here, we would encourage the use of a posterior stabilised implant as the box would add some protection against the anterior bone loss on the distal femur from removing the femoral component. However, if there is significant bone loss anteriorly then a revision component with a stem might be needed to achieve adequate fixation.

Top Tip: If using femoral augments, do not rely only on boxed components for fixation but always use either a short cemented or a cementless stem to ensure durable fixation.

(ii)

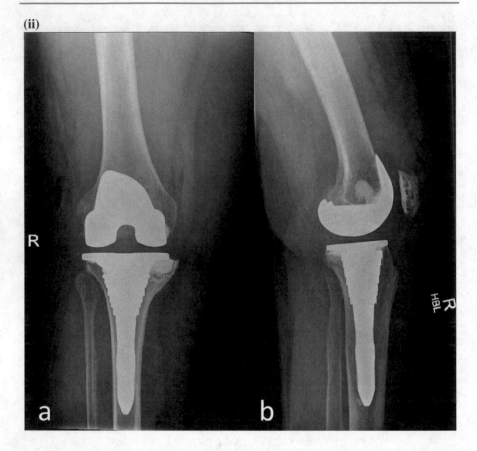

Fig. 2.10 (continued)

(i)

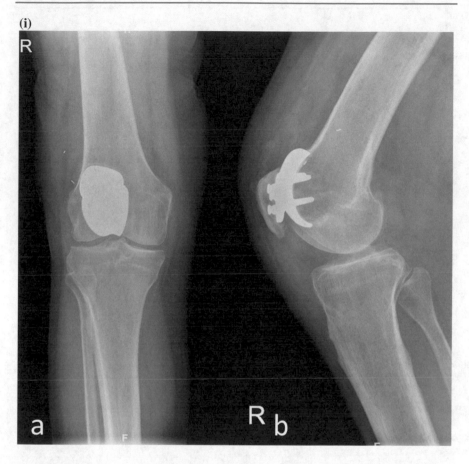

Fig. 2.11 i 68 years old woman with a symptomatic worn PFJA and minimal bone loss. **ii** Postoperative radiographs following a revision with a primary implant

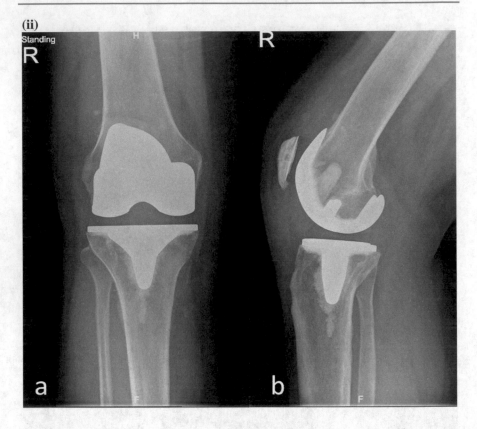

Fig. 2.11 (continued)

(i)

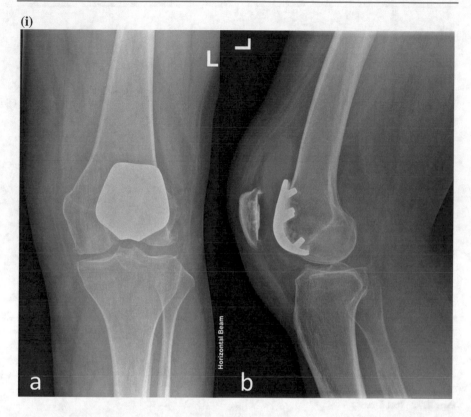

Fig. 2.12 i Preoperative radiographs of a symptomatic 59 years old lady with PFJA. **ii** Postoperative radiographs at 2 years following revision with a primary PS implant

(ii)

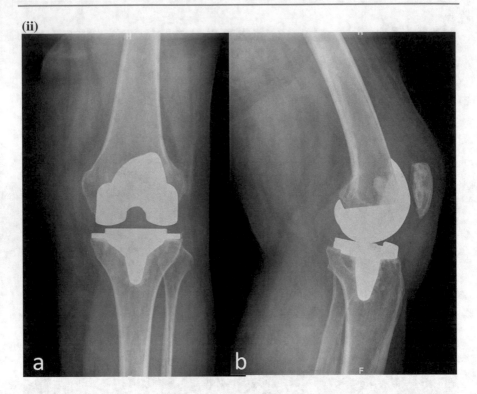

Fig. 2.12 (continued)

2.8 Previous Patellectomy

Patellectomy, now a largely historical operation, was traditionally performed as a salvage procedure for severely comminuted patella fractures, recurrent patellar dislocation or degenerative arthritis of the patellofemoral joint [11–13]. Patients with patellectomy have significant functional limitations with knee instability, pain, abnormal gait, difficulty ascending stairs, and loss of terminal extension [14]. Poor clinical outcomes have been reported following TKA for patients with previous patellectomy [15].

A number of techniques have been described to improve the outcomes of patients with patellectomy undergoing TKA with varying success. These include autograft bone reconstruction using bone graft sewn into the previous anatomical position of the patella with a subsynovial pouch for stabilisation [16], allograft reconstruction of the patella using a whole patella-quadriceps tendon allograft [17], and the use of a prosthetic trabecular metal patella implant [18, 19]. Although some stability can be achieved using a patella implant if residual bone is present, early loosening and failure was encountered when soft tissue was used for fixation to the implant [20].

We have recently described a novel *Tubeplasty* technique [21], developed by Jeffrey Gollish, with satisfactory outcomes based on *Insall's* isolated proximal re-alignment for PFJ instability. Here, in the context of TKA, the knee is approached in the usual fashion. The extensor mechanism is invariably thinned centrally and tends to sublux and track laterally with attenuated medial tissues. The lateral margin of the extensor mechanism is then identified and followed up to the lateral inter-muscular septum; bluntly dissecting vastus lateralis off the intermuscular septum. The vastus lateralis is then separated from the iliotibial band all the way distally to the interval between the patella tendon and iliotibial band to allow sufficient mobilisation of the extensor mechanism. The *Tubeplasty procedure* is performed by folding the lateral half of the extensor mechanism tendon under the central half of the rectus portion of the extensor mechanism forming a semi-tube. This results in thickening of the extensor mechanism tendon and central patella tracking. The VMO is then advanced and brought across to the reconstructed *(tubed)* central portion of the extensor mechanism. The tubeplasty procedure compensate for the thinned central portion of the extensor mechanism tendon and has the advantage of relying on normal native tissues with the main aim of improving extensor mechanism tracking during functional range of motion. Further, it has the added benefit of improving the mechanics of extension, as the tube matures into a thick well-defined structure, increasing the lever arm of the quadriceps (Fig. 2.13; see Chap. 14 on patella dislocation for further details).

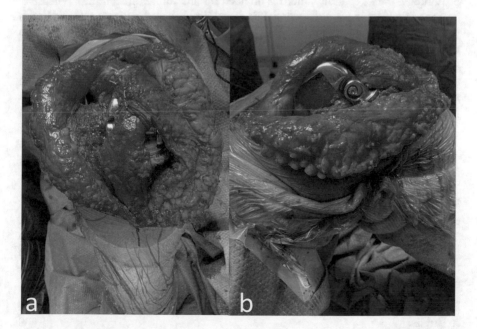

Fig. 2.13 Clinical photographs for a complex reconstruction in a case with previous patellectomy and extensor mechanism dislocation; **a, b** in flexion following *Matar's procedure* with patella tubeplasty (see Chap. 14 for more details)

We do use a PS design in those patients for mechanical reasons rather than a need for constraint as they are more tolerant to any anterior slide which can be exaggerated by weakened quadriceps. This also achieves reasonable function without any soft tissue reconstruction procedures [22].

Top Tip: **In patients with previous patellectomy, always ensure central extensor tracking and use a PS implant.**

2.9 Patella Baja and Alta

Anything that we do to help the patellofemoral joint will have an impact on the tibiofemoral joint. In *patella baja* scenarios, we have yet to find a reliable way of improving this situation as even osteotomy techniques do not change the fact that the patella tendon is short; raising it proximally may lead to impingement. So, if patients have longstanding and well-adapted baja with good range of motion then they are likely to enjoy similar range postoperatively and the issue here is exposure and implantation as discussed earlier. If, on the other hand, it is an acquired baja due to technical errors or recent surgery then patients would be unhappy with impingement and reduced range of motion and joint line alterations might be necessary; this must be balanced against tibiofemoral joint stability.

Patella alta is less of an issue as access is easier with a long patella tendon and providing it tracks centrally, there is no need for any further procedures. What may be more problematic is congenital PFJ instability which is often associated with patella alta. Remember, until the patella engages in the trochlear groove it is at high risk of dislocating or maltracking if not central. You may occasionally find that lowering the patella button might add some security. Finally, if you do decide to alter the joint line in either case then do so on both sides (tibial and femoral cuts) to minimise the impact on the tibiofemoral joint and the collaterals within the frame principle; 2–3 mm at most.

2.10 Previous Septic Arthritis

These are very challenging cases for two reasons; firstly, with pyogenic infections and subsequent chondrolysis, stiffness is a major issue with difficulty exposure and access. Early extensile maneuverers such as a tibial crest osteotomy is advised early on. Secondly, the bone quality is poor due to lack of loading which has an effect on achieving adequate fixation. Further, preoperative tissue samplings for microbiology are advised with the use of antibiotic-loaded cement.

Top Tip: **Always have a salvage option on standby in cases with previous septic arthritis.**

2.11 Primary Hinged TKA

Indications for primary hinged TKA are many but in this context include Charcot joint, elderly patients with significant valgus and deficient collaterals. Once the deformity is corrected with bony cuts, the extensors are invariably tight. Remember that most hinges have a fixed posterior axis of rotation; like a clamshell. Hinges cope well with instability but have implications on the extensors. Any excessive load on already tight extensors with a clamshell mechanism will lead to disastrous fatigue failure; patella fracture, dislocation or tendon failure (Fig. 2.14). So, it is important to ensure that you do not overstuff the PFJ, know your implant thickness and resect enough bone. This is one of the rare occasions where the joint line is no longer sacrosanct; gravity flexion intraoperatively and soft tissue tension testing with trials in situ are good guides. This is more so with valgus knees in elderly frail

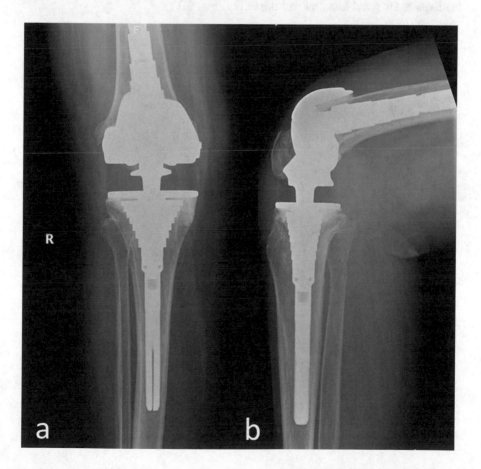

Fig. 2.14 Example of a failed hinged rTKA with an overstuffed PFJ and raised joint line at time of reconstruction and the inevitable, but preventable, complication of a failed extensor mechanism

patients with a pre-operative short and tight extensor mechanism (see Chap. 10 on hinge implants for further details).

Top Tip: **Do not overstuff the PFJ with a posterior fixed axis of rotation hinge implant; the extensors will fail.**

Charcot joints are not painful and only operated on to restore some ability to stand or function. The rule is to think about it in diabetic patients, investigate it, and hinge it! (Fig. 2.15). Other examples where hinges are needed are salvage for supracondylar fractures in elderly frail patients, using a distal femoral replacement to ensure immediate weight-bearing and rehabilitation to minimise medical complications (see Chap. 16 for further details) (Fig. 2.16). Finally, in the rare scenarios of skeletal dysplasia one would have to consider custom-made implants as the varied anatomy and deficient ligaments make any attempted soft tissue balancing inadequate for good function and durability (Fig. 2.17).

(i)

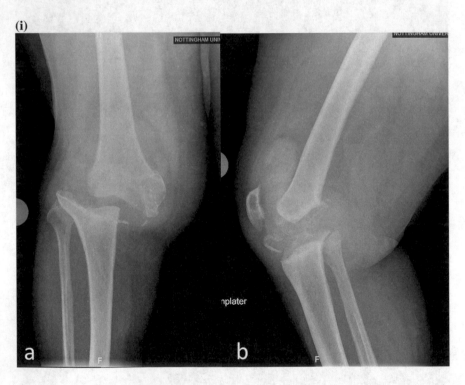

Fig. 2.15 i Preoperative radiographs of a Charcot joint in a 49-year old man. **ii** Postoperative radiographs with reconstruction using a rotating-hinge (fully cemented)

(ii)

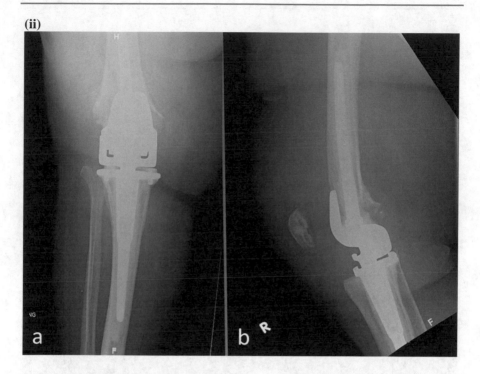

Fig. 2.15 (continued)

2.12   What About Patient Specific Instrumentation (PSI)?

As we have previously shown looking at published RCTs in primary TKA, PSI made no real impact on outcomes [23]. However, in the context of complex primary TKA, particularly in the presence of metal work where conventional jigs cannot be used, PSI does have a role and can be a very useful adjunct. It is worth noting, however, that the food and drug administration (FDA) clearance for most PSI systems currently mandates the use of a neutral mechanical axis or only limited correction ($\pm 3°$ from mechanical axis) but not enough to account for severe extra-articular deformity. So, if you have an angular deformity where PSI could really help within the collateral frame principle, PSI would want to restore that deformed limb to neutral mechanical axis which may not be desirable in those cases [24]. The argument here is about whether you will accept some residual deformity when reconstructing a longstanding deformed knee aiming to achieve a balanced knee and not necessarily a mechanically aligned knee. Each case must be treated on its own merits. However, practical experience has taught us that patients with a lifelong deformity have adapted to prefer a well-balanced knee with residual deformity than an unbalanced knee in neutral mechanical alignment. (Figs. 2.18 and 2.19).

(i)

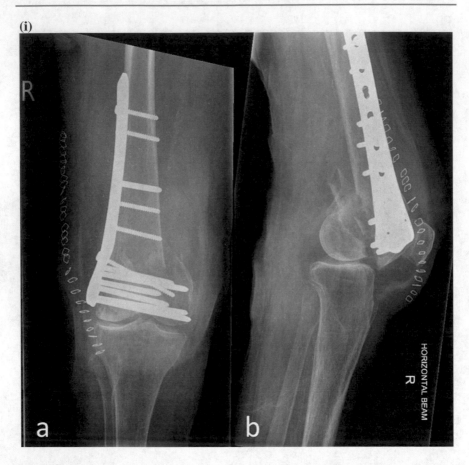

Fig. 2.16 i Example of failed attempted fixation of a supracondylar femoral fracture in a 90-year-old. ii Salvaged with a complex primary TKA using a DFR implant with immediate weight-bearing and rehabilitation

(ii)

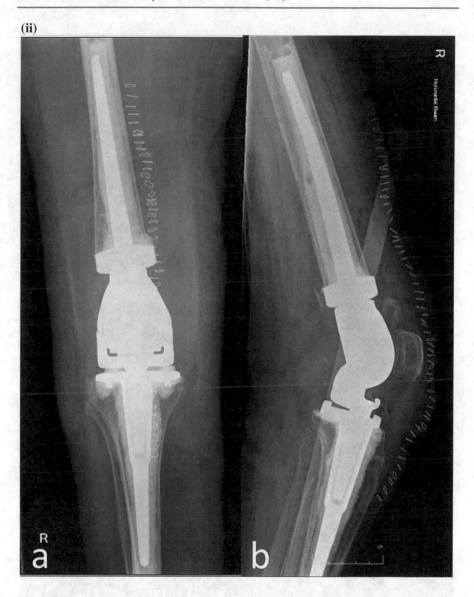

Fig. 2.16 (continued)

In summary, complex primary TKA can be challenging with a variety of clinical scenarios encountered. Understanding and anticipating the complexity with detailed preoperative planning is crucial to ensure good outcomes.

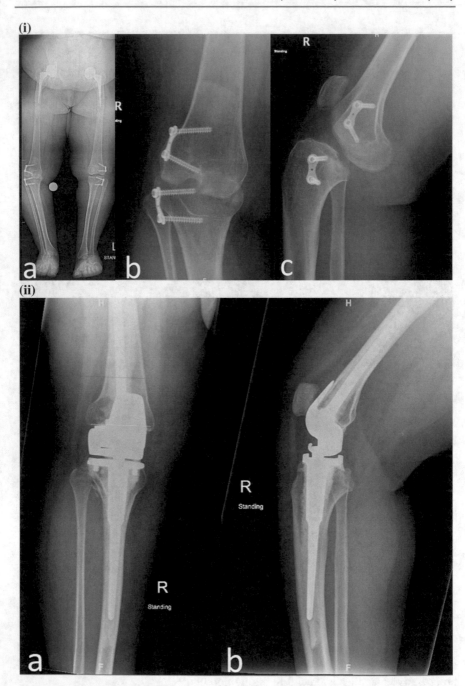

Fig. 2.17 **i** Mechanical alignment, anteroposterior and lateral radiographs of right knee in a 24 years old woman with skeletal dysplasia with short stature and a painful unstable knee; she had previously had bilateral epiphysodeses. **ii** Postoperative radiographs at 4 years following knee reconstruction with a custom-made hinge knee implant with restored function and satisfactory outcomes

(i)

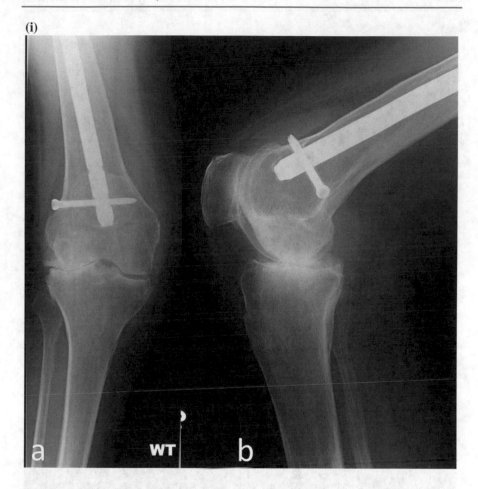

Fig. 2.18 i Preoperative radiographs of a 68 years old man with advanced symptomatic OA and previous ipsilateral femoral intramedullary nail for femoral fracture. **ii** Postoperative radiographs following a primary TKA using PSI cutting guides

(ii)

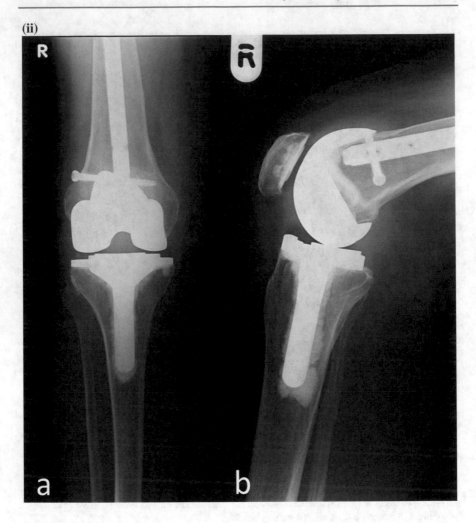

Fig. 2.18 (continued)

(i)

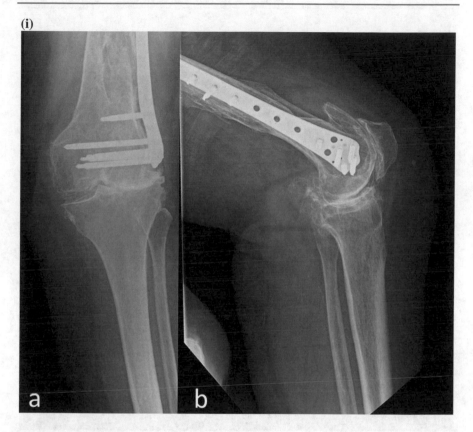

Fig. 2.19 **i** Preoperative radiographs of 88 years old woman with advanced symptomatic OA of her right knee with ipsilateral total hip implant and previous supracondylar femoral fracture which was plated few years ago. **ii** Preoperative radiographs of the femur. **iii** Operative images of the PSI cutting guides and implants used; CT-based. **iv** Operative images demonstrating the application of the PSI positioning guides (**a**, **b**) on the femur and tibia (**c**, **d**). Once pinned in situ, the cutting jigs can then be applied of the pre-determined size. **e** Operative images demonstrating the implant at final stages leaving the lateral plate in situ. Two screws had to be taken out but the reminder of the plate offered the extramedullary protection negating the need for stemmed implant. **v** Postoperative radiographs following complex primary using PSI with a primary PS femoral component and stemmed tibial component. The plate was retained and only couple of screws were removed

(ii)

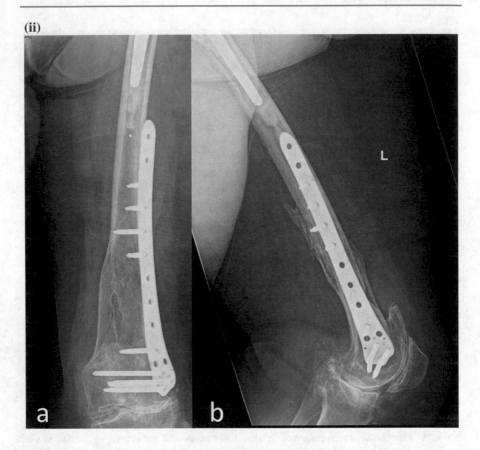

Fig. 2.19 (continued)

(iii)

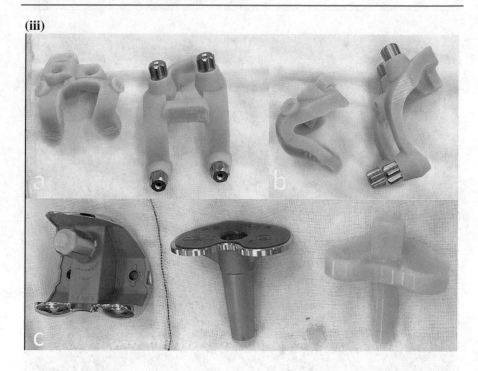

Fig. 2.19 (continued)

(iv)

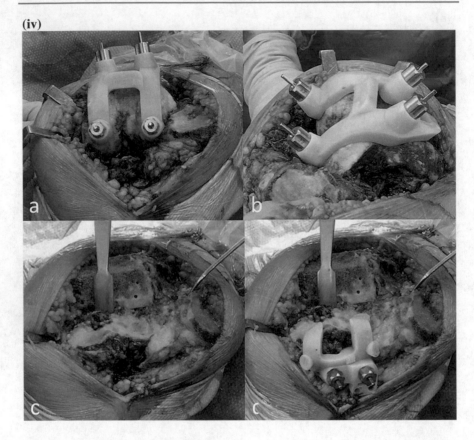

Fig. 2.19 (continued)

(v)

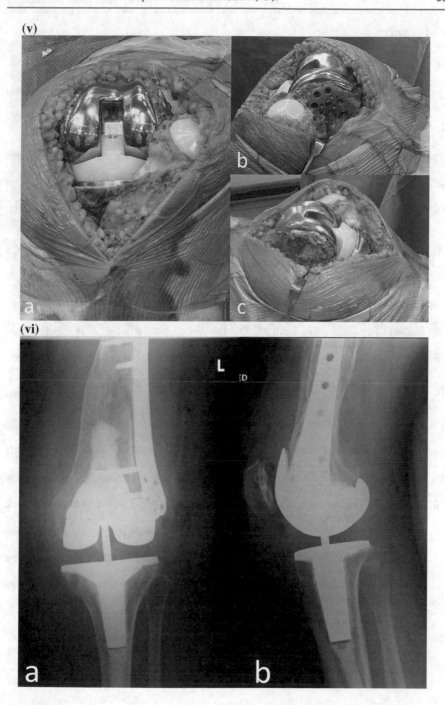

(vi)

Fig. 2.19 (continued)

References

1. Martin JR, et al. Complex primary total knee arthroplasty: long-term outcomes. J Bone Joint Surg Am. 2016;98(17):1459–70.
2. Badawy M, Fenstad AM, Furnes O. Primary constrained and hinged total knee arthroplasty: 2- and 5-year revision risk compared with unconstrained total knee arthroplasty: a report on 401 cases from the Norwegian Arthroplasty Register 1994–2017. Acta Orthop. 2019;90 (5):467–72.
3. Mancino F, et al. Satisfactory mid-term outcomes of condylar-constrained knee implants in primary total knee arthroplasty: clinical and radiological follow-up. J Orthop Traumatol. 2020;21(1):22.
4. Watts CD, et al. Morbid obesity: increased risk of failure after aseptic revision TKA. Clin Orthop Relat Res. 2015;473(8):2621–7.
5. D'Apuzzo MR, Novicoff WM, Browne JA. The John Insall Award: morbid obesity independently impacts complications, mortality, and resource use after TKA. Clin Orthop Relat Res. 2015;473(1):57–63.
6. Kosashvili Y, et al. Distal femoral varus osteotomy for lateral osteoarthritis of the knee: a minimum ten-year follow-up. Int Orthop. 2010;34(2):249–54.
7. Cerciello S, et al. Total knee arthroplasty after high tibial osteotomy. Orthopedics. 2014;37 (3):191–8.
8. Closkey RF, Windsor RE. Alterations in the patella after a high tibial or distal femoral osteotomy. Clin Orthop Relat Res. 2001;389:51–6.
9. Scuderi GR, Windsor RE, Insall JN. Observations on patellar height after proximal tibial osteotomy. J Bone Joint Surg Am. 1989;71(2):245–8.
10. Neri T, Myat D, Parker D. The use of navigation in osteotomies around the knee. Clin Sports Med. 2019;38(3):451–69.
11. Kelly MA, Brittis DA. Patellectomy. Orthop Clin North Am. 1992;23(4):657–63.
12. Reiley RE, DeSouza LJ. Patellectomy. an alternate technique. Clin Orthop Relat Res. 1974; (103):170–7.
13. Orso CA, Crisci V. Patellectomy in the treatment of knee arthrosis. Minerva Ortop. 1967;18 (9):578–82.
14. Sutton FS Jr, et al. The effect of patellectomy on knee function. J Bone Joint Surg Am. 1976;58(4):537–40.
15. Asadollahi S, et al. Total knee arthroplasty after patellectomy: a meta-analysis of case-control studies. Knee. 2017;24(2):191–6.
16. Buechel FF. Patellar tendon bone grafting for patellectomized patients having total knee arthroplasty. Clin Orthop Relat Res. 1991;271:72–8.
17. Busfield BT, Ries MD. Whole patellar allograft for total knee arthroplasty after previous patellectomy. Clin Orthop Relat Res. 2006;450:145–9.
18. Kwong Y, Desai VV. The use of a tantalum-based Augmentation Patella in patients with a previous patellectomy. Knee. 2008;15(2):91–4.
19. Nasser S, Poggie RA. Revision and salvage patellar arthroplasty using a porous tantalum implant. J Arthroplasty. 2004;19(5):562–72.
20. Ries MD, et al. Porous tantalum patellar augmentation: the importance of residual bone stock. Clin Orthop Relat Res. 2006;452:166–70.
21. Matar HE, Bawale R, Gollish JD. Extensor mechanism reconstruction "Tubeplasty" in total knee arthroplasty with previous patellectomy: surgical technique and clinical outcomes. J Orthop. 2020;21:14–8.

22. Cameron HU, Hu C, Vyamont D. Posterior stabilized knee prosthesis for total knee replacement in patients with prior patellectomy. Can J Surg. 1996;39(6):469–73.
23. Matar HE, et al. Overview of randomized controlled trials in total knee arthroplasty (47,675 Patients): what have we learnt? J Arthroplasty. 2020;35(6):1729-1736.e1.
24. Sassoon A, et al. Systematic review of patient-specific instrumentation in total knee arthroplasty: new but not improved. Clin Orthop Relat Res. 2015;473(1):151–8.

Assessment of Painful Total Knee Arthroplasty

3

If I had an hour to solve a problem, I'd spend 55 minutes thinking about the problem and 5 minutes thinking about solutions.

Albert Einstein

3.1 Introduction

Total knee arthroplasty is a reliable and cost-effective operation for end-stage degenerative joint disease. Despite its success and longevity, unfavourable long-term pain outcomes have been reported by 10 to 34% of patients. In the best quality studies, an unfavourable pain outcome was reported in about 20% of patients following TKA [1]. The reason for dissatisfaction is multifactorial including ongoing knee pain, limited function, and failure to meet preoperative expectations [2, 3]. With the ever-increasing demand for TKA worldwide, the number of unhappy knees presenting to revision knee clinics is estimated to increase substantially [4, 5].

The most common failure modes, aside from periprosthetic joint infection (PJI), are aseptic loosening, instability, and malalignment. With the introduction of improved polyethylene in the early 2000s, polyethene related-wear in contemporary knees is less prevalent [6]. Infection, loosening and instability are by far the most common modes of failure in most national registries, with some more prevalent than others [6–8].

A systematic way of evaluating problematic knees is essential to ascertain whether a revision surgery, a major undertaking, would solve patients' problems. Every practice or institute would have their own pathways or algorithms to investigate patients. Here, we try to shed lights on some practical aspects of

H. E. Matar et al., *Revision Total Knee Arthroplasty*,
https://doi.org/10.1007/978-3-030-81285-0_3

evaluating patients presenting to revision knee clinics rather than a comprehensive review of the merits of well-known investigations or diagnostic criteria which have been covered extensively in the literature [9–11].

3.2   Clinic Assessment

Detailed history, clinical examination and plain radiographs form the basis for establishing and understanding the mechanism of failure in the majority of cases. A management plan should be formulated at this point with additional investigations only to confirm and answer a specific diagnostic question that would alter the surgical plan.

We have to understand the indication for the index procedure; minimal OA on preoperative radiographs is a major finding in a lot of unhappy knees [12]. It has been shown that patients with complete joint space collapse enjoy significantly better outcome scores following TKA compared to those with less severe changes [13]. Similarly, concurrent ipsilateral hip OA or a degenerative spine can also cause knee pain and has been found to be associated with post-operative dissatisfaction, particularly when this has not been discussed as part of the consenting process [14, 15].

The onset of symptoms and relation to time of index surgery is often revealing when a patient has ongoing pain, issues with wound healing, or even discharge postoperatively which would strongly suggest infection. Here, the diagnosis is made clinically from the first visit and some confirmatory blood tests or joint aspiration to identify the infecting organism are only adjuncts to provide a documented evidence both to the patient and the surgeon and help to tailor a targeted antibiotic therapy. On the other hand, a new symptom many years after implantation in a previously well-functioning knee points towards a recent failure; either loosening or less commonly haematogenous infection. PJI should always be considered when evaluating an unhappy knee through history, examination, blood tests and aspirations when appropriate.

Top tip: If a patient had a rip-roaringly arthritic knee and a justified TKA but has never been happy, infection is the most likely culprit.

Once infection is ruled out, there are many potential causes of a painful TKA. The common scenarios seen in clinical practice, however, are loosening, instability, and referred pain. Less commonly, extra-articular causes around the knee such as neuralgic pain, soft tissue pain and impingement (such as popliteus) can cause trouble. These are diagnoses of exclusion.

Classically, start-up pain on weight-bearing that settles a bit after few steps indicates occult loosening. Instability pain is non-specific and often associated with an effusion because of recurrent synovial irritation. The pain is often felt anteriorly due to overloading of the anterior structures and tissues as most cases are anteroposterior (AP) instability. Here, the pain is most pronounced on loading the knee in a semi-flexed position; stairs, standing from sitting and apprehension where patients lose confidence and do not lead with the affected knee as they lack trust in it. These are good clinical indicators that there are instability issues at play.

Anterior Knee Pain: this is a contentious topic in the literature particularly around patella resurfacing with opposing views [16–18]. However, patella resurfacing aside, we believe that anterior knee pain is generally a sign of patellofemoral joint (PFJ) and extensor mechanism overload. This pertains to femoral rotation, malalignment and tibiofemoral instability which can all manifest in PFJ overload. This is probably why secondary patella resurfacings seldom solve the problem—we simplify the cause to an unresurfaced patella, while in fact patients have instability which drives the femur anteriorly putting too much load on the extensor mechanism and PFJ. Take for example a video fluoroscopic view of the knee—once the knee flexes beyond 70–80°, you find that the patella is no longer articulating with the femoral component but actually it is the extensor hood that does so in this position [19]. The most important implant-related factor in patella-femoral pain is the trochlea design, and having an adequate groove for tracking which would minimise patella related pain or issues, irrespective of whether it has been resurfaced or not [20].

Secondary patella resurfacing: This is only indicated if patients have evidence of complete obliteration of the articular cartilage on a skyline view, usually affecting the lateral facet, in a knee that in all other aspects is functioning well i.e. well-balanced throughout range of motion and particularly in mid-flexion. This needs to be further supported by clinical history that demonstrates a functioning knee before the patella cartilage had worn out and that this is a new problem that has developed over time. This could be elicited by enquiring about PFJ symptoms with the absence of symptoms in walking on flat surfaces but problematic during walking on inclined slopes where they are engaging their PFJ (Figs. 3.1 and 3.2).

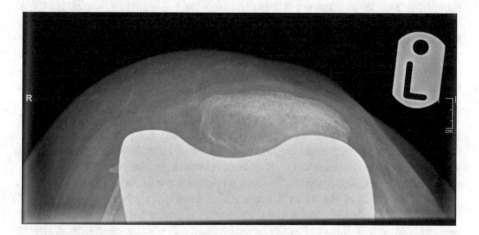

Fig. 3.1 Example of a skyline view of a left knee with a native patella which had become symptomatic presenting with anterior knee pain, there is evidence of loss of articular cartilage particularly on the lateral facet

Top tip: The majority of anterior knee pain in a painful TKA is due to PFJ overload and not isolated patella pain.

Effusion in TKA: It is important to keep in mind that some effusion and swelling following TKA could last for up to 2 years to dissipate, sometimes it never does so. Also, a lot of well-functioning TKAs will have a degree of small effusion which is by no means a pathological finding unless it is accompanied by other symptoms. Only a brave surgeon would revise a knee within 2 years of surgery unless there is a infection, clear mechanical issue or catastrophic ligamentous failure. Equally, when evaluating a painful TKA that is completely dry, then extra-articular causes of pain are far more likely.

Top tip: In most cases, a painful but dry TKA is a reassuring sign that suggests an extra-articular cause of pain.

Stability: The majority of painful TKAs are stable in full extension as the posterior capsule stabilises the joint in extension. Similarly, at 90° flexion most painful knees with intact collaterals are stable. Isolated posterior instability, recurvatum, is rare and implies complete posterior capsular disruption necessitating the use of hinged implants. However, it is in mid-flexion where most instability is elicited; this is the most common type of instability in unhappy TKAs.

Mid-flexion instability is a multifactorial problem; partly due to surgical technique; in particular how we address flexion and extension gaps. Conceptually, we (as orthopaedic surgeons) tend to describe everything in two planes, we do this for fractures (AP and lateral) and also for deformity around the knee. Most surgeons tend to over-release ligaments to correct deformity. For example, take a knee that has varus AND fixed flexion deformity. There is in fact no such thing! It is all the same deformity, it is amalgamated together, but that description is ingrained in our thought-process throughout our training as surgeons. Subsequently, we tend to think about correcting the varus by releasing medial structures and tissues, and we do something else to correct the fixed flexion contracture. However, as we outlined in previous chapters, it should all be posteromedial work; removing the osteophytes and posteromedial capsular release off the proximal tibia. We also over-resect the distal femur increasing the extension gap to address the 'fixed flexion'. While this may work in balancing the posterior capsule in extension, once we put the knee in 20–30° flexion and make the posterior capsule redundant, we are now faced by medial instability due to over-released structures that would normally stabilise the knee in mid-flexion. So, by not recognising where the deformity is at the start of the operation we make erroneous decisions to fix it and end up with a problem that is quite difficult to solve. A gap balanced approach would minimise some of those issues.

The other driver of instability is implant's design particularly for minimising AP translations. This can be controlled with increased conformity between the femur and the tibia. Whilst this conformity is well tolerated as we near extension, it is well established that in knee flexion tibiofemoral rotation must be allowed. Too much conformity in flexion will stress the fixation interfaces and put the longevity of the implant at risk.

Two design philosophies have evolved including a single radius knee and multi radii designs with each having its pros and cons. For a single radius design to work, it must allow rotation in flexion which is delivered through a reduction in tibio-femoral conformity. The negative impact of this however, is the reduced ability of the implant to provide stability in mid-flexion and gait. On the other hand, multi radii designs are very conforming throughout range of motion which improves stability throughout range. However, when transitioning from one radius to another a paradoxical anterior slide has been demonstrated [21]. We have a catch-22 situation as surgeons between optimising implant design to give us stability but also increasing constraint which in turn affects its longevity by transmitting shear stresses to the implant-cement-bone interfaces. Single-radius designs have non-conforming poly inserts making them inherently unstable while multi-radii designs have 'jumps' in radii at 30° or 45° which can cause mid-flexion instability.

Painful rTKA: The same assessment process also applies to painful rTKA, however multiply revised cases are different with soft tissue scarring and there is a truth to the fact that knees will tolerate a limited number of surgeries with less chance of fixing the problem with salvage options. In general, causes of pain after rTKA are broadly similar to a painful primary with the addition of end of stem pain.

Examination under Anaesthetics (EUA): this is a valuable tool in assessing a painful TKA. A lot more information can be gained when the patients are relaxed and apprehension is taken out of the equation. End points become readily recognisable, it also allows us to aspirate the joint at the same time or even consider diagnostic injections of local anaesthetics in some cases.

Malalignment: the big problem is *'unbalanced malalignment'* which can lead to instability. In this context, it is a broad term that includes flexion of the femoral component or oversizing and overhang (causing popliteus impingement syndromes), or an overhanging tibial component irritating the iliotibial band on the lateral side or the MCL, PFJ overstuffing, patella clunk with the patella catching the box of the femoral component, persistent deformity with thrust, and rotational malalignment where in severe cases you can see the foot pointing in the wrong direction. On the other hand, sometimes we can have *'balanced malalignment'* which tend to present with premature failure due to malalignment but not necessarily a painful knee which is a different issue. Sagittal malalignment is readily identifiable from plain radiographs; axial malalignment requires some cross-sectional imaging such as CT.

Top tip: We would caution against patella realignment procedures in the presence of rotational malalignment—consider it in terms of the train (patella) and the track (trochlear flange); it's never the train that is the problem. The train always follows the track.

Computed tomography (CT): Can be used to identify subtle loosening, axial malrotation, and to assess bone loss particularly with boxed designs. However, all implants create a halo of scatter around them, even with metal artefact reduction sequences, and therefore CT should be interpreted with caution as we see some exaggeration of bone loss or lack of osteointegration.

Ultrasound: might be useful for extraarticular causes around the knee particularly in painful rTKA cases such as iliotibial band irritation or pes anserinus bursitis or pain. Guided trigger point injections can be diagnostic as well as therapeutic in some cases.

Bone scans: a negative bone scan is helpful reassurance for the surgeon and the patient. A positive one, however, is difficult to interpret. Therefore, a judicious use of this modality is needed. In some cases, such as consideration of secondary patella resurfacing in otherwise well-functioning knee, there is usually increased uptake in the patella with the rest of the knee being fairly normal (Fig. 3.2). However, changes on bone scan following a primary TKA can last years. Therefore, there is very little value to be gained from a bone scan within 2 years of surgery.

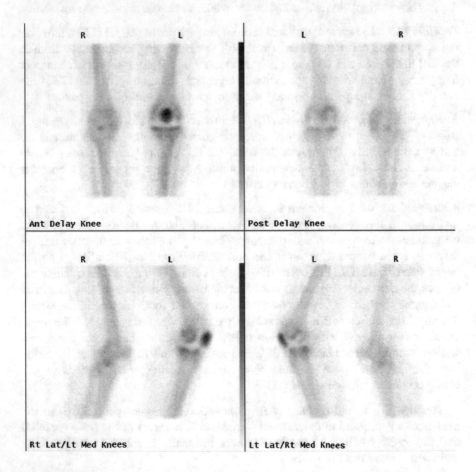

Fig. 3.2 Example of a bone scan in a 63 years old patient with a painful left TKA showing fairly normal uptake around the prosthesis with no evidence of increased activity around either components. The patella had not been resurfaced and show high uptake in an otherwise mechanically well aligned and balanced knee

Manage Patients' Expectations and MDTs: Not only at the time of initial assessment but throughout waiting for investigations—particularly coming to a tertiary centre where they expect you to sort their problem out. Finally, a multi-disciplinary team approach is crucial for the efficient and successful running of a revision knee service where complex cases can be discussed, second opinions can be sought, and other specialists such as microbiologists and orthoplastic surgeons can provide their input in the planning stages to standardise care and improve patients' outcomes.

In summary, when assessing majority of patients with painful TKA, a thorough clinical history, examination and plain radiographs are all what is needed to formulate management plans. Confirmatory investigations are only to confirm and document the clinical impression.

References

1. Beswick AD, et al. What proportion of patients report long-term pain after total hip or knee replacement for osteoarthritis? A systematic review of prospective studies in unselected patients. BMJ Open. 2012;2(1):e000435.
2. Becker R, et al. Expectation, satisfaction and clinical outcome of patients after total knee arthroplasty. Knee Surg Sports Traumatol Arthrosc. 2011;19(9):1433–41.
3. Toms AD, et al. The management of patients with painful total knee replacement. J Bone Joint Surg Br. 2009;91(2):143–50.
4. Singh JA, et al. Rates of total joint replacement in the United States: future projections to 2020–2040 using the national inpatient sample. J Rheumatol. 2019;46(9):1134–40.
5. 17th Annual Report of the National Joint Registry for England, Wales, Northern Ireland, the Isle of Man and the States of Guernsey. [cited 2020 23rd Oct]. https://reports.njrcentre.org.uk/Portals/0/PDFdownloads/NJR%2017th%20Annual%20Report%202020.pdf.
6. Lum ZC, Shieh AK, Dorr LD. Why total knees fail-A modern perspective review. World J Orthop. 2018;9(4):60–4.
7. Le DH, et al. Current modes of failure in TKA: infection, instability, and stiffness predominate. Clin Orthop Relat Res. 2014;472(7):2197–200.
8. Mathis DT, et al. Reasons for failure in primary total knee arthroplasty—an analysis of prospectively collected registry data. J Orthop. 2021;23:60–6.
9. Kalson NS, et al. Investigation and management of prosthetic joint infection in knee replacement: a BASK surgical practice guideline. Knee. 2020;27(6):1857–65.
10. Kalson NS, et al. Revision knee replacement surgery in the NHS: a BASK surgical practice guideline. Knee. 2021;29:353–64.
11. Kalson NS, et al. Clinical prioritisation of revision knee surgical procedures: BASK working group consensus document. Knee. 2021;28:57–63.
12. Gunaratne R, et al. Patient dissatisfaction following total knee arthroplasty: a systematic review of the literature. J Arthroplasty. 2017;32(12):3854–60.
13. Liebensteiner M, et al. Patient satisfaction after total knee arthroplasty is better in patients with pre-operative complete joint space collapse. Int Orthop. 2019;43(8):1841–7.
14. Dibra FF, et al. Don't forget the hip! Hip arthritis masquerading as knee pain. Arthroplast Today. 2018;4(1):118–24.
15. Malahias MA, et al. Association of lumbar degenerative disease and revision rate following total knee arthroplasty. J Knee Surg. 2020.
16. Longo UG, et al. Patellar resurfacing in total knee arthroplasty: systematic review and meta-analysis. J Arthroplasty. 2018;33(2):620–32.

17. Abdel MP, Parratte S, Budhiparama NC. The patella in total knee arthroplasty: to resurface or not is the question. Curr Rev Musculoskelet Med. 2014;7(2):117–24.
18. Matar HE, et al. Overview of randomized controlled trials in total knee arthroplasty (47,675 Patients): what have we learnt? J Arthroplasty. 2020;35(6):1729-1736.e1.
19. Williams D, et al. The relationship between alignment, function and loading in total knee replacement: in-vivo analysis of a unique patient population. J Biomech. 2020;112:110042.
20. Napier RJ, et al. A prospective evaluation of a largely cementless total knee arthroplasty cohort without patellar resurfacing: 10-year outcomes and survivorship. BMC Musculoskelet Disord. 2018;19(1):205.
21. Clary CW, et al. The influence of total knee arthroplasty geometry on mid-flexion stability: an experimental and finite element study. J Biomech. 2013;46(7):1351–7.

Indicated for Revision Total Knee Arthroplasty

Indications for Revision Total Knee Arthroplasty

4

> We cannot solve problems by using the same kind of thinking
> we used when we created them.
>
> *Albert Einstein*

4.1 Introduction

Over the last four decades, there has been considerable innovation in the field of TKA in terms of implant design, materials, instrumentation, and surgical techniques. Long-term survivorship data of TKAs from national registries and large case series have demonstrated excellent longevity with ever-increasing demand on TKAs. In a review of studies reporting beyond 15 years survivorship with all-cause survival of TKA construct, pooled survival-estimate from 47 registry-based studies (299,291 TKAs) at 25 years was 82.3% (95% CI 81.3–83.2) [1].

In a review of 52 studies including registry-based studies with 333,727 primary TKA and 12,907 rTKA and cohort studies with 54,777 primary TKA and 2,145 rTKA, the annual revision rate was 0.49% (95% CI; 0.41 to 0.58) [2]. Worldwide, the projected volume of primary and revision TKA will place an immense burden on future health care systems over the next few decades in many developed countries and advanced economies [3–7].

In the United States, between 2005 and 2006, 60,355 rTKA were performed, with the most common indications being infection (25.2%), implant loosening (16.1%) and implant failure/breakage (9.7%) [8]. In a subsequent study between 2009 and 2013, 337,597 rTKA were reported with infection again being the most common indication for revision (20.4%), followed by mechanical loosening (20.3%) [9]. Similar trends have emerged over the last few years in many healthcare settings with infection and aseptic loosening being the most common causes of failure of contemporary TKAs [10–13]. Overall, there has been a substantial reduction in implant-related failures such as polyethylene wear. Most short- to medium-term failures are currently due to infection, instability, and malalignment [14–17].

In this chapter, will discuss some of the contemporary indications for revision providing a summary of our practical experience and views on the current challenges in rTKA. Periprosthetic joint infection will be discussed in a dedicated chapter (see Chap. 16).

4.2   Our Series

In our series between 2003–2019, using a prospective local database and nationally collected data through the National Joint Registry (UK-NJR), we performed 1,298 consecutive rTKA on 1,254 patients. Forty-four patients had bilateral revisions. There were 985 aseptic revisions in 945 patients (75.4%) and 313 septic revisions in 309 patients (24.6%). Aseptic loosening and infection were the leading indications for our revision workload in a tertiary centre (Table 4.1) [18].

Top Tip: If you revise a knee without understanding what's wrong with it, you may end up with a different X-ray but the same outcome!

4.3   Polyethylene Wear

Historically, loosening due to polyethylene delamination failure and the processes that ensued was the dominant mechanism of failure (Figs. 4.1 and 4.2). Operatively, significant lysis is usually found in the posterior femoral condyles which can be

Table 4.1 Indications of rTKA in our series

Indication	Number of rTKA (%)
Aseptic loosening	511 (39.37)
Septic revisions (single and two-stages)	309 (23.8)
Instability	207 (15.95)
Stiffness	59 (4.55)
Conversion of uni to total	50 (3.85)
Periprosthetic fractures	37 (2.85)
Malalignment	37 (2.85)
Poly wear	35 (2.7)
Secondary patella resurfacing	31 (2.39)
Component dissociation	14 (1.08)
Implant fracture	8 (0.61)
Total	1,298

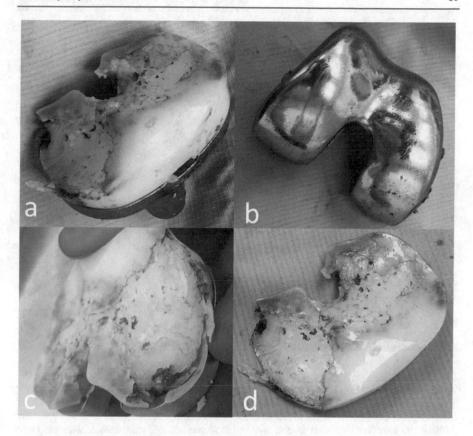

Fig. 4.1 Example of a catastrophic polyethylene delamination failure

quite hard to see on plain radiographs. Incidentally, this is the one area where adequate cementation is hard to achieve in primary TKA. Simply, as we implant the femoral component, it is a sliding motion onto the posterior condyles which shears off the cement layer, and it is very difficult to get reliable pressurisation in this area. In most revision cases, we tend to find a lot of debris and thick synovium in the posterior condylar area which forms a sheet of granulation tissue extending down the posterior capsule onto the tibia; it is always very important at the time of revision surgery to clear the posterior space.

The lysis also invades the area under the anterior flange which becomes loose, and with no physiological loading, bone resorption takes place. The distal femur does not loosen as easily as we tend to get good cement interdigitation when we pressurise and impact the component unlike the posterior condyles.

In polyethylene delamination, a thin layer in the surface separates from the deeper layers. It was most commonly seen in inserts sterilised by gamma irradiation in air where free radical damage has oxidised the polyethene [19]. In their landmark paper, *Dr Gerard Engh* and colleagues from the Anderson Orthopaedic Research

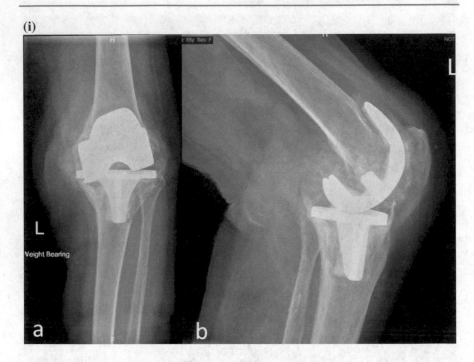

Fig. 4.2 i Preoperative radiographs of a failed left knee with significant bone loss, loosening as a result of catastrophic polyethylene failure in 85 years old woman. **ii** Postoperative radiographs at 2 years follow up following revision with a cemented rotating hinge due to the significant instability and the implant design (femoral component) which allows options to restore joint line without the need for augments in this system. Frail patients with osteopenic bone are better managed with a cemented implant

Institute looked at the influence of tibial baseplate surface finish and sterilisation methods of the polyethylene insert. They reported 5 to 10 years outcome on 365 CR Anatomic Modular Knee primary total knee arthroplasties performed from 1987 to 1998. Osteolysis was 4 times more likely with gamma irradiation in air than gamma irradiation in nitrogen, osteolysis was 2.6 times more likely with titanium baseplates than with cobalt-chrome base plates, and knee hyperextension (causing impingement) increased the risk of osteolysis [20]. Retrieval studies also demonstrated that there is a complex interplay between the baseplate surface finish and the locking mechanism design; a polished baseplate with a robust locking mechanism had the lowest incidence of backside damage and linear wear [21]. The improved manufacturing, sterilisation and packaging processes of polyethylene have also led to a substantial decrease in polyethylene related failures.

In primary total hip arthroplasty, randomised controlled trials of highly crossed-linked polyethylene (HXLPE) demonstrated better wear characteristics compared with conventional polyethylene at 5-,10- and 15-year follow-ups [22]. However, this has not been the case in primary TKA. Data from the Kaiser

(ii)

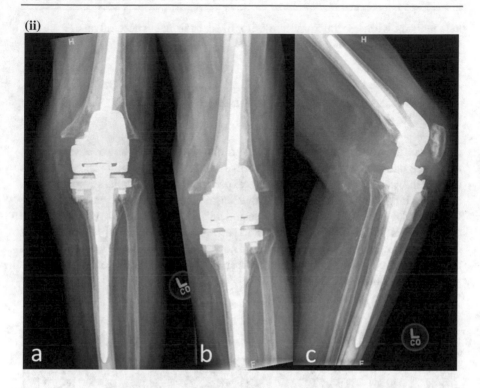

Fig. 4.2 (continued)

Permanente Total Joint Replacement Registry showed no differences in risk of revision for HXLPE (n = 11,048) compared with conventional polyethylene (n = 60,841) in conjunction with a cobalt-chrome tibial tray at 5 years follow-up [23]. Similarly, data from the NJR of conventional polyethylene (n = 513,744) compared with HXLPE (n = 36,914) showed no overall survival benefit of HXLPE after a maximum duration of 12 years follow-up, however HXLPE may have a role in specific "higher demand" groups such as patients < 60 years of age and/or those with a BMI of > 35 kg/m^2 [24]. Vitamin-E infused HXLPE and antioxidant polyethylene inserts are also in current use with early data suggesting some fatigue damage resistance and oxidation resistance [25]. However, it remains to be seen whether these new innovations will have an impact on long-term implant survivorship.

From a practical perspective, polyethylene inserts have got much better with the elimination of the oxidative degradation that we used to see and polyethylene wear is no longer a major cause of failure. Currently used conventional polyethylene inserts have overall better resistance to wear and multidirectional motion. This may get even better with antioxidant-infused and cross-linked polyethylene in the future. From an implant point of view, we do generally have much better locking mechanisms with less micromotion with fixed bearings. These advances are big steps forward in ensuring the longevity of TKAs.

4.4   Fixation and Aseptic Loosening (Figs. 4.3, 4.4, 4.5 and 4.6)

Cemented fixation is still the gold standard and widely used, however cementless knees are on the rise, particularly in North America and Australia. There are units around the world which have extensive experience with cementless implants with excellent long-term results [26–28]. However, national registries data including the UK, Sweden, Australia and New Zealand all show superior survivorship with cemented TKA [29]. This is in contrast to series published by high-volume users of cementless implants. It is worth noting, however, that registries present data on cementless knees of different manufacturers as a whole; some cementless knees perform better than others [30].

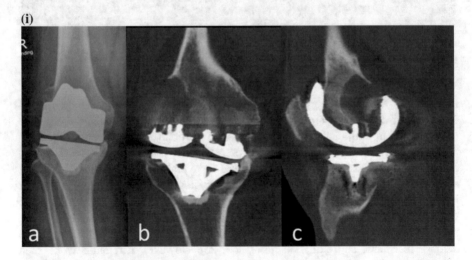

Fig. 4.3 i Example of a loose failed TKA with the common pattern of tibial tray collapsing medially and the knee collapsing into varus. The lateral femoral condyle had also collapsed with a large osteolytic lesion; (b-c) CT images demonstrating the extent of the femoral bone loss. ii Intraoperative photograph **a** demonstrating the large defect in the lateral femoral condyle; **b** circumferential press-fit metaphyseal sleeve preparation, the defect was cleared and cemented as a void filler while implant fixation achieved by metaphyseal/epiphyseal fixation and supported by a press-fit stem. iii Postoperative photographs following reconstruction with metaphyseal sleeves both sides and a condylar revision with a VVC insert

(ii)

(iii)

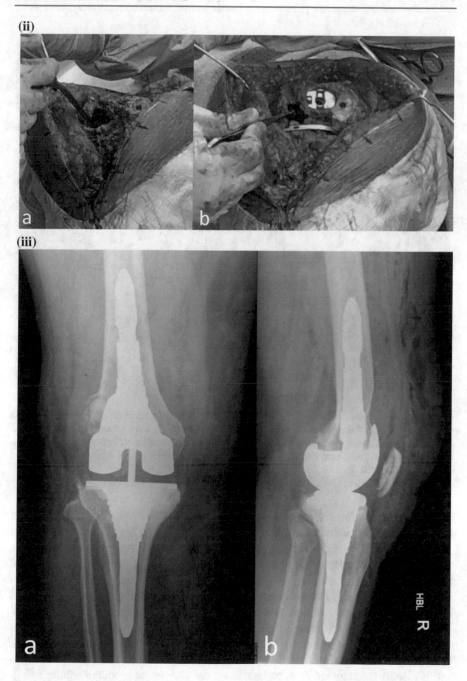

Fig. 4.3 (continued)

(i)

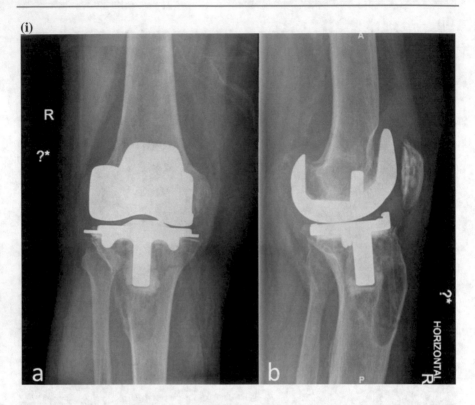

Fig. 4.4 i Preoperative radiographs of a failed right TKA in a 73 years old man with significant osteolysis affecting the proximal tibial secondary to polyethylene wear presenting with pain and instability symptoms. **ii** Postoperative radiographs at 1 year following reconstruction with hybrid fixation technique using cemented tibia and cementless femoral sleeve. **iii** Follow up radiographs at 7 years with well-fixed implant and satisfactory clinical outcome

Cemented fixation works well but we do see early failures with fixation given that we are predominantly only 'surface cementing' with a flat surface on the tibia. Cementation technique is very important here in order to minimise those issues. As far back as 2000, it has been shown that application of the cement to the implant undersurface early in the doughy state of the cement increased the fixation strength of the cement-implant interface. So, cement should be applied to the components early before applying it to the bone while it is sticky with adhesive properties [31]. We also know that the mixed cement in its working phase is incompatible with aqueous liquids such as saline or blood which reduces its bonding strength [32]. Blood laminations in the cement can also reduce its mechanical strength [33]. Lipid infiltration at the implant–cement interface may also cause premature failure [34]. We can influence these aspects as surgeons with our technique ensuring that we have a washed/dried bed in order to remove fat and lipid content and get pressurised

(ii)

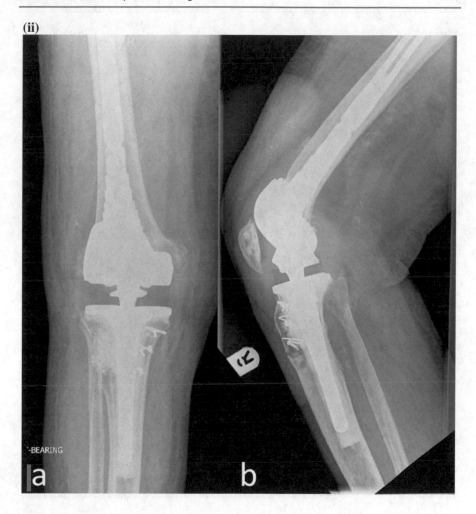

Fig. 4.4 (continued)

cement into bone porous structures and cement the keel which has been shown to further strengthen the bond in the cement-implant interface [35].

However, the weak link remains the cement-implant interface. In a study of 149 rTKA for aseptic loosening of the tibia (2005–2017), implant failure was more prevalent at the implant-cement (94%) than the cement–bone interface (6%) with two distinct patterns of failure; almost 65% of patients developed varus collapse and 35% of patients developed failure between the implant–cement interface without angulation [36].

Cement viscosity is an area where a lot of discussion and variation continues worldwide. In the UK and most European countries, high viscosity cement is the most commonly used while most North American surgeons use low or medium

(iii)

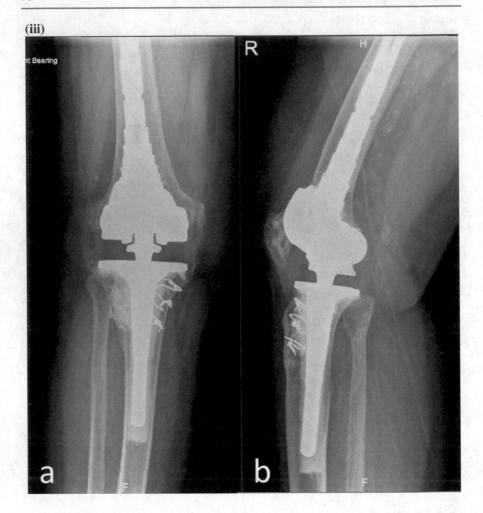

Fig. 4.4 (continued)

viscosity cement. We routinely use antibiotic-laden, high viscosity cement. Although low viscosity cement may flow better into porous bone, it tends to flow out of the prosthesis. A sticky high viscosity cement with adhesive properties at time of applying to the prosthesis would also ensure better bond in the implant–cement interface, it gives good protection keeping the interfaces dry and clean of any debris or laminations and ultimately increases the pull-out strength. Line to line preparation as opposed to leaving a larger cement mantle around the keel also increases the pull-out strength [35, 37].

Moving the knee while the cement is setting can be detrimental. This is because most contemporary knee designs are more kinematic with the dwell point changing in an anteroposterior direction as we progress with range of motion, so there is no

(i)

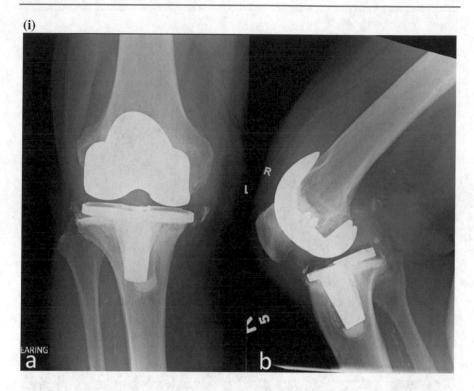

Fig. 4.5 i Preoperative radiographs of a failed right knee with aseptic loosening in a 73 years old man with a cemented CR implant and a fractured tibial tray as a fatigue failure under cyclical loading. **ii** Postoperative radiographs at 2 years follow up with a condylar revision implant (varus-valgus-constraint) with a cementless metaphyseal tibial sleeve and a short cemented femoral stem (hybrid fixation technique)

constant dwell point that would keep the cement pressurised. If you rock the tibia early on by moving the joint through range of motion, it starts to suck in the lipid or blood which can then spread across the interface and may weaken the pull-out strength of the implant.

All cemented fixation will eventually fail as the weak link remains the implant–cement interface, which we can improve by strengthening the bond on the under-surface of the implant to better transmit the load to the other interface onto bone. However, it is again a catch 22-situation. What is the compromise? Do we want implants to last or to have the ability to revise them easily? Would we rather have a very well-fixed implant with biological fixation that can last a lifetime but would be incredibly difficult to extract should revision be required?!

Hugh Cameron is a pioneer of cementless biological fixation and began working on porous metals in 1971 with experiments to define the parameters of porous metal which ultimately led to the development of the AML hip stem. A number of clinical problems were encountered and overcome leading to the introduction of the ICLH

(ii)

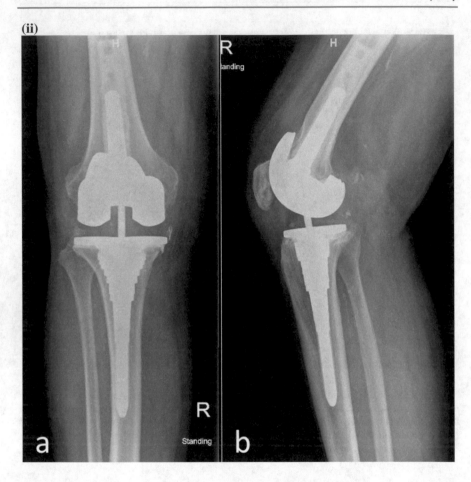

Fig. 4.5 (continued)

knee, the Tricon with its different editions and upgrades and the Profix which was first implanted in 1995. The learning points here were that the femoral component should be an opening-wedge, which allows some errors, because on loading, it is forced tighter onto the bone. If it is parallel sided there is no room for errors at all. *Profix* was parallel sided, as opposed to the opening-wedge original *Tricon*, where simply femoral loosening did not occur. The problem, however, is the tibia. This is because it is loading on a flat fairly flexible surface, there must be some horizontal motion on vertical load due to the *Poisson ratio*. A flat surface component can be used, but there is no margin of error, and compression screws are useful to suck the plate tight to the bone. Alternatively, the *Profix* modular roughened surface heavily fluted metaphyseal stem had excellent results; no loose tibiae were encountered with or without screws. Of note, if screws are used in the design of the tibial component, the posterolateral screw may protrude into the arch between the tibia

(i)

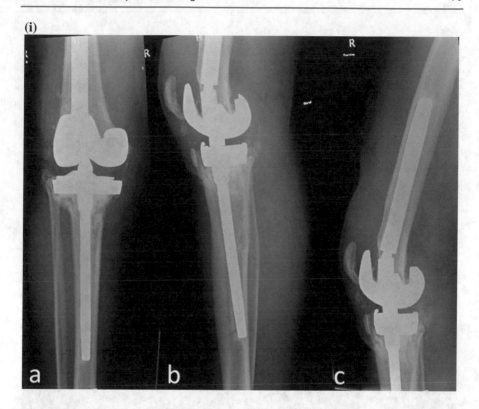

Fig. 4.6 i Preoperative radiographs of a failed right revision TKA (Kinemax, Stryker) with loosening and proximal tibial collapse and significant bone loss in both distal femur and proximal tibia. There is also an intra-medullary implant fracture at the modular junction between stem and femoral component. **ii** Mechanical alignment views with failed bilateral knees (revision right, primary left), pelvic obliquity is noted with apparent shortening of the right extremity with different joint line levels. **iii** Postoperative radiographs following right revision TKA with salvage endoprostheses using distal femoral and proximal tibial replacements. **Iv** At 3 years follow up following left sided revision TKA with a condylar revision (VVC) hybrid fixation with sleeved tibia and short cemented femoral component. **v** At 5 years follow up with good functional outcomes, the hydroxyapatite (HA) coated collar is ingrown which also provides a secondary point of fixation

and fibula and care should be taken to avoid any injury. In a systematic review of the *Profix*, 8 studies were included with 987 patients (1152 knees) and the overall estimated implant survival was 98.6% at 5 years and 94.2% at 10 years using revision for any reason as an endpoint. Mean/median preoperative Knee Society knee scores improved from 39.2/24.7 at baseline, to 91.4/92.1 at last follow-up [38].

Similarly, impressive results have been reported with the LCS RP Knee with 98% survivorship at 15 years [39]. In his series of 500 TKAs of LCS RP (all with cementless tibial trays), *David Beverland* reported survivorship of 97.4% at a mean

(ii)

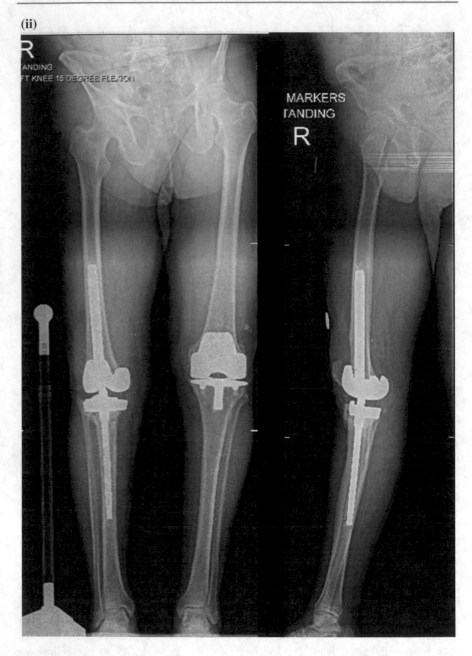

Fig. 4.6 (continued)

(iii)

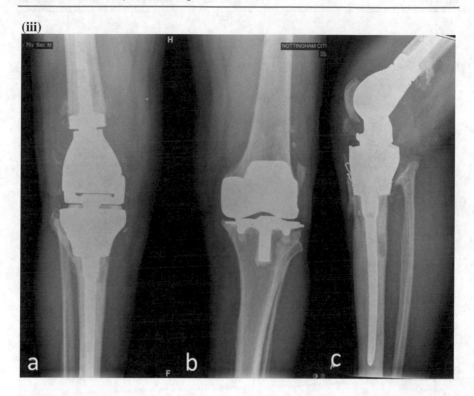

Fig. 4.6 (continued)

follow up 18.1 years (17–21.8) using any cause revision as an endpoint. Thirteen knees required revision: 3 for infection, 3 bearing only revisions for spinout, 3 for tibial tray subsidence, 2 secondary patella resurfacings, 1 aseptic loosening, and 1 for suspected aseptic loosening that was ultimately found to be well fixed [40].

So, why do we see this discrepancy between registry data, which favours cemented fixation, and high-volume cementless users? The answer to this is that there is no margin for error with cementless knees. As a surgical technique, it is less forgiving which makes teaching and training for junior surgeons more challenging. Improved instruments from different manufactures have made this transition easier but it remains the case that if the component rocks even a little bit it will not work.

(iv)

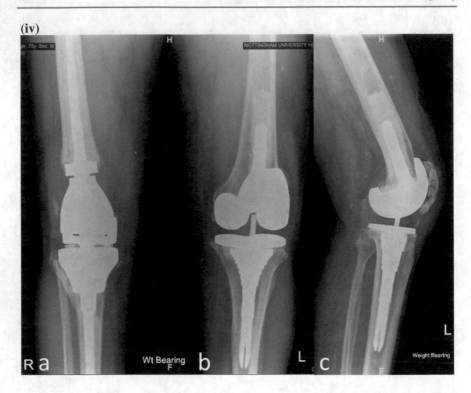

Fig. 4.6 (continued)

What about stress shielding with cementless fixation? This has not been as much of an issue with knees as it has been with hips. In knees, we are not bypassing anything, it is essentially a primary re-surfacing. So, whether we load the bone with a biological interface/porous coat finish or a thin layer of cement makes little difference. In fact, theoretically we get better results with the posterior condyles as they are still loaded [40].

So, with good polyethylene and cementless durable biological fixation, which is likely to become more prevalent in the future, indications for revision will be limited to instability (largely surgical errors), infection, and wear in the very long-term. The problem remains in extraction, but should we be worried about that? We can still get them out, and the more we have to do it the better we will get at it. Here, more centralised and tertiary revision workload in high volume units is advantageous. Again, it is the question of whether we want to have well-fixed implants in the majority of patients who would function well and never need any revisions providing they are well-balanced which is the primary surgeon's main duty, versus implants which are easier to take out at revision surgery, but perhaps may not have as good longevity. A few of those cementless knees (1–2%) will have to be revised for infection and a few more for other indications (trauma, malalignment.... etc.). This is a choice that surgeons will have to make moving

(v)

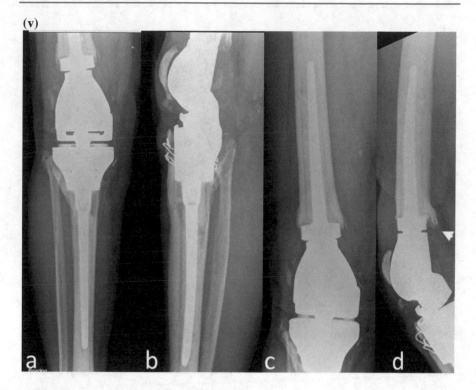

Fig. 4.6 (continued)

forward as the burden of revision knees is likely to increase substantially in the future based on current projections.

4.5   Instability (Figs. 4.7, 4.8 and 4.9)

Early instability is usually related to surgical technique. Here we need to work out whether it is caused by malalignment or related to soft tissue failure. Later instability could be due to grossly loose TKA, then it will be unstable but that does not mean you necessarily also have soft tissue or ligament failure.

Top tip: Posterior instability (recurvatum) is rare, practically, a posterior capsular failure or MCL failure always requires a hinged implant.

Mid-flexion instability: Examination under anaesthetic (EUA) can be helpful in evaluating subtle instability particularly in mid-flexion. We must work out the cause of the instability to be able to reverse it and fix it rather than going directly to increased levels of constraint. The tibial height influences both flexion and extension, so you do not have to necessarily revise it with few prerequisites. If it is

(i)

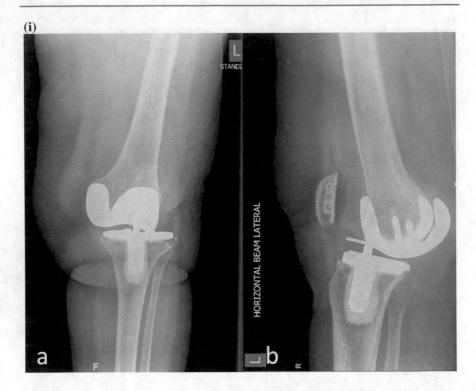

Fig. 4.7 i Preoperative radiographs of a failed left knee in 76 years old lady with instability and posterior capsular failure. **ii** Postoperative radiographs following revision using hinge implant with metaphyseal sleeves at 8.5 years follow up

well-fixed, well-aligned, compatible with the new femoral component and can accept a revision insert, it can potentially be retained. We do, however, prefer to take it out as it makes exposure and clearing the posterior space easier.

It is really on the femoral side that mid-flexion instability can be corrected. Here, we need to go back to a balanced approach, expose the knee, take the component out, clear all granulation tissue particularly at the back of the knee, curette out all scar and thickened tissue from the posterior capsule, and hyperflex the knee to be able to expose the posterior femoral condyles. This allows the posterior vessels to fall back. Then, you feel around the posterior condyles and you will notice the thickened granulomatous soft tissue which starts to encroach posteriorly. Stick to bone at the posterior condyles and lift off scar tissue at its most anterior projection by using a diathermy to expose both posterior condyles (Fig. 4.10). This develops a dissection plane between the scar tissue and the native bone and then the posterior capsule. Once this plane is identified, you can use a curette to further develop it, sweeping the thickened tissue off the bone down to the posterior capsule, proximal to distal to its insertion onto the proximal tibia. Very often, this granulation tissue will also have invaded the interface between the tibia and the tibial component.

(ii)

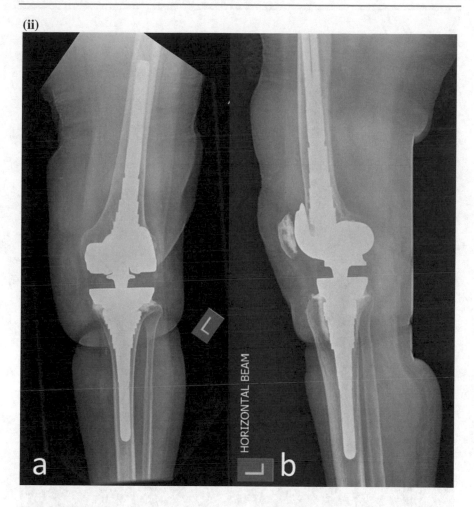

Fig. 4.7 (continued)

Once you are at the level of the proximal tibia you can then resect this tissue that you have peeled off. Failure to address the posterior space will have significant impact on the extension gap. It is easier to start on the medial side due to the medial parapatellar exposure giving earlier sight of this area, but it is imperative that the totality of the posterior space is cleared. If you start seeing clear fat, you should be concerned that you have probably breached the posterior capsule in close proximity to the neurovascular structures.

Top tip: When clearing the posterior space of scar and granulation/thickened tissues, we prefer not to use nibblers but rather we need to dissect the scar tissue from the posterior capsule which must be left intact.

(i)

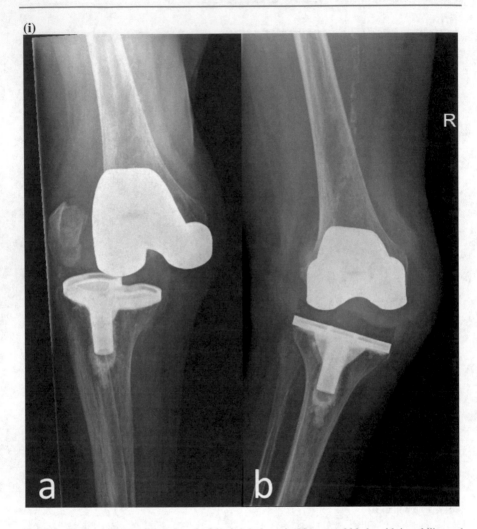

Fig. 4.8 i Preoperative radiographs of a failed right knee in 82 years old lady with instability and MCL failure. **ii** Postoperative radiographs following revision with a cemented fixed hinged implant at 3 years follow up

The next step is to re-establish the AP dimension of the femur which is based on the femoral size and positioning; here most systems have a great deal of versatility in deploying offsets and augments to ensure adequate balancing of flexion gap by restoring adequate posterior condylar offset, based on a stable tibial platform. In most cases you have to distalise the femur by using distal augments to lower the joint line. Then we assess the extension gap.

(ii)

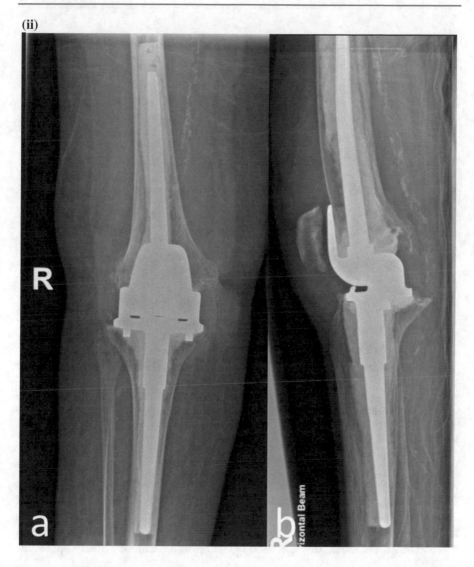

Fig. 4.8 (continued)

Our philosophy here is that once the components are out and soft tissue clearance is done, we virtually place the joint line then set the implants to fit the joint line. If we know we will need distal augments, then we initially prepare for those augments to restore the joint line. We do not know *accurately* how much bone was taken at time of primary or how much bone was lost by debridement and extraction, or how much remodelling there may have been. In the absence of a reliable, reproducible, and easy to use operative technique, we use the meniscal scars which are fairly constant even in salvage cases to restore the joint line. A common mistake

(i)

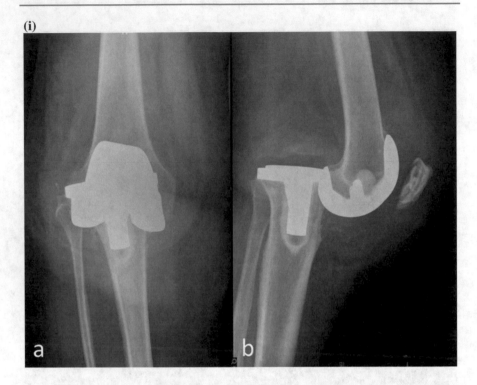

Fig. 4.9 i Emergency department radiographs of a dislocated CR-TKA in a 48 years old woman with high BMI following a traumatic fall. **ii** Postoperative radiographs following revision surgery with a fixed hinged design. Choice of implant in this case was dictated by her small canal diameters and the system available

is to cut the bone back to healthy margins and then decide that you need joint line distal to that by 5 or 10 mm based only on the augment you have in the system. Our approach is the other way around, locate your planned joint line then reconstruct to it. *(see chapter of surgical reconstruction for further details).* In those cases where the collaterals are intact, this approach is similar to a balanced primary approach.

4.6 Stiffness

The challenge here is to understand why it is stiff; primary stiffness (true arthrofibrosis) is rare and difficult to diagnose preoperatively unless you see a progressively shortening patella tendon on sequential radiographs. More commonly, however, we see unbalanced stiff knees or 'unstable stiff knees' due to malrotation, malpositioning, or sizing errors. Instability often causes irritation, synovitis and a subsequent inflammatory response with recurrent effusion,

(ii)

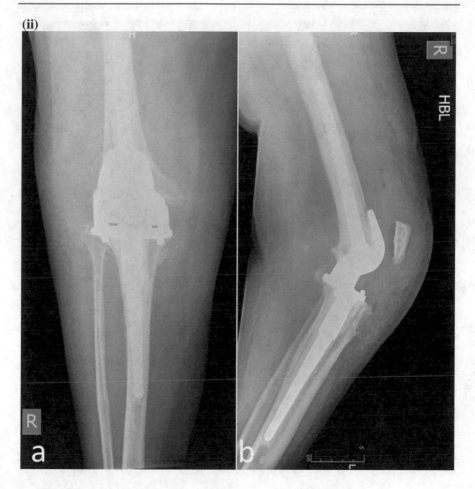

Fig. 4.9 (continued)

progressive fibrosis and stiffness. Anything that can cause a haemarthrosis is a risk. One of the main challenges in revising stiff knees is exposure. Consider an early tibial crest osteotomy for severe stiffness to gain safe exposure; you often need to do extensive releases and a hinged implant may be necessary. In all cases, an extensive synovectomy is needed; the medial and lateral gutters are easy to clear, don't forget to excise the scar behind the patella tendon which tend to cause tethering to the proximal tibia; it is important to clear it all out so you can safely slide the patella laterally and if the knee is really stiff consider osteotomy.

Top tip: Unless you can find a surgical cause for stiffness that can be corrected at time of revision then rTKA outcomes and prognosis are very guarded.

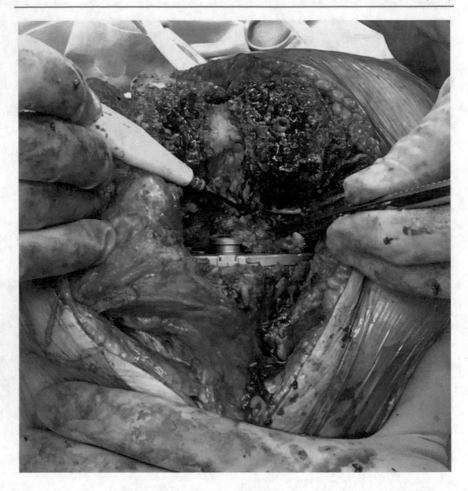

Fig. 4.10 Intraoperative clinical photograph demonstrating the technique described to clear out the posterior space of scar and granulation tissues peeling it off the posterior condyles

In summary, there are varying indications to revise a poorly performing TKA. Understanding why a knee is not functioning well and being able to fix the problem is an essential prerequisite before embarking on revision surgery.

References

1. Evans JT, et al. How long does a knee replacement last? A systematic review and meta-analysis of case series and national registry reports with more than 15 years of follow-up. Lancet. 2019;393(10172):655–63.
2. Chawla H, et al. Annual revision rates of partial versus total knee arthroplasty: A comparative meta-analysis. Knee. 2017;24(2):179–90.

3. Klug A et al. The projected volume of primary and revision total knee arthroplasty will place an immense burden on future health care systems over the next 30 years. Knee Surg Sports Traumatol Arthrosc. 2020:1–12.
4. Inacio MCS, et al. Increase in total joint arthroplasty projected from 2014 to 2046 in Australia: a conservative local model with international implications. Clin Orthop Relat Res. 2017;475(8):2130–7.
5. Inacio MCS, et al. Projected increase in total knee arthroplasty in the United States - an alternative projection model. Osteoarthritis Cartilage. 2017;25(11):1797–803.
6. Kalson NS, et al. Provision of revision knee surgery and calculation of the effect of a network service reconfiguration: an analysis from the national joint registry for England, Wales, Northern Ireland and the Isle of Man. Knee. 2020;27(5):1593–600.
7. Patel A et al. The epidemiology of revision total knee and hip arthroplasty in England and Wales: a comparative analysis with projections for the United States. A study using the National Joint Registry dataset. Bone Joint J. 2015; 97-b(8):1076–81.
8. Bozic KJ, et al. The epidemiology of revision total knee arthroplasty in the United States. Clin Orthop Relat Res. 2010;468(1):45–51.
9. Delanois RE, et al. Current epidemiology of revision total knee arthroplasty in the United States. J Arthroplasty. 2017;32(9):2663–8.
10. Koh CK, et al. Periprosthetic joint infection is the main cause of failure for modern knee arthroplasty: an analysis of 11,134 Knees. Clin Orthop Relat Res. 2017;475(9):2194–201.
11. Abdel et al. Contemporary failure aetiologies of the primary, posterior-stabilised total knee arthroplasty. Bone Joint J. 2017; 99-b(5):647–52.
12. Labek G, et al. Revision rates after total joint replacement: cumulative results from worldwide joint register datasets. J Bone Joint Surg Br. 2011;93(3):293–7.
13. Sharkey PF, et al. Why are total knee arthroplasties failing today–has anything changed after 10 years? J Arthroplasty. 2014;29(9):1774–8.
14. Pietrzak J, et al. Have the frequency of and reasons for revision total knee arthroplasty changed since 2000? Comparison of two cohorts from the same hospital: 255 cases (2013–2016) and 68 cases (1991–1998). Orthop Traumatol Surg Res. 2019;105(4):639–45.
15. Sadoghi P, et al. Revision surgery after total joint arthroplasty: a complication-based analysis using worldwide arthroplasty registers. J Arthroplasty. 2013;28(8):1329–32.
16. Le DH, et al. Current modes of failure in TKA: infection, instability, and stiffness predominate. Clin Orthop Relat Res. 2014;472(7):2197–200.
17. Thiele K, et al. Current failure mechanisms after knee arthroplasty have changed: polyethylene wear is less common in revision surgery. J Bone Joint Surg Am. 2015;97 (9):715–20.
18. Matar HE et al. Septic Revision Total Knee Arthroplasty Is Associated With Significantly Higher Mortality Than Aseptic Revisions: Long-Term Single-Center Study (1254 Patients). J Arthroplasty. 2021.
19. Bell CJ, et al. Effect of oxidation on delamination of ultrahigh-molecular-weight polyethylene tibial components. J Arthroplasty. 1998;13(3):280–90.
20. Collier MB et al. Osteolysis after total knee arthroplasty: influence of tibial baseplate surface finish and sterilization of polyethylene insert. Findings at five to ten years postoperatively. J Bone Joint Surg Am. 2005; 87(12):2702–8.
21. Sisko ZW, et al. Current total knee designs: does baseplate roughness or locking mechanism design affect polyethylene backside wear? Clin Orthop Relat Res. 2017;475(12):2970–80.
22. Matar HE et al. Overview of Randomized Controlled Trials in Primary Total Hip Arthroplasty (34,020 Patients): What Have We Learnt? J Am Acad Orthop Surg Glob Res Rev. 2020; 4(8): e2000120.
23. Paxton EW, et al. Is there a difference in total knee arthroplasty risk of revision in highly crosslinked versus conventional polyethylene? Clin Orthop Relat Res. 2015;473(3):999–1008.

24. Partridge TCJ, et al. Conventional versus highly cross-linked polyethylene in primary total knee replacement: a comparison of revision rates using data from the national joint registry for England, Wales, and Northern Ireland. J Bone Joint Surg Am. 2020;102(2):119–27.
25. Spece H, et al. Reasons for revision, oxidation, and damage mechanisms of retrieved vitamin E-stabilized highly crosslinked polyethylene in total knee arthroplasty. J Arthroplasty. 2019;34(12):3088–93.
26. Drexler M et al. Cementless fixation in total knee arthroplasty: down the boulevard of broken dreams - opposes. J Bone Joint Surg Br. 2012; 94(11 Suppl A):85–9.
27. Napier RJ, et al. A prospective evaluation of a largely cementless total knee arthroplasty cohort without patellar resurfacing: 10-year outcomes and survivorship. BMC Musculoskelet Disord. 2018;19(1):205.
28. Mont MA, et al. Long-term implant survivorship of cementless total knee arthroplasty: a systematic review of the literature and meta-analysis. J Knee Surg. 2014;27(5):369–76.
29. Porter M. The registries: what do they tell us about knee arthroplasty? A narrative review of six national arthroplasty registers. Orthopaedics and Trauma. 2021;35(1):30–8.
30. National Joint Registry National joint Registry for England, Wales, and Northern Ireland; 17th annual report. 2020. 18/01/2021]. Available from https://reports.njrcentre.org.uk/Portals/0/PDFdownloads/NJR%2017th%20Annual%20Report%202020.pdf.
31. Shepard MF, Kabo JM, Lieberman JR. The Frank Stinchfield Award. Influence of cement technique on the interface strength of femoral components. Clin Orthop Relat Res. 2000 (381):26–35.
32. Rudol G, et al. The effect of surface finish and interstitial fluid on the cement-in-cement interface in revision surgery of the hip. J Bone Joint Surg Br. 2011;93(2):188–93.
33. Tan JH, et al. Compression and flexural strength of bone cement mixed with blood. J Orthop Surg (Hong Kong). 2016;24(2):240–4.
34. Mason JB. Lipid infiltration. In AAOS Annual Meeting 2018.
35. Billi F et al. Techniques for improving the initial strength of the tibial tray-cement interface bond. Bone Joint J. 2019; 101-b(1_Supple_A):53–8.
36. Martin JR et al. Where Is the "Weak Link" of Fixation in Contemporary Cemented Total Knee Replacements? J Arthroplasty. 2021.
37. Refsum AM, et al. Cementing technique for primary knee arthroplasty: a scoping review. Acta Orthop. 2019;90(6):582–9.
38. Viganò R, et al. A systematic literature review of the Profix in primary total knee arthroplasty. Acta Orthop Belg. 2012;78(1):55–60.
39. Hopley CD, Crossett LS, Chen AF. Long-term clinical outcomes and survivorship after total knee arthroplasty using a rotating platform knee prosthesis: a meta-analysis. J Arthroplasty. 2013; 28(1):68–77.e1–3.
40. McMahon SE, et al. Seventeen to twenty years of follow-up of the low contact stress rotating-platform total knee arthroplasty with a cementless tibia in all cases. J Arthroplasty. 2019;34(3):508–12.

Challenges of Surgical Exposure

5

If you only pray when you're in trouble.... you're in trouble!

Anonymous

5.1 Introduction

Getting adequate exposure is the first and most important step in rTKA surgery. This means we should be able to visualise the knee joint and safely remove the components with minimal bone loss, while protecting skin, ligaments, neurovascular structures and the extensor mechanism, allowing us the ability to balance and reconstruct the joint using a stable and durable construct. In this chapter we will present our approach to exposure in rTKA with a practical case demonstration for our preferred extensile approach.

Skin incision: Use the old incision where possible. When you have multiple longitudinal incisions it has been suggested that you should use the most lateral as the blood flow tends to be lateral to medial [1]. However, if the incision is too lateral it may compromise the exposure. So, when in doubt check first with a plastic surgeon. The main point here is to avoid developing superficial skin flaps. Dissection should be down to the extensor mechanism and then raise thick full-thickness skin flaps. Do not put too much tension on your skin flaps, by trying to do it through minimally invasive approaches—revision surgery requires adequate exposure. Always extend the incision proximal and distal by a couple of centimetres to the old incision which helps you identify soft tissue planes better by getting back to virgin territory. You can raise the skin flaps with a knife but our preference is to use diathermy with an insulated tip set at a low energy setting.

H. E. Matar et al., *Revision Total Knee Arthroplasty*,
https://doi.org/10.1007/978-3-030-81285-0_5

Arthrotomy: the workhorse approach is a medial parapatellar; it is well-established, it is extensile, it is familiar and gives excellent exposure. We would caution against using mid-vastus, sub-vastus or lateral approaches for revision cases.

Synovectomy: the collaterals are sacrosanct, so synovectomy is performed in knee extension, starting with the medial side which is easier to reach. We lift the scar tissue off the distal femur and dissect it off the under-surface of vastus medialis obliquus leaving its fascia intact. Then continue around the medial side of the component exposing all its interfaces; here the aim is to re-establish the medial gutter.

We then move on to the lateral gutter, which is more difficult, and better done with the surgeon standing on the contralateral side. Start with the patella clearing the scar tissue from its medial edge and follow it proximally leading you to the suprapatellar pouch and distally clearing all the scar tissue from the patella tendon, you also need to clear the extensor mechanism from any adherent anterolateral scar tissue.

If it is tight, flex the knee and remove the polyethylene insert early, before coming back to extension and dividing any fibrous transverse bands from the femur to the extensor mechanism which would allow you more access to clear the remaining scar tissue. Then flex the knee once again and sublux the patella laterally to get better access to the femoral component and clear tissues adherent to it, before removing the femoral component, taking care to minimise bone loss.

Then put the knee back in extension. Now that you have removed at least 9 mm thickness of the femoral component, and 5–10 mm of polyethylene (assuming it is a primary implant in situ), you will have better access to finish clearing out and re-establishing the lateral gutter. Coming back to flexion, we clear the notch of scar tissue and then we should have a good view of the tibia, allowing it to be subluxed forward for implant removal. Re-establishing the lateral gutter is an important step of a successful exposure and we often find ourselves continually going from flexion to extension clearing out more of the lateral side after each component is removed, while ensuring that it is done safely protecting the important lateral stabilisers. The aim is to get a mobile extensor mechanism with no adherence to the femur laterally.

Posterior space: having removed the components and cleared the medial and lateral gutters, you will have an excellent view of the posterior space. The task now is to clear all scar tissue and granulation tissue adherent to the posterior capsule. Further, when you do a refreshing cut to the tibia, very carefully with retractors in place posteriorly, cut all the way to the posterior cortex, tilt the saw up and it will lift off but do not pull it out, as it lifts off you will see scar tissue attached to it, grab it with a bone grabber or bone forceps and excise it with the scar tissue attached using a cutting diathermy; the medial side is easier to get to first and you can work your way around it, this helps to further clear out the posteromedial and posterolateral corners. As previously mentioned (earlier chapter), curette out all scar and thickened tissue from the posterior capsule, and hyperflex the knee to be able to expose the posterior femoral condyles. This allows the posterior vessels to fall back and if you feel around the posterior condyles and you will notice the soft tissues starting to encroach posteriorly. If you start seeing clear fat, you have probably gone too far and you will be close to the neurovascular structures. Stick to bone at the posterior condyles and lift off the scar tissue in the AP direction using a diathermy exposing both condyles, then you can use a curette to further develop this plane, sweeping it off the bone down to the posterior capsule, proximal to distal. The medial side is easier to start with, and once the tibial component has been removed, you can see the proximal tibial border and where you are heading with the dissection, gently teasing the thick scar tissue off the posterior capsule which will peel off once you are in the right plane. Once you are at the level of the proximal tibia your freshening tibial cut will further identify the posterior scar tissue allowing for clearance of the posterior space.

Extensile approach: the aim is to be able to clear the gutters adequately and remove the components safely while protecting the extensor mechanism throughout. If this cannot be achieved through the steps outlined above, then an extensile approach is required to achieve those goals. Our preferred technique is a tibial crest osteotomy rather than proximal extensor mechanism manoeuvres. This is because the access you will always struggle to get in rTKA is at the posterolateral aspect of the joint. Therefore, proximally based manoeuvres proximal to the patella such as quads snip or turndown will not logically optimise exposure for this aspect of the knee. Tibial crest osteotomy, however, facilitates access to the lateral side of the joint at both tibial and femoral levels, it protects the extensor mechanism particularly in cases of severe stiffness or patella baja, it is reliable and reproducible, it has a low complication and a high union rate [2–6].

5.2 Tibial Crest Osteotomy

This osteotomy was originally described by *Dolin* in 1983 [7], and further developed by *Whiteside* and others [5]. The idea here is to allow a bone fragment to rotate on its longitudinal axis allowing the patella to be moved laterally along with the extensor mechanism. It is crucial to maintain the lateral soft tissue attachment intact (fascia, muscles of the anterior compartment) to maintain blood supply and stability. The osteotomy should be thick enough to prevent fragmentation, long enough to ensure large contact area for bone-to-bone healing and stability, and wide enough to leave the zone of injury away from the patella tendon insertion. Excellent outcomes have been reported in the literature for this approach with low rate of complications and high union rate [3, 4, 6]. In fact, when the osteotomy was performed on re-revision cases in whom prior osteotomy had been performed in one series, the osteotomy healed in all cases [2].

5.2.1   Our Technique

Indications: severe patella baja (Fig. 5.1), 2nd stage reconstruction from a static spacer (fusion nail), stiff knees, and inability to get adequate exposure to safely remove components in situ.

Length: between 10–15 cm, with a wide surface area for better healing and stability (Fig. 5.2).

Osteotomy: find your tibial tubercle, work above it to free the tendon clearing any scars behind it, and extend the skin incision distally exposing the adequate length of the tibial crest. Measure it and mark it with a diathermy. Aim to leave a transverse bridge or rim of bone proximally adjacent to the joint line. This helps to guide reduction, prevent any proximal migration and gives a second interface for healing.

Next, using a 2.5 mm drill bit, make multiple drill holes medial to lateral spaced apart along the line of the osteotomy, 1 cm apart in the correct plane where you want it to open, going through both medial and lateral cortices, that plane should be tapered at the end to prevent stress risers (Fig. 5.2). Then, use a very thin short saw blade on the medial side to connect the drill holes. We us an oscillating saw with 0.4 mm blade thickness, just connecting the dots on the medial, but not to the

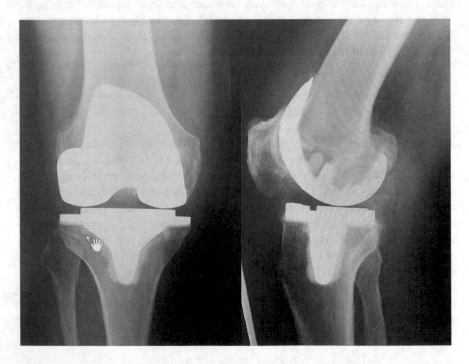

Fig. 5.1 Example of a stiff knee with primary arthrofibrosis, severe patella baja and 40° arc of motion.

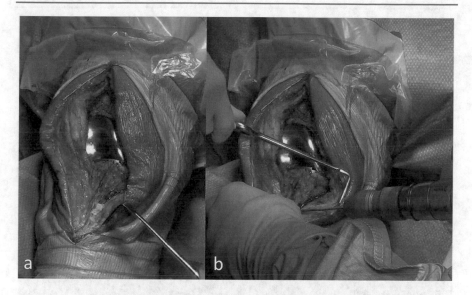

Fig. 5.2 Intraoperative clinical photographs **a** following arthrotomy and synovectomy, the skin incision is extended distally, the tibial crest osteotomy site is planned and exposed, marked with a diathermy; **b** Sequential, 1-cm apart, *bicortical* drill holes are then made using a 2.5 mm drill bit

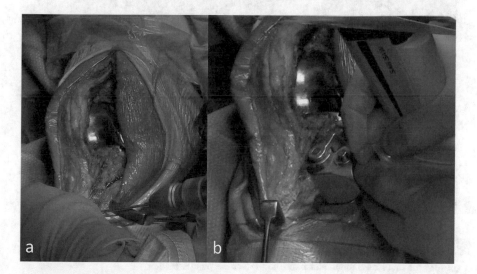

Fig. 5.3 Intraoperative clinical photographs **a** completing the drill holes down to the tapered end of the planned osteotomy; **b** using a fine blade (0.4 mm thickness) cutting the medial cortex only connecting the drill holes

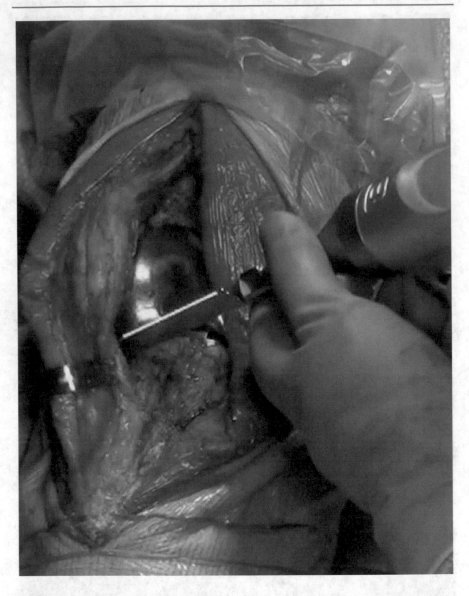

Fig. 5.4 Intraoperative clinical photograph demonstrating the creation of a proximal rim of bone close to the joint line with a reciprocating saw to help reducing the osteotomy at the end and prevent proximal migration. Make sure to protect the patella tendon

lateral, side (Fig. 5.3). Using a reciprocating saw (Fig. 5.4), make a transverse cut behind the patella tendon adjacent to the joint line which would later help reduction, stability and prevent proximal migration.

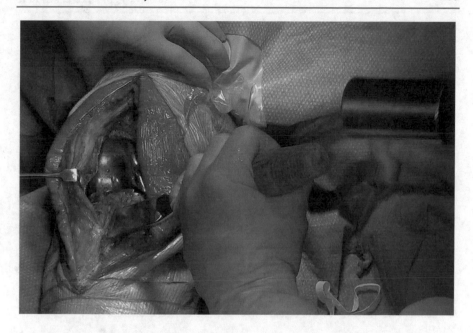

Fig. 5.5 Using a 1-inch broad osteotomy, complete the osteotomy all the way to the lateral cortex and leave the osteotome in situ

Then multiple broad (1 inch) osteotomes are inserted and we keep tapping until we get to the lateral side, finally separating the lateral cortex with the osteotome. The previously performed drill holes control the lateral extension of the osteotomy by creating a controlled failure in this cortex and prevent propagation or inadvertent fracture in the posterolateral tibia. This leaves the under-surface and the lateral edge irregular which makes it easier to key back in and gives it more stability than a flat on flat fixation. Lift all the osteotomes up at once and the crest osteotomy will open up (Figs. 5.5 and 5.6). Again, make sure you leave the periosteal and soft tissue sleeve attached laterally which aids with stability of the fragment and ensures preservation of blood supply to the bony fragment allowing reliable healing.

Once it is lifted and retracted laterally with the extensor mechanism attached, you will see some scarring tissue on the joint line adherent to the proximal tibia that you could not clear earlier in the lateral gutter and you can complete the soft tissue clearance in preparation for later reconstruction. The osteotomy can be then rotated laterally giving you excellent exposure (Fig. 5.7) and allowing the knee to flex beyond 90 degrees.

Fixation: With the trial components in, bring the osteotomy back in place and secure it temporarily with sutures to check the tension in flexion. Once you are happy, fixation is next once the definitive implants are assembled and ready. We prefer to use cerclage wires for fixation, although other techniques can be used. We prefer to use three drill holes in the medial proximal tibia, pass the wires through

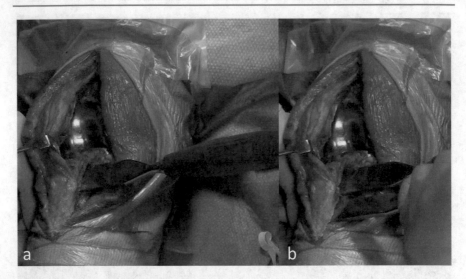

Fig. 5.6 Leaving the first osteotome in situ (**a**); **b** a second osteotome is used in the same fashion and simultaneously lifting both osteotomes at once to release the tibial crest

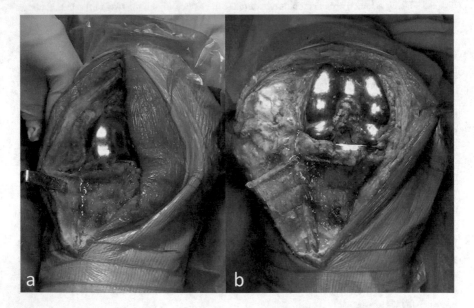

Fig. 5.7 a, b The osteotomy is completed and retracted laterally with the attached extensor mechanism with intact lateral soft tissue attachments giving excellent view to the joint

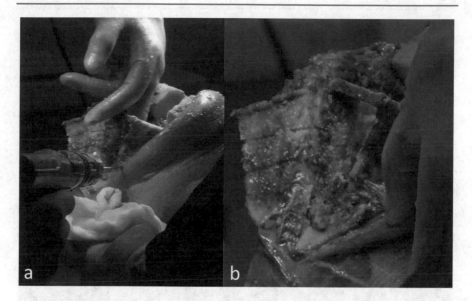

Fig. 5.8 a, b Following joint preparation and trials; wiring the osteotomy before final implantation using 2.5 mm drill bit through the medial cortex (**a**); three drill holes are needed to pass the wires (**b**)

adjacent to the posterior tibial cortex so they will be behind the definitive prosthesis once it is in and bring those wires out of the osteotomy hole (Figs. 5.8 and 5.9). Once the definitive prosthesis is implanted, then drill holes through the crest and pass the three wires (you need at least two, we use three in case one snaps as it is tightened) before knotting them medially, as posteromedial as possible. The ends are folded down and the soft tissue envelope closed over the top (Figs. 5.10, 5.11 and 5.12). This way the wires are pulling on the crest bone ensuring bone to bone contact rather than circumferentially strangulating the patella tendon and soft tissues. The lateral intact soft tissue attachment maintains lateral tension, the wires will give you medial tension ensuring stability with bone to bone contact for it to heal, and the proximal rim will lock it back in place. If you overtighten the wires and one snapped, the remining two should suffice, if you snap two…then you might be able to use a screw if you have space or you will need alternative ways to fix it such as *Ethibond* sutures, but we strongly advise you to take care when tightening the wires to avoid this happening.

Complications: if your crest is fragmented, providing the lateral soft tissues are intact, you can still use a cerclage wire of the fragments as above. The proximal part of the osteotomy with the extensor mechanism is usually strong but the inferior part where it is tapered is weaker.

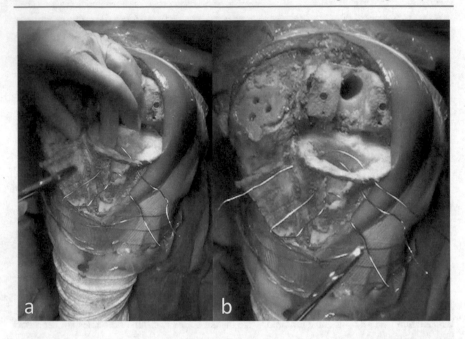

Fig. 5.9 **a** three wires are passed from medial tibial cortex and positioned posteriorly adjacent to the posterior cortex then passed through the lateral cortex **b** definitive implant can then be inserted in the usual fashion

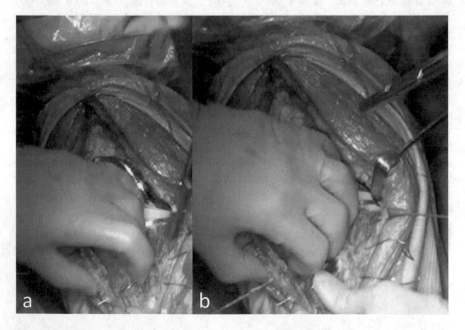

Fig. 5.10 **a** following implantation, the wires are drilled and passed through the crest osteotomy to ensure bone-on-bone reduction; **b** the drill bit is passed lateral to medial and the wire is then fed medial to lateral

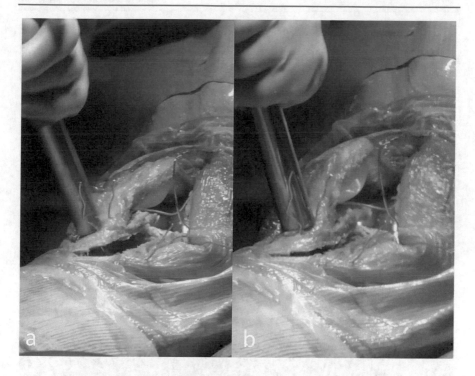

Fig. 5.11 a, b the crest is reduced and gently punched in place with the proximal rim keying in helped by the rim of bone left proximally adjacent to the joint line

Postoperatively: no special requirements are needed for routine osteotomy in terms of weight-bearing or splinting; routine rehabilitation and early flexion is encouraged.

Metalwork prominence: over the years we had to remove wires in one or two cases in thin elderly patients, so it is a rare but recognised complication. We do not use screws to fix the osteotomy as we use sleeves for our tibial fixation but if you have enough space screws are an alternative.

Outcomes: over the years, we have had excellent outcomes with this technique with reliable healing within 6 months or so (Fig. 5.13). The reported outcomes in the literature are also very favourable for this technique.

In summary, for difficult exposure in rTKA, tibial crest osteotomy is a reliable and safe technique offering extensile exposure and protecting the extensor mechanism with excellent union rate and clinical outcomes.

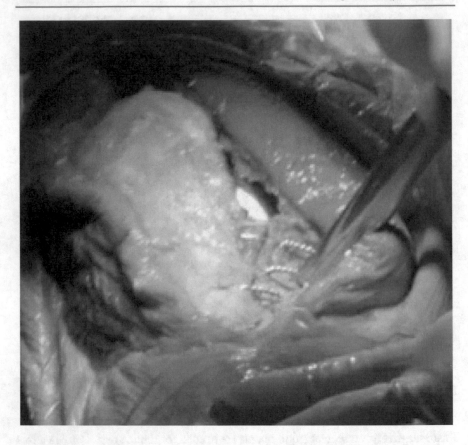

Fig. 5.12 The wires are tightened and knotted on the medial side and punched flat to the bone to prevent irritation underneath the medial soft tissues which are then sutures on top

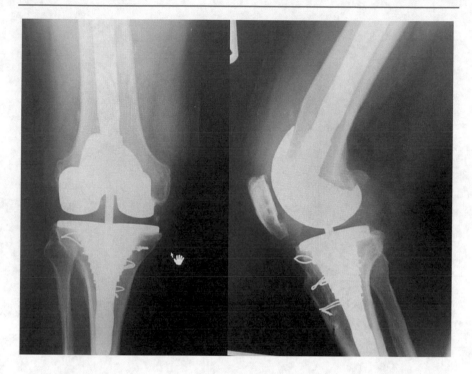

Fig. 5.13 Postoperative radiographs at 6 months follow up with a healed osteotomy

References

1. Haertsch PA. The blood supply to the skin of the leg: a post-mortem investigation. Br J Plast Surg. 1981;34(4):470–7.
2. Chalidis BE, Ries MD. Does repeat tibial tubercle osteotomy or intramedullary extension affect the union rate in revision total knee arthroplasty? A retrospective study of 74 patients. Acta Orthop. 2009;80(4):426–31.
3. Le Moulec YP, et al. Tibial tubercle osteotomy hinged on the tibialis anterior muscle and fixed by circumferential cable cerclage in revision total knee arthroplasty. Orthop Traumatol Surg Res. 2014;100(5):539–44.
4. Punwar SA, Fick DP, Khan RJK. Tibial Tubercle Osteotomy in Revision Knee Arthroplasty. J Arthroplasty. 2017;32(3):903–7.
5. Whiteside LA, Ohl MD. Tibial tubercle osteotomy for exposure of the difficult total knee arthroplasty. Clin Orthop Relat Res. 1990;260:6–9.
6. Zonnenberg CB, et al. Tuberositas osteotomy for total knee arthroplasty: a review of the literature. J Knee Surg. 2010;23(3):121–9.
7. Dolin, M.G., *Osteotomy of the tibial tubercle in total knee replacement. A technical note.* J Bone Joint Surg Am, 1983. **65**(5): p. 704–6.

Removal of Well-Fixed Components

6

Wisely and slow; they stumble that run fast
William Shakespeare

6.1 Introduction

Implant removal is a crucial step in revision knee surgery. When performed safely, efficiently and with minimum bone loss, successful reconstruction can smoothly follow as planned preoperatively. If on the other hand, exposure is not adequate, or the surgeon is not familiar with the implant to be removed or the best techniques to do it, removal can be time-consuming, may result in iatrogenic bone loss or soft tissue and ligament damage which may complicate reconstruction [1–3]. Patience is definitely a virtue at this stage. In this chapter we describe our practical approach and tips to successful implant removal of both primary and revision components, as well as metaphyseal sleeves.

6.2 Prerequisites for Implant Removal

Getting adequate exposure is the main prerequisite for safe removal of implants with minimal bone loss. Ensure that you have the ability to recreate the gutters and have clear access to both sides of the femoral component. If you are struggling to get access, an early decision to use an extensile approach such as a tibial crest osteotomy protects the extensor mechanism, improves exposure and saves time. In cemented implants, the main philosophy is to break the cement-implant interface and lift the implant off the cement mantle (Fig. 6.1). In cementless implants, on the

© The Author(s), under exclusive license to Springer Nature Switzerland AG 2021
H. E. Matar et al., *Revision Total Knee Arthroplasty*,
https://doi.org/10.1007/978-3-030-81285-0_6

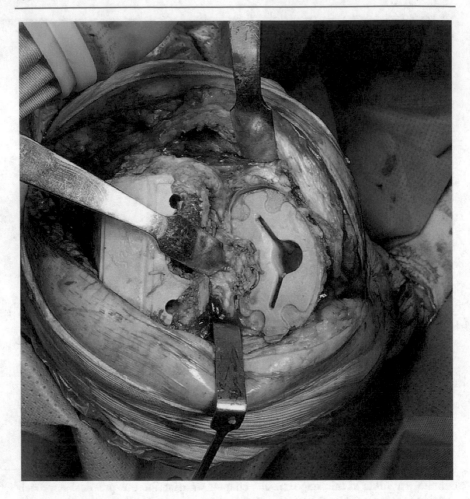

Fig. 6.1 Intraoperative clinical photograph of a revision knee following removal of cemented implant; demonstrating the philosophy of breaking the cement-implant interface and lifting the implant off the cement mantle

other hand, there is only one interface to address; that between implant and bone. Loose implants are easy to knock out once soft tissues and scars have been cleared with a clear path for extraction. This will be evident in most cases on preoperative radiographs and as you are exposing the joint you would see movement of the components which will come out with minimal effort. Well-fixed implants, on the other hand, require detailed preoperative planning and understanding of the implants in situ. When taking an implant for the first time, make sure you contact the manufacturer to enquire about the implant, design, interfaces, points of fixation, instruments for removal…. etc. Always have alternative plans on standby with salvage options particularly when revising a revision component.

6.3 Removal of Cemented Primary TKA

Exposure is the first step as discussed previously, and we must have strategies for extensile approaches. For us, this is through a medial parapatellar approach and a tibial crest osteotomy when needed. We cannot emphasise enough the importance

(i)

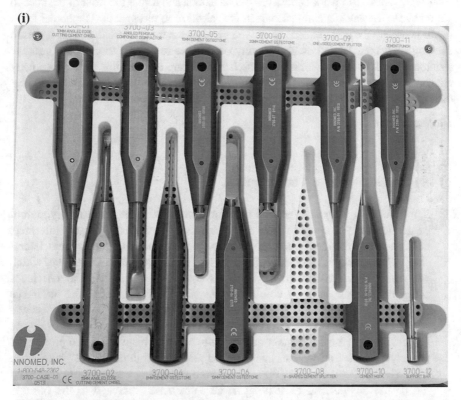

(ii)

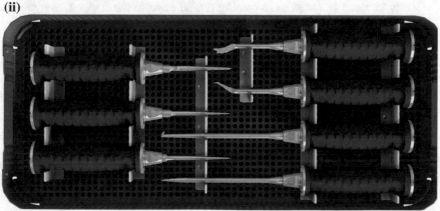

Fig. 6.2 i Example of cutting osteotomes of different sizes, shapes and angles to aid implant removal. **ii** Another example from the HP Knee Extraction Instrumentation (DePuy)

of clearing the gutters to get good access to both sides of the femoral components; the medial side is easier but we also have to get access to the lateral femoral component for all interfaces which means getting the extensor mechanism far enough out of the way laterally to access the anterior flange, the chamfers and the distal femur. In CR designs, we also have to clear the notch.

On the tibial side, medial and anteromedial access is relatively straightforward. However, you have to work behind the patella tendon and across the front of the knee to get access to the anterolateral tibia which is achievable in most cases. The harder bit to get to is usually the posterolateral tibia. The more access we get here the easier it gets to use angled, reverse angled or back-cutting osteotomes to be able to clear any residual fixation (Fig. 6.2). As previously discussed in exposure chapter, tips to facilitate early exposure includes removal of the poly to de-tension the knee, and soft tissue and scar clearance in the gutters with the aim of getting better access posterolaterally.

Our sequence:

(a) Exposure
(b) Insert out
(c) Re-establish medial and lateral gutters
(d) Femur
      We expose the interfaces around the component taking any residual synovium or granulation tissue out, so we can clearly see the implant–cement interface, cement–bone interface, and the bone underneath on both medial and lateral side. Sometimes, we are faced with hard scar tissue around that interface, which we remove with either a saw blade or osteotome to expose the interfaces properly. The aim is to be able to get the saw blade parallel to the interfaces (Fig. 6.3). We use a small oscillating saw (0.4 mm) blade and work on the cement-implant interface with the aim of debonding the implant from the cement and leaving the cement on the bone surface. This will help to protect the underlying bone and we can later remove this cement under direct vision once all the components are out (Fig. 6.1). Avoid separating cement from bone and hitting the component, as leaving some cement still attached to the bone is likely to result in some bone coming out attached to the implant, and we are aiming to reduce iatrogenic bone loss (Fig. 6.4).

      Top tip: When working on the interfaces during component removal, never angle your saw or osteotome into the bone, always be parallel or angle towards the prosthesis.

      We use the saw for this step as it gives you better control as those blades are thin and short, making it more accurate and efficient than a flexible osteotome which tends to be quite long and flimsy by nature, it has a long lever arm which makes it easier to divert out of the plane and into soft bone. Further, the oscillating saw blade cuts through the interface allowing better control of the plane and direction rather than hitting an osteotome (Figs. 6.3 and 6.5). We start on the anterior flange on the medial/lateral side, then the anterior chamfer. You

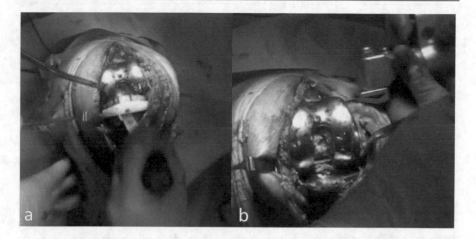

Fig. 6.3 Following synovectomy and exposure of the femoral component and identifying all interfaces; **a** remove the poly which would take some of the tension off and helps to clear out the lateral gutter; **b** using an oscillating saw (0.4 mm thickness blade) starting on either the medial or lateral side separating the implant–cement interface working systematically from the anterior flange all the way around to the posterior chamfer

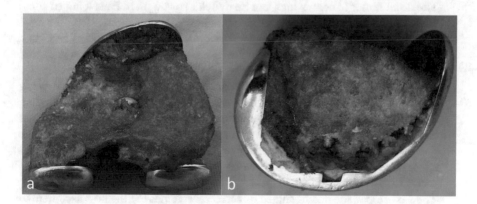

Fig. 6.4 Example of a bad surgical technique with significant iatrogenic bone loss where the implant was hit rigorously by a disimpactor before the cement-implant interface was disrupted

can get a long way under the anterior flange medially, this is an easy place to start as fixation is often poor anteriorly, so you can develop the plane of implant-cement separation easily. The distal chamfer, on the other hand, is an area that gets better fixation, but once you establish your way in and you understand the internal dimensions of the component you can angle your saw blade to fit the internal geometry of the component at the correct interface.

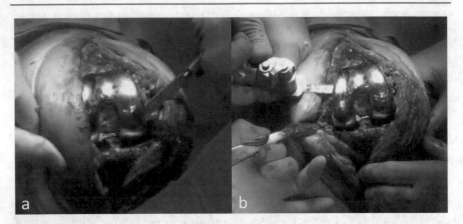

Fig. 6.5 a Flexible osteotomes are also used once the plane of separation created by the oscillating saw; **b** same process completed on the medial side

Top tip: always remain parallel to the components and bias the direction of your cut towards the implant.

The distal femur is next, which can be difficult as you often have a lug of some sort to the component which can catch and block the saw blade. Here, we have to work around it either by using a narrower saw blade or a fine osteotome. In a CR design, the distal cut can also be accessed from the notch with angled osteotomes which aids this process. Then we get to posterior chamfer where we apply the same principles. Posterior condyles are not readily accessible being hidden by the collateral ligaments but do not generally get a very good fixation. We work on this interface being mindful of the proximity of the collaterals in this area. In our experience, as long as we clear off most of the other areas, the posterior chamfer, if not able to clear in fear of damaging collaterals, does not cause bone loss when extracting the component as the cemented fixation here is weak.

The next step is the notch, angled or offset osteotomes are the best used here to clear around the notch and particularly around the lug areas which we could not get to from the outer surfaces.

Top tip: Have a low threshold to change saw blades as they wear out quickly.

The medial side is next: either switch sides or your experienced assistant can perform this step repeating the same process (Fig. 6.6).

Usually when this process is completed all around the femoral component, it would loosen it sufficiently to then use a punch (Fig. 6.6) to gently tap it out placed on the anterior flange with the handle on the distal femur as parallel as possible to the flange, looking all around it making sure no adherence from either side with the help of an assistant.

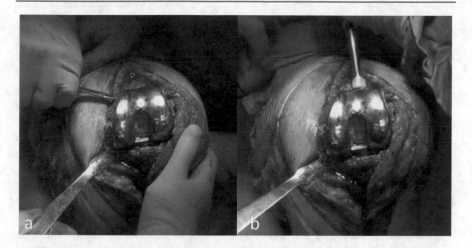

Fig. 6.6 a Flexible osteotome is again used on both sides to ensure complete separation of the implant–cement interface; **b** with a clear path for extraction and once we are sure that the implant–cement interface is separated thoroughly, a femoral impactor (punch) is used to disimpact the femoral component

If it is still fixed at this stage, our next step is to use flexible osteotomes. We have already created the space with the short saw blade, we use it to advance the thin flexible osteotome further in separating the cement-implant interface. We have more control here and we clear the rest going all the way round identifying areas that need further separation. Clearing any soft tissue that block the direct extraction path is important not to overlook. By this stage, in our hands, the vast majority of primary cemented femoral components would come out with minimal bone loss. The key is to be patient and thorough in separating the interfaces and only then attempt to disimpact with a punch.

Top Tip: In removing cemented TKA components, do not hit the components unless you are sure you've loosened all around the cement-implant interface.

Boxed primary PS components often do not have lugs, so we can get all the way around the distal femur to the inside of the box, we cannot do much about the area directly adjacent to the box. However, it is usually smooth with no cement pocket on it so as long as we have thoroughly separated the implant–cement interface throughout then it will generally dis-impact in a similar fashion to a CR femur. It is slightly more problematic if there is a combination of lugs and a box, however, as the lugs will prevent complete separation of the cement-implant interface on the distal surface. It is important to make sure everything else is clear as there is no way of accessing this area before you try to dis-impact. The other area where it might be a bit tricky is femoral components which have a little chip-cut to recess the trochlea, this is usually difficult to clear as well because simply we cannot get to it. Reassuringly, this area, if there was to be bone loss, is where the box and boss for the revision component will be and it will make no difference as fixation for the final revision femoral component is achieved posteriorly and distally. By the time you have reamed and prepared for the box, you will have lost that bit of the bone anyway. So, chip-cut areas are difficult to get to clear, but if a bit of bone is lost it should not be detrimental to subsequent reconstruction.

Now, we have successfully removed the femoral component, hopefully with cement still left on the distal femur. We leave that cement on for now, it gives a firm distal femoral surface against which we can place retractors until we complete removal of the tibial component.

(e) Tibia

We use the broadest retractors we have against the distal femur to distribute the load and prevent any iatrogenic bone collapse in order to sublux the tibia forward. We make sure we have cleared all soft tissue circumferentially around the tibial tray, identify and expose the interfaces by sharp dissection; implant-cement, cement-bone and bone. Then using the small oscillating saw blade, from anteromedial to posteromedial and anterolateral as posterolateral as possible and around the keel (Fig. 6.7), between the implant and the cement. Then again, using flexible osteotomes to complete the separation, once we completed the initial step with a saw creating the plane of separation, this again gives good control and handling of the flexible osteotomes.

Then we use back-cutters in the posteromedial and posterolateral corners as much as possible. Then we use stacking osteotomes with the broadest osteotomes on the set (the wallpaper scraper) into the interface on top of the cement, tap in gently to the keel and we will then start to see the tibial tray lifting off, then we put a second osteotome on top and tap it in again and the tibial

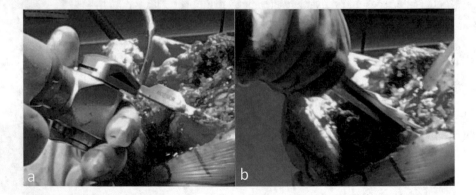

Fig. 6.7 a Example from a different case with well-fixed tibial component; here following removal of the loose femoral component, an oscillating saw blade is used to work on the well-exposed and identified implant–cement interface; b once separation is complete, stacked broad osteotomes are wedged in to lift the tibial component off its cement mantle

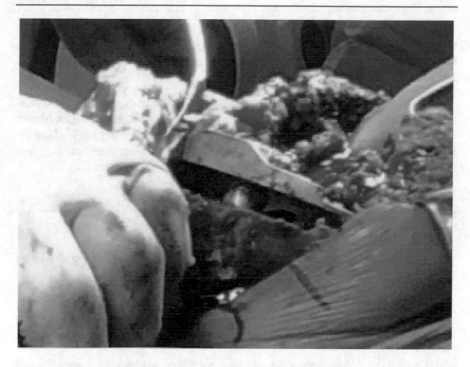

Fig. 6.8 With a clear path for extraction, the tibial component is removed with a punch impactor

component will pop out of its mantle (Fig. 6.8). We grab it with pliers and pull it out once we make sure the path of extraction is clear with enough retraction on the distal femur to protect the posterior condyles.

Again, patience is needed throughout this process. The most difficult part is the posterolateral corner, always ensure that no soft tissue/scar/granulation tissue is tethering the area and preventing access and work on it until you release and separate the implant–cement interface (Fig. 6.9).

(f) Cement removal

We use sharp osteotomes to remove surface cement with the aim of creating little splits (cement is weak in tension) on the top surface to create cracks in the cement which loosens the cement and allows it to be taken out. The difficult area is that of the transition between surface area and keel/stem area, this has to be gently broken with splitters and osteotomes separating the surface cement from the keel cement. The keel cement can be removed again using splitters longitudinally creating multiple splits under direct vision with frequent saline washing to clear out the canal. Finally coming to the cement plug, if it is well-fixed we drill through it which lessens the hoop stresses in the cement and will split it. Once one piece of the plug is out, the rest will come out soon after.

Top tip: **Proper cement splitters are very useful tools; they create radial splits in columns of cement, you can then use chisels to go behind the cement longitudinally pushing the cement centrally into the cement cavity with minimal leverage.**

Challenges in removing primary components: If any component has a stem on either side, you need to know your implant. Older designs had grit blasted under-surfaces of the component and they can present great problems because the implant–cement interface is much stronger that cement–bone interface and very difficult to separate. Be prepared for salvage options in those cases.

6.4 Removal of an All-Poly Tibial Component

Again, the same principles apply here with the added advantage of being able to cut through the keel as well.

6.5 Patella Removal

If it is well-fixed and in reasonable condition we would not take it out even if it was from a different manufacturer to the new implant [4]. If we do need to change it because it is loose, badly worn or in infected cases, we clear all the soft tissues around it and identify and expose the button-cement interface. We can either a patella cutting jig to guide the saw blade or usually a free-hand technique would suffice, cutting with a thin saw blade directly under the button. The latter will come out leaving three pegs in situ. Under direct vision, we either drill into them and pick them out or tease them out with a double ended dissector *(McDonald), or* small nibblers. The main thing here is to keep all the bone and cement layer intact.

6.6 Cementless Primary (Fig. 6.9)

Theoretically these are more difficult to remove, as the only bond here is between implant and bone with no protective secondary interface. The first thing to understand with cementless implants, whenever possible, is the metal composition of the fixation substrate which can affect how you get them out safely particularly with reference to the pegs. You must also understand where the ingrowth surface is on the implant. This is particularly relevant to the tibia where any central cone or keel, if fully coated could lead to significant difficulty in removal. If this is the case, we would have a low threshold for performing a crest osteotomy to get access to this interface to prevent catastrophic bone loss on removal.

(i)

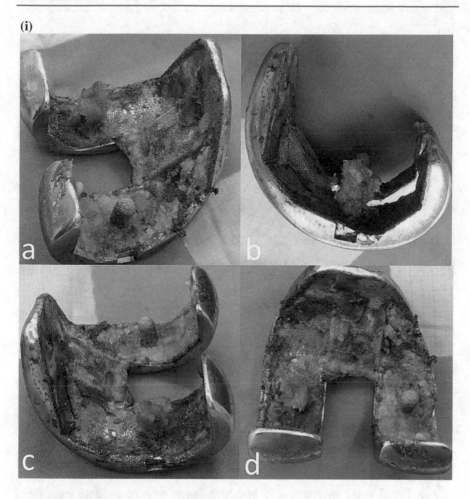

Fig. 6.9 i Example of removing a cementless primary femoral component with minimum bone loss. **ii** Example of removing a cementless primary tibial component with minimum bone loss. **iii** Example of removing a cementless patella component with minimum bone loss

Tantalum-backed tibial components, although they are usually very well ingrown, can be addressed by cutting through the pegs with a reciprocating saw, then using a sharp osteotome you can break the rest of the pegs. So, as outlined above we firstly use an oscillating saw with a thin blade to create the plane of separation, then when we get to the pegs we use a combination of reciprocating saw and sharp osteotome to get through. The posterolateral peg is again the most difficult to get to; in either posterolateral peg in a 4-peg tray or the lateral peg in 2-peg tray. We ensure that we get through all pegs before attempting to extract.

(ii)

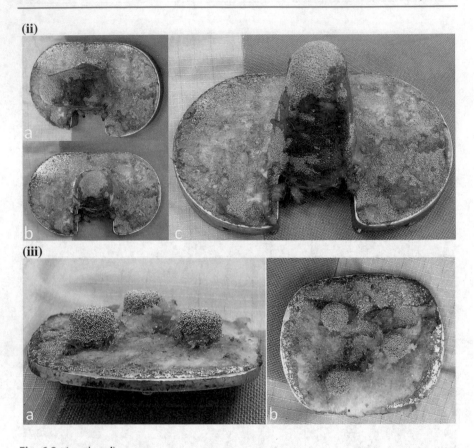

(iii)

Fig. 6.9 (continued)

Top tip: **If using osteotomes to break the pegs on a cementless tray, force can be transmitted through the tray to the bone behind it and cause fracture. Stabilise the tray with an axial pressure through a tibial impactor or similar device to minimise parting energy to the posterior cortex.**

Other implants may not have any pegs but a fully coated cone such as the LCS; the dilemma here is that on plain radiographs we might see some lucent lines around it and think it is loose and easy to get out. This is usually due to stress shielding and all fixation points around the central cone are intact. Again, here, we have to go all around the tray separating as much as possible breaking the bond between implant-bone interface. The cone in this case is cobalt-chrome and we cannot cut through it. We therefore have to plan for reconstruction beforehand anticipating metaphyseal bone loss and consider adjuncts such as metaphyseal sleeves which is our preferred technique. The important point here is to maintain an intact rim of bone on the tibia for sleeve fixation.

Another variant is the 4-peg cobalt-chrome tray such as the Cementless Attune RP. The coating on the central cone in these implants is not all the way down, at least a saving grace! But the pegs are all coated, here again, we make sure to clear the whole periphery with *angled* or *back-cutting osteotomes* behind the posterior pegs. For that we need excellent exposure, clearance and the ability to work posterocentral to posteromedial and posterolateral. We inevitably have some metaphyseal bone loss, and we factor that in our plan for reconstruction. If we are struggling to get access, we consider an extensile approach early i.e. tibial crest osteotomy.

On the femoral side, it is a similar process to cemented implant in that we need to work all around it with a combination of an oscillating saw and flexible osteotome to break the bond between implant and bone. Although we anticipate and plan for potentially more bone loss compare with a cemented implant.

Cementless knees are gaining popularity and it is inevitable that we will face dealing with infected cases, not acutely where a DAIR procedure can be utilised, but perhaps a few years post implantation through haematogenous spread. Other scenarios are likely to present where well-fixed cementless knees have to be taken out. As we take more of these out, we will develop better skills to deal with these cases. However, as a community of arthroplasty surgeons, we do need to develop better techniques and instrumentation to help extracting those implants. Modern knees are increasingly using materials that we can cut through with a combination of saws and osteotomes. Also, the fixation pegs on some new designs are not solid but have a hollow interior. They are strong in terms of load transmission but are *'cut-able'*. These include porous tantalum [5] and porous titanium [6] being manufactured through plasma spray or three-dimensional (3D) printed technology [7, 8].

6.7 Removal of Revision Components

The same first principles apply with the difference being the presence of stems, sleeves, and intramedullary fixations. Understanding the implant system that we are trying to remove is of paramount importance. The difficulty lies in getting access and that we cannot change the angle of extraction, particularly on the tibial side. The other issue is getting the insert out. In most systems, there is a locking bolt into the tibial tray, so we cannot slide the poly out but we have to translate the tibia anteriorly to clear a path for extraction.

Most implants will come out as one construct, others can be taken out sequentially by taking the surface replacement component out first and the stem secondarily. The latter option is only possible if it is a Morse taper connection and not a screw thread connection. Stems in revision implants are usually positional stems and not fixation stems, which is in contrast to sleeves which are used for fixation purposes. Stems are generally not ingrown but rather made with a roughened titanium surface and splines for extra stability. So, they are not *ingrown* along their length but might have some *ongrowth* at best in junctional areas. Most revision knee systems have extraction devices that can be attached to the end of the stem and removed with a slap hammer. In rare cases, some hip revision techniques in stem extraction can be useful such as using K-wires driven into the splines or circumferentially around a broken stem to get enough length for a mole wrench engagement.

Top tip: When removing revision implants, understand the system well, get any extraction instruments for the system and have adequate exposure.

A challenging scenario in removing cemented stems in revision components, which would be evident on preoperative radiographs, is if the diameter of the stem is wider than that of the boss. This leaves cement on the junction between the two and makes safe removal unattainable. The stem must be either parallel or narrower than the boss for it to be extracted safely.

Top tip: When using cemented stems, never use a stem thicker than the thickness of the boss. Also, be wary of a cemented offset stem for the same reason.

Similar challenges can be seen in cemented offset adaptors, in those circumstances, unless you can disimpact the femoral component from the offset adaptor to get access to clear the cement in between, it cannot be taken out without significant bone loss. Fortunately, this is a rare scenario, but we do occasionally see it. Cemented stems do not require offset, they can be placed eccentrically in the canal within the mantle. Always have a salvage megaprosthesis option on standby.

6.8   Removal of Metaphyseal Sleeves

Sleeves offer excellent fixation and well-ingrown sleeves are difficult to remove. Contemporary sleeve systems are compatible with salvage options in cases of re-revision. The only real indication for removing a sleeve is chronic infection. Theoretically, they may be loose although in one infected case we had, it was indeed well ingrown (Fig. 6.10).

In the femur, they are located above the box extending proximally into the femoral canal. On the tibia, although they are adjacent to the joint surface, they are covered by the tibial tray. Although we have been using metaphyseal sleeves for almost 20 years, we have only had a few cases where we had to remove them. The following tips apply to the systems we used over the years (S-ROM, TC3 and Attune):

1. Clear the cement and loosen the surface replacement like a primary TKA using oscillating saw and flexible osteotomes...etc.
2. *Femoral side*; disengage the Morse taper between the femoral component and the sleeve.
(a) In S-ROM and TC3, this can be achieved only by a direct blow to the femoral component once the cement interfaces are cleared. There are especially designed splitters that can be used but getting them into the junction is very difficult. An anterior femoral window might be an option.

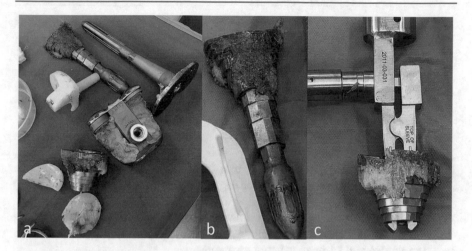

Fig. 6.10 Example of a metaphyseal sleeve removal in an infected rTKA case. The patient had undergone 2-stage revision for infection and was reconstructed with a sleeved prosthesis on the tibia. The infection had recurred a year later; a DAIR procedure was attempted but failed. The only option was therefore to repeat the 2-stage procedure. **a** Rotating Platform bearing could not be removed so the poly was sectioned to allow it to rotate and be lifted out; the tibial stem was < 14 mm so could be extracted through the sleeve using a tuning fork to break the Morse taper between tibial tray and sleeve (**b**). The sleeve was then extracted from the top using osteotomes and the sleeve extractor (**c**). On the femoral side, the femoral component was separated from the sleeve and again the sleeve was extracted using osteotomes and slap hammer. As noted below, the sleeves were osseointegrated even with chronic infection in this case

(b) In the newer Attune system, the Morse taper can be disengaged from the joint surface by going up through the boss with a specially designed instrument that screws onto the femoral component utilising a pin up against the sleeve which is then attached to large levers to introduce a load that would break the Morse taper and disengage the femoral component from the sleeve.

(c) Now we have an ingrown sleeve with a stem above, and can use flexible osteotomes or K-wires gently to work around it and remove the ingrowth from the coating. Have a model sleeve available to guide you where the ingrowth is to aid this step.

(d) The extraction device is then threaded into the sleeve and extracted with a slap hammer; for S-ROM and TC3 a hook device is available for extraction. Alternatively, a mole-wrench with attached slap hammer can be used.

(1) *Tibial side*; there is a gap between the tray and the top of the sleeve. Identify and expose this gap. A splitter is then introduced to disengage the tibial tray from the sleeve.

(a) In S-ROM and TC3, a tuning fork-like splitter is tapped in, it acts as a wedge and pops the tray out.

(b) In the Attune system, a newer splitter with levers is used applying a distraction force and disengaging the Morse taper.

(c) In both cases, the stem attaches to the tray, so the tray and stem are removed as one leaving the ingrown sleeve behind. Here, this is dependent on the surgeon not oversizing the tibial stem, otherwise the stem cannot simply pass through the sleeve if it has a larger diameter than 14 mm. In those cases, you may need an extensive crest osteotomy to work around the sleeve anteromedially and anterolaterally. Or use a *Midas Rex* metal cutter instrument to drill out the stem connection to the under-surface of the tibial tray to be able to remove the tray and leave the stem behind, then remove the sleeve as above followed by the stem.

(d) There is a dedicated sleeve removal tool for the tibia which has jaws that open up distal to the sleeve and allow for the attachment of a slap hammer (Attune)

Top Tip: Anticipate problems in sleeves that have been implanted for a long time due to cold welding; disengaging the Morse taper might prove a bone destructive process so have salvage strategies.

To conclude, the safe removal of implants with minimal bone loss is a crucial step in revision knee surgery and it paves the way for an efficient and successful reconstruction. Ensure you gather all relevant information preoperatively particularly for the less familiar cementless components or revision systems. The overarching principle for this step is that patience is indeed a virtue.

References

1. Uggen JC, Engh CAJ. Getting out the well-fixed knee: all hands on deck. Sem Arth. 2013;24:160–6.
2. Firestone TP, Krackow KA. Removal of femoral components during revision knee arthroplasty. J Bone Joint Surg Br. 1991;73(3):514.
3. Mason JB, Fehring TK. Removing well-fixed total knee arthroplasty implants. Clin Orthopaed Relat Res. 2006;446:76–82.
4. Lonner JH, et al. Fate of the unrevised all-polyethylene patellar component in revision total knee arthroplasty. J Bone Joint Surg Am. 2003;85(1):56–9.
5. De Martino I, et al. Total knee arthroplasty using cementless porous tantalum monoblock tibial component: a minimum 10-year follow-up. J Arthroplasty. 2016;31(10):2193–8.
6. Winther NS, et al. Comparison of a novel porous titanium construct (Regenerex®) to a well proven porous coated tibial surface in cementless total knee arthroplasty-a prospective randomized RSA study with two-year follow-up. Knee. 2016;23(6):1002–11.
7. Sultan AA, et al. Cementless 3D printed highly porous titanium-coated baseplate total knee arthroplasty: survivorship and outcomes at 2-year minimum follow-up. J Knee Surg. 2020;33 (3):279–83.
8. Kamath AF, et al. Cementless fixation in primary total knee arthroplasty: historical perspective to contemporary application. J Am Acad Orthop Surg. 2020; Publish Ahead of Print.

Principles of Surgical Reconstruction: Back to the Beginning… Again

7

An expert is someone who knows some of the worst mistakes
that can be made in their subject, and how to avoid them.

Werner Heisenberg (Nobel laureate)

7.1 Introduction

Outcomes and durability of revision total knee arthroplasty (rTKA) are influenced
by a number of factors: achieving good fixation, restoring kinematics as near the
native knee as possible, and ensuring stability in the joint throughout its range of
motion [1–3]. In other words, function, stability and fixation. If we get those three
elements correct, we will have a durable construct and a happy patient. All these
three domains are inextricably linked. However, in this chapter our focus is on the
principles of joint reconstruction.

7.2 Philosophy of rTKA

Our philosophy in reconstructing the knee joint at the time of revision surgery is
exactly the same as for primary TKA. We all agree that in every revision situation
we will have no cruciate ligaments, we may have compromised bone stock but at
least still some tibia and femur to work with, and for condylar revisions we have to
have intact collateral ligaments. So, we are back to the 'frame principle' for all
condylar revisions. Our aim is to position the joint within that collateral frame to
restore the joint line in both flexion and extension and to get balanced gaps
throughout range of motion in flexion, extension and very importantly mid-flexion.

Therefore, balanced gaps and a correct joint line leads us to a stable joint throughout range of motion. A well-balanced, stable joint with a restored joint line is how good kinematics are achieved. What is different from a primary TKA in this context is the lack of virgin bone with its normal bony landmarks. If the collaterals are compromised, particularly the MCL, then we are into hinged implant territory as a condylar revision will certainly fail.

7.3   Our Approach to Condylar Revisions

For a successful condylar revision, we must have a stable tibial platform, a stable femoral platform and intact collateral ligaments. At this point, we have achieved adequate exposure and we have removed the old implants with minimal bone loss. Here, we might have a number of problems using anatomical landmarks as a building block for our reconstruction. This is because we do not know for certain, in a reliable and reproduceable, easy to teach way, how much bone was taken at the time of primary TKA. A lot of decisions may have been made at that point that ultimately led to the current failure. So, if we build the reconstruction based on those decisions we may again have a suboptimal outcome. Therefore, we need a strategy to ensure that we can build a stable construct irrespective of those variables that would give us stability, restore joint line, durable fixation with good kinematics for a successful outcome.

The first premise is that the medial and lateral collaterals are intact. Secondly, we believe that clearing the posterior space of all scar and granulation tissue is a key step in joint reconstruction and often overlooked. The aim is to get as clear a soft tissue envelope as possible, akin to a primary case. Once we have a clear posterior space and intact collateral ligaments, then how is this different from a balanced approach in a primary TKA? The only difference is that we have to address bone loss on both femoral and tibial sides.

We do not accept the premise that most revisions are lax in flexion; why should that be the case unless the collateral ligaments are attenuated or incompetent. The collaterals are the tether linking the proximal tibia to the distal femur. What are the reasons revision knees appear slack in flexion during surgery?

Firstly, there is usually posterior condylar bone loss which gives an apparent increase in the flexion space. The use of posterior femoral augments to compensate for this bone loss will allow restoration of the joint line in flexion and lead to a balanced and well-tensioned flexion space.

Secondly, as previously discussed there is usually significant posterior capsular thickening with granulation type tissue spanning the posterior space from the posterior femoral condyles to the posterior aspect of the proximal tibia. This tightens the knee by being a posterior tether when the knee is put into extension. It is for this reason that we believe posterior capsular clearance is an important early step in revision TKA.

So, we would argue that revisions are not lax in flexion but instead tight in extension. It is these two factors together which are often responsible for the mismatch between flexion and extension gaps. The proximal tibia has equal effects on both, what we can do to rectify the mismatch is on the femoral side (posterior condyles) and posterior capsule.

Top Tip: Being meticulous in clearing the posterior space is a major factor in achieving equal gaps.

This is compounded by the focus on the joint line in extension. If we only rely on anatomical landmarks to restore the joint line in extension before adequately clearing out the posterior space, we may need to decrease the tibial insert thickness to allow the knee into full extension with our pre-determined joint line. The knee would be stable in extension but as soon as we flex the knee making the posterior capsule redundant, we become increasingly reliant on the collateral ligaments for stability in mid-flexion and flexion, but with an undersized tibial insert these structures will not be appropriately tensioned once the tight posterior capsule is negated leading to mid-flexion and flexion instability. Most surgeons, in this scenario, would use offset to posteriorize the femoral component or would accept that all revisions are slack in flexion and use a prosthesis with a high post to control stability; this is suboptimal in terms of delivering better kinematics and patients' outcomes. This approach, however, will not address the mid-flexion space resulting in ongoing instability and an increased requirement for constrained revision implants. Although, most revision implants do cope with some flexion instability, we strongly believe that it is better to follow the basic principles of a balanced approach in revision surgery in keeping with the frame principle as outlined.

Top Tip: Revisions are not lax in flexion, but rather tight in extension. The key is to close the flexion space down by addressing posterior condylar bone loss and to fix the extension tightness by clearing out the posterior scar.

7.4   Flexion First Approach

The aforementioned argument boils down to adequate exposure of the joint and reconstructing the joint on the frame principle. The sequence of reconstruction with the prerequisites of intact collateral ligaments and clear posterior space, similar to a primary TKA, is first *an absolutely stable tibial platform*. In our approach, this is achieved through the tibial broach, tibial sleeve, and trial tibial base plate.

Secondly, to complete the only missing side of the frame, is the question of where to position the femoral component to balance the knee in flexion, extension, and mid-flexion by respecting the joint line. Our starting point is to get some stability for the femoral construct within the intramedullary canal. We then need to decide what size femoral component we are planning to use. Things to consider when making this decision are (a) previous radiographs of the native knee; (b) the preoperative radiograph of the current implant looking at the mediolateral and posterior offset of the component and make a judgement of whether it is well-sized, oversized or undersized; (c) looking at the mediolateral size of the remaining distal femur and the corresponding anteroposterior diameter of the appropriate size femoral component without overhang either medially or laterally. The patient's own anatomy will dictate the femoral component's size. Pre-operative templating using widely available software can be beneficial at this stage.

So far, we have some stability in the femoral canal and an estimation of the size of the femoral component. Now we can gap balance using either a cutting block or cut-through trials or any other device your preferred revision system provides. We then position the correct size femoral component as posterior as possible without creating a femoral notch and check the flexion space in flexion. Once the correct size femur is appropriately positioned to restore the posterior condylar offset (as posterior as possible) our options to further alter the flexion gap on the femoral side are exhausted. This will tell us the thickness of the insert needed to get a stable flexion gap. Here, we can still do secondary checks by using anatomical landmarks such as the distance from the epicondyles or meniscal scars. This flexion gap ultimately has to be equal to the extension gap.

Once we are happy with our posterior space clearance and our joint line in flexion, we turn our attention to the extension space. We ignore the existing distal femoral bone cuts and estimate the extension joint line. In practice, we intentionally leave the trial femoral construct approximately 4 mm (corresponding to the thinnest distal augment on our revision system) proud of the estimated joint line, expecting the extension space to be tight. We then measure the extension space and compare to the flexion space already established. We then advance the femoral construct incrementally to open the extension gap making regular checks to achieve flexion extension balance. At all times, we cross check with anatomical landmarks and soft tissue tension to maximise accuracy. We have now restored the joint line with respect to the soft tissue envelope throughout the range of motion by positioning the implant within an intact collateral frame. This is no different to the gap balanced approach to a primary TKA.

Once the joint line is established, the native femoral bone is prepared from that joint line using augments distally and posteriorly to ensure bony contact.

This technique of leaving the construct intentionally proud ensures that with advancement of the construct to open the extension space enhances intramedullary fixation. The reverse to this technique is not practical. Imagine if we position the femoral construct in exactly where we think the joint line should be in flexion, and we prepared the femur for a press-fit stem or sleeve and then discovered that the extension gap is slack, distalising the construct even by couple of millimetres could jeopardize the press-fit due to the conical shape of the distal femur.

The advantage of this flexion first approach is that we are not driven by anatomical landmarks which are not consistent in revision cases or through bony cuts that rely on refreshing the remaining bone surfaces and are arbitrary in terms of restoring kinematics. Instead, this approach relies on a clear posterior space and intact collateral ligaments, irrespective of the amount of bone loss we have; with a stable tibial platform and finally by positioning the appropriately sized femoral component flush on the anterior femoral cortex which dictates flexion gap. This will in turn dictate the extension gap. Then we can replace bone defects with augments bringing the bone to the component ensuring that the augments are referenced off the joint line and not the other way around.

Now, we have a stable tibial platform, intact collateral ligaments and the fourth bar of the frame is connected with the femoral component. Secondary checks of kinematics, stability and anatomical landmarks (when available) are made to ensure that the joint line has been appropriately restored.

7.5 Caution

If a surgeon chooses to undersize the femur to compensate for posterior femoral bone loss, there is a danger the flexion gap will be balanced by increasing insert thickness rather than restoring posterior condylar offset. If this is not recognised and the extension gap is noted to be tight due to the thickness of the poly insert, there is a risk the surgeon will significantly raise the joint line in extension to balance the knee. This will lead to patellofemoral problems and suboptimal tibiofemoral kinematics.

Top Tip: Correct femoral component sizing and positioning are imperative for a successful outcome in a flexion first balanced workflow.

7.6 What About Collateral Ligaments' Attenuation?

The absolute contraindication of a condylar revision (VVC) is an incompetent or absent MCL. From our own practical experience, we do not find that the MCL stretches or attenuates in the majority of condylar revision cases. We do, however, see cases with an incompetent MCL, particularly in elderly female patients with neglected valgus deformities. MCL competency is therefore in our view, a binary situation; it is either intact or not.

Most TKAs fail with a medial tibial collapse ending up in a degree of varus deformity. In this situation, the lateral side can attenuate; it is not the LCL per se but rather the lateral soft tissue complex. So, let us accept that there might be a degree of lateral attenuation in some cases and examine the impact on the gap balanced approach. It may lead to excessive external rotation of the cutting block in flexion. This will be apparent intraoperatively. On the lateral side, dynamic stabilisers such the ITB can help stabilise the joint in gait. A judgment call is needed as to whether the lateral structures are sufficiently competent to be compatible with a condylar revision or whether a hinged implant is needed.

7.7 Augments and Bone Loss

On the tibial side, bone loss dictates the need for augments in relation to where the joint line needs to be. It is usually due to medial tibial bone loss that might require an augment. This will be clear from the preoperative radiographs. It is important to create a stable tibial platform with augmentation or tibial sleeves or cones. If you are using an augment, it is important to consider the impact of tibial rotation on the patellofemoral joint and post impingement in the revision settings. Ideally, a desired revision system allows a stable tibial platform to be established and rotation to be set at the end of the procedure.

On the femoral side, we know where the joint line needs to be and we know where the remaining bone is, so we need to connect the two bringing the bone to the component. This is in contrast to building the joint line from the native bone. Whilst both will require augmentation, joint line restoration should take priority and should be governed by the soft tissue envelope rather than the existing residual bone.

Significant posterior condylar bone loss is a challenging situation which can lead to either compromised fixation or flexion instability. It is important to have enough posterior condylar fixation to resist rotational torque on the femoral construct. Failing to achieve this will lead to premature loosening. There is a limit to the amount of augmentation which can be used which leads to a temptation to undersize the femoral component to ensure bony contact. This potentially leads to an unbalanced reconstruction with flexion instability. In practice, we believe it is imperative to protect the joint line regardless of bone loss and look to enhance fixation within the metaphysis where there is invariably good bone stock. Out preference is to use metaphyseal sleeves which resist rotational torque and deliver durable fixation; others may use cones or bone grafts, or in other systems with a massive flexion–extension mismatch the only bailout option may well be a hinged implant.

7.8 How Do We Restore Posterior Femoral Offset?

If you are a long press-fit stem user, the net effect as the stem engages the isthmus is to anteriorise the entry point and this in turn anteriorises the femoral component. You would need to add offset to get to the outcome we are describing. That is why offset works; not because it is closing down the flexion gap, but rather because it allows the femoral component to be positioned where it should be independent of the stem position. If you are using a cemented stem reconstruction, this is less of a worry as you can position the femoral component where it needs to be using an undersized cemented stem which will not dictate your femoral component position. For femoral sleeves, there are two ways of approaching this: either broach last or broach more posteriorly. In the former, we position the femoral component where it needs to be, defining the axis of this position, and broach to that axis. The latter technique is preferred as we slightly posteriorize the entry point, this is a different philosophy to the long press-fit preparation where you need to go more anterior to get proximal cortical engagement and then use an offset. With sleeves we are shortening the intramedullary construct as most of the fixation is in the metaphysis. So, for a sleeve we prepare with a posterior entry point and broach more posteriorly which will negate the need for offset. Our preference is to broach to get some stability, then position the femoral component, do the checks, and then we can upsize the broach from this position to optimise fixation without impacting component position.

7.9   Constraint and the Balanced Approach

By default, all revision condylar systems have a degree of constraint. For the purist, however, when we have a frame with intact collaterals, constraint is theoretically not needed. Increased varus-valgus constraint (VVC) is helpful to surgeons dealing with a compromised soft tissue envelope or difficulty in balancing the knee properly. If the balanced approach is applied with intact collateral ligaments, a posterior stabilised construct alone is sufficient because we are re-establishing the joint line and the gaps akin to a primary TKA. Here, VVC acts as an additional comfort to surgeons, with extra stability and certainty if there are any concerns about attenuation of the lateral structures. If, on the other hand, we have an absent or incompetent MCL, then VVC is doomed to failure. The other practical aspect here is that most systems do not have a stemmable posterior-stabilised femur; you have to use a revision femur but you can pair this with a posterior-stabilised articulation. If you are a fixed-bearing revision surgeon, you should give serious thought to that option as otherwise you are abolishing the rotational freedom.

The VVC constraint is delivered by a post in a box which gives the side-to-side stability, but it also restricts rotation. So, with the VVC constraint comes a degree of rotational constraint (fixed bearing VVC systems generally allow for 1–4° of rotation) which is potentially detrimental to the fixation interfaces. So, it is very important to understand the revision system used with the impact of a VVC constraint on rotational constraint. This could be avoided by using a rotating platform (RP) articulation which dissipates the rotational torque and protects the fixation interfaces while at the same time keeping the advantages of a VVC insert. The downside of an RP bearing is that it is less tolerant to any flexion instability with the potential for spin-out. We ensure our flexion gap is stable and routinely use an RP-VVC articulation for the advantages it offers in terms of extra stability, without the downside of having rotational constraint that can transmit to the fixation interfaces. It is indeed a delicate balancing act and it has to be understood within the features of the revision system used.

Top Tip: with VVC constraint comes a degree of rotational constraint which is potentially detrimental to the fixation interfaces – particularly with fixed-bearing inserts.

7.10   Patellofemoral Joint

If we get the joint line correct, and if we get the femoral rotation correct and with balanced gaps, the kinematics of the patellofemoral joint would follow. Practical considerations here are to keep the patella button from the primary TKA if at all possible unless it is badly worn. If so, then remove it but maintain the bone stock. Clear the cement carefully and cement a new button. Some systems have round rather than offset patella buttons which have the advantage of being able to turn the peg holes to fit. Make sure it is tracking without any lateral pulling force, revisit the lateral gutter and ensure it is clear from any scarring or granulating tissue causing any tethering. In our practice, we also resurface native patellae in revision cases to reduce the risk of box engagement.

In conclusion, our workflow in condylar revisions relies on the *frame principle* similar to a primary TKA with good surgical exposure, clearing the posterior space, establishing a stable tibial platform, balancing the knee in flexion with intact collateral ligaments, followed by balancing the knee in extension, setting femoral rotation, performing femoral bone cuts and implantation.

7.11   Case Demonstration (Figs. 7.1, 7.2, 7.3, 7.4, 7.5, 7.6, 7.7 and 7.8)

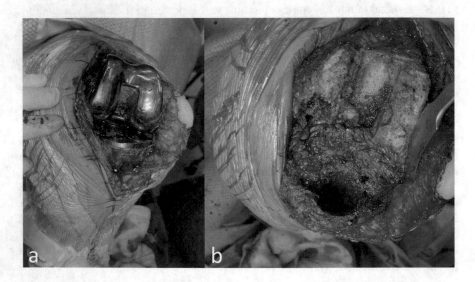

Fig. 7.1 Clinical photographs **a**) following exposure and **b**) removal of components with minimal bone loss and preparation of the tibia for a metaphyseal sleeve

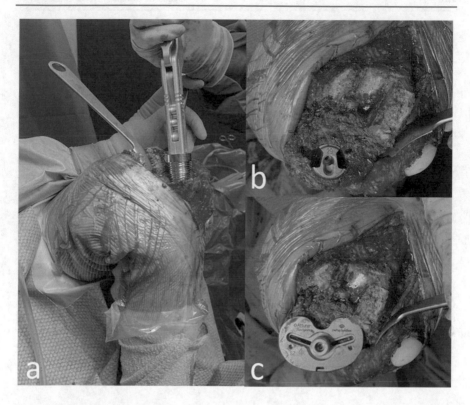

Fig. 7.2 Tibial preparation is performed through three simple steps: **a**) broaching for a sleeve (press-fit); **b**) a tibial refreshing cut off the broach; **c**) a trial tibial tray of appropriate size is assembled

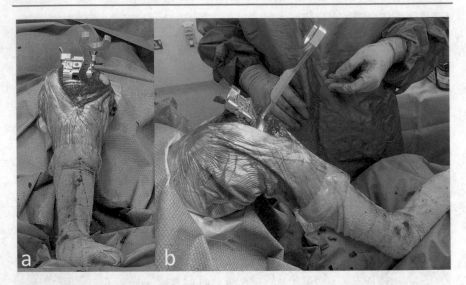

Fig. 7.3 Femoral preparation is performed; reaming the femoral canal to the appropriate diameter stem then attaching the appropriately AP sized cutting block; (**a-b**) balancing the knee in 90° flexion with a stable tibial platform and intact collateral ligaments (*frame principle*) and a spacer block establishing a balanced flexion space. Femoral rotation will be set later once the knee is balanced in both flexion and extension

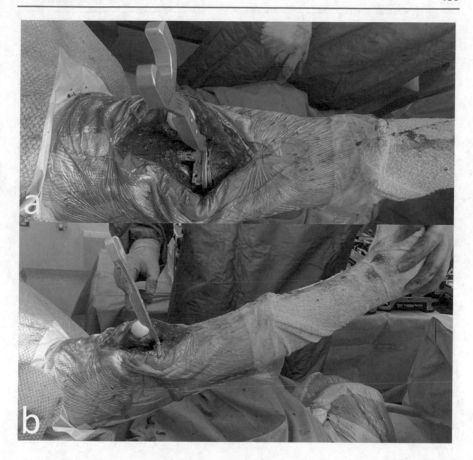

Fig. 7.4 Once the knee balanced in flexion, the extension gap is checked (**a, b**)

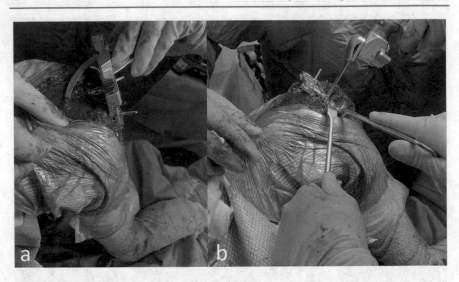

Fig. 7.5 a) The final step before making any bony cuts is setting femoral component rotation in flexion based on flexion balance with secondary checks using an angel wing device; **b)** bony cuts are completed on the femoral side and measuring for augments as necessary

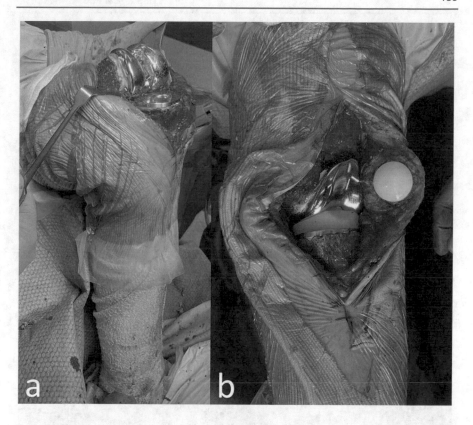

Fig. 7.6 **a**) Deep flexion view with definitive components implanted (hybrid fixation in this case) with sleeved tibial component and short-cemented femoral stem; **b**) extension view with a balanced knee

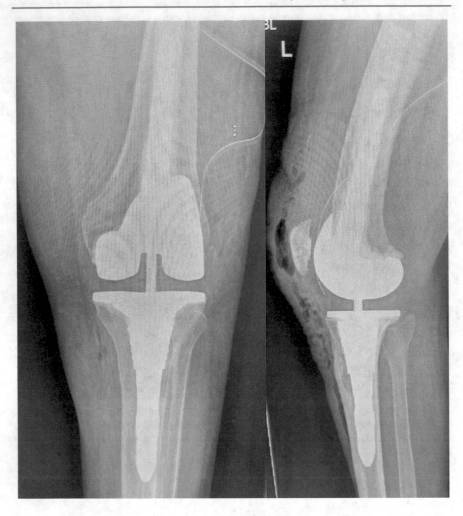

Fig. 7.7 Postoperative radiographs with hybrid fixation with cemented femoral stem and a sleeved tibial component with a mobile bearing VVC insert

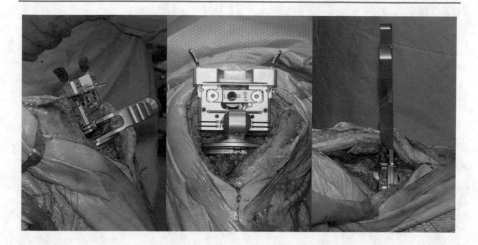

Fig. 7.8 Other similar devices can be used (horseshoe) in a balanced approach

References

1. Ghomrawi HM, et al. Patterns of functional improvement after revision knee arthroplasty. J Bone Joint Surg Am. 2009;91(12):2838–45.
2. Fehring TK, et al. Stem fixation in revision total knee arthroplasty: a comparative analysis. Clin Orthop Relat Res. 2003;416:217 24.
3. Edwards PK, et al. Are cementless stems more durable than cemented stems in two-stage revisions of infected total knee arthroplasties? Clin Orthop Relat Res. 2014;472(1):206–11.

Fixation in Revision Total Knee Arthroplasty

8

It is not only the beauty of a building you should look at; it is the construction of the foundation that will stand the test of time.

David Allan Coe

8.1 Introduction

Outcomes and durability of rTKA are influenced by a number of factors; construct stability, joint line restoration, restoration of kinematics, managing bone defects and implant fixation [1–3]. The latter continues to be a subject of debate in the literature although the need to use stems to enhance implant fixation in condylar revisions is universally agreed. Stemmed components offload stresses at the damaged metaphyseal interfaces, bypass bone defects, and provide additional prosthetic surface area for fixation [2, 4, 5]. Three fixation techniques are described in the literature for modular rTKA; *cementless fixation* of all components and stems, *cemented fixation* of all components and stems and *hybrid fixation* where cement is used for both "surface fixation" of the components with either cementless press-fit stems or a cemented stem on either tibial or femoral sides [6–8]. However, most contemporary rTKA systems use either hybrid or fully cemented techniques. In cases of significant metaphyseal bone loss, adjunctive fixation with sleeves or cones has shown excellent long-term outcomes [9–11]. This chapter will focus on the philosophies of different fixation techniques and our preferred approach to not only achieve durable fixation but also to help in joint reconstruction using tibial metaphyseal sleeves to reliably establish a stable tibial platform with the *frame principle*.

8.2 Philosophy of Fixation Techniques

The principle of fixation in rTKA is having a stable fixation of implant to bone, just like in primary TKA, and ideally that fixation should be at or close to the joint line. In revision settings, although the bone adjacent to the joint line can be compromised, we still have to get fixation concentrating near the joint line and adjunctively at the metaphyseal and diaphyseal segments.

On the femoral side, as previously discussed, we position an appropriately sized femoral component and bring the bone to the component, optimising fixation with augments. This is of paramount importance particularly augmenting the posterior femoral condyles to ensure rotational stability of the femoral component at the joint line. Augments are used to bridge gaps and there is a limit to how much reliable fixation we can get at the augmented component-bone interface. So, we need to supplement this surface fixation by also getting secure canal fixation.

Mechanically speaking, with all the load (axial, torsional torque, constraint..... etc.) that goes through the femoral component, the question is how can we make the fixation as robust and stable as it can be? Consider press-fit cementless stems with diaphyseal engagement: they are splined and fluted long stems, not ingrowth stems, and often drive you to need offset. The downside here is that we then have a short segment of fixation proximally at the diaphysis, with some fixation at the joint line but very little else in between. If we then have any micro motion of the component with such a long lever arm, this will translate to motion at the short fixation segment and lead to early loosening and failure. So, mechanically, using a long press-fit stem when we have compromised distal femoral bone is not robust enough for long-term durability. Bringing the fixation closer to the joint line i.e. shortening the lever arm of fixation is more intuitive. This is achieved by getting metaphyseal fixation in addition to the epiphyseal fixation.

Top Tip: Get durable fixation near the joint line, but also get fixation at the joint line particularly at the posterior femoral condyles with augments even when using femoral metaphyseal sleeves.

On the tibial side, similar to the femoral side, the best stability of the construct is achieved by having the fixation interface as close as possible to the joint line to resist rotational torque. Just like in a primary, we do not simply cement a round cone in the canal because it is rotationally unstable, we use a keel which provides stability. In revision cases, if there is significant bone loss, augments can fill the space but then will need a stem below it: either long press-fit or cemented stems. The fixation is then all along the length of the stem which is different from the femoral side due to its multifaceted articulation and complex geometry with its five interfaces. The tibia is a flat surface with a flat tray and often central bone loss by the time the tibial component is removed. So, a keel will be largely unsupportive with only a stem below it. If an augment is used, then we are relying on the stem for the tibial fixation. The issue here is rotational stability of the construct particularly when using augments which are again flat-surfaced supported by a slim cortical rim in most cases. So, a long press-fit stem is used to provide stability of the construct. However, we are back to a longer lever arm for the construct and in a constrained articulation the rotational torque will eventually lead to mechanical loosening.

A good real-life example to further illustrate this mechanical point is seen in rugby for instance. In a rugby scrum, all the load goes through the prop forwards who are the broadest, heaviest and stockiest of players with all their power close to engagement point. You will never see a forward prop who is tall and thin and can be easily knocked over!

Top Tip: the closer we get our fixation to the joint line the more we negate the effects of a long lever arm on the construct.

8.3   Metaphyseal Fixation

Shortening the lever arm of the construct means that we need to bring the fixation closer to the joint line i.e., to the metaphysis. There are three techniques to achieve metaphyseal fixation; metaphyseal sleeves, cones or short cemented stem constructs. The latter two overlap in principle as they provide a closed reconstructive canal where metaphyseal fixation can be obtained. Sleeves on the other hand are an integral part of the component and offer robust metaphyseal fixation.

The concept of metaphyseal sleeve fixation is to use an intramedullary device to enhance metaphyseal and diaphyseal fit, promote intramedullary load sharing, fixation into intact bone, and to bypass stress risers in situations of bone deficiencies. It was featured, amongst other modifications, in the third generation S-ROM mobile-bearing hinge total knee prosthesis (DePuy, Warsaw, IN) in response to the high failure rates seen in earlier hinge designs. Metaphyseal sleeves are stepped and coated with titanium beads allowing for bone ingrowth [12, 13] and fixed with a Morse taper junction to either the femoral or tibial component. In 2001, Jones & Barrack et al. [14] reported on their combined series of modular, mobile-bearing hinged knee arthroplasties with metaphyseal sleeves for salvage cases with good midterm outcomes and notable success of the sleeves. Hence, further engineering developments have resulted in the use of metaphyseal sleeves with semi-constrained mobile-bearing revision implants. Since then, the use of metaphyseal sleeves has gained popularity with numerous clinical series demonstrating excellent osseointegration and survivorship at short- to medium-term and more recently medium- to long-term follow up [9, 15–18].

The metaphyseal bone is well-vascularised and often spared the damage seen in epiphyseal bone during revision surgery. This offers advantages for cement interdigitation or implant osseointegration [19]. Once ingrown, sleeves transfer the load to the metaphysis, protecting the epiphyseal fixation and improving the rotational stability of the construct. It is superior in doing so compared to fluted cylindrical stems [20]. Furthermore, sleeves have the added advantage of being used as instruments during surgery. Similar to the preparation of the proximal femur during uncemented hip arthroplasty, the canal is reamed and broached to achieve rotational and axial stability. Once the metaphysis is filled, this offers a stable cutting platform negating the need for pinning jigs and cutting guides. The bony cuts can be made, efficiently ensuring appropriate alignment, directly off the metaphyseal broach attached to a trial stem of desired length.

8.4   What About Metaphyseal Cones?

Trabecular metal cones (Zimmer, Warsaw, IN), and also more recently with other materials from different manufacturers, are effectively cutting down the amount of cement needed with the advantage, over cement alone, in getting ingrowth into the bone. They provide excellent stability in the cone-bone interface and secondly by getting cement interdigitation in the cement-cone interface. So, here the void is filled with a metal cone and then the construct is cemented into the cone. Although cones made of porous tantalum have favourable porosity, a high coefficient of friction and low stiffness with a high rate of osteointegration [21], they require fixation or "unitisation" to the revision components by an added cemented interface. Therefore, they act more like a "metallic bone graft" and are separate to implant fixation.

8.5   What About a Short-Cemented Stem Construct?

Whilst there is good evidence to support the use of a short-cemented construct on the femoral side, it is different on the tibial side. In our series, we have reported excellent outcomes of hybrid fixation technique using short cemented femoral stems and tibial metaphyseal sleeves with a rotating platform. We have reported high survivorship of short cemented femoral stems in condylar revisions without significant femoral metaphyseal bone loss in 72 consecutive patients (72 knees) with minimum 5-year follow-up; at mean follow-up of 6.87 years (median 6.7; range 5–11.8), only two patients required revision for infection. Using 'any cause implant revision' as an end point, implant survivorship for this construct was 97.2% at median 6.7 years [22]. Our experience indicates that in rTKA with good femoral condylar bone stock, high survivorship with a short cemented femoral stem in conjunction with a mobile bearing and a tibial sleeve can be achieved. This has the advantage of reducing the length of the revision construct and ensuring durability by keeping the fixation close to the joint line.

However, it is different on the tibial side. Here, the central support for the keel is often lost. The remaining bone is often of poor-quality, the reliance is therefore on cement to support the keel and then in turn on the cement–bone interface for fixation with the remaining concerns in resisting rotational torque. Our preferred technique on the tibia is to use a metaphyseal sleeve. Similar to the femoral side, the sleeve is an integral part of the construct fixing the implant to bone, it fills the metaphyseal segment providing rotational stability, it is not simply a void filler and it gives durable ingrowth biological fixation. Furthermore, it is load-bearing and because of its tapered geometry it generates hoop stresses loading the proximal tibial bone in a radial manner particularly near the joint line creating an ideal environment for durable fixation. When we then couple metaphyseal sleeves with a rotating platform, long-term survivorship has been excellent in multiple series including our own [9, 15, 16, 18, 20].

8.6   Our Indications for Metaphyseal Sleeves

We always use a sleeve on the tibial side in our practice because it gives the best fixation, and simplifies the surgical procedure with a completely stable tibial platform to build the reconstruction. On the femoral side we use them in selected cases with significant metaphyseal bone loss. In most routine revision cases, there is usually enough distal femoral bone for surface epiphyseal fixation of the implant and in those cases, we use a short-cemented femoral construct. If, however, the bone quality near the joint line is poor affecting stability of the component then we use metaphyseal sleeves.

The Anderson Orthopaedic Research Institute (AORI) classification system, developed by *Engh*, is widely used to classify bone loss both pre- and intra-operatively [23]. Smaller defects (AORI-I) can be managed with cement or localised bone grafts. Larger defects with damaged or deficient metaphyseal bone (AORI-II/III) can be managed with metal augmentation (sleeves or cones), structural allografts or impaction grafting and in severe cases with condylar replacing prostheses when the defect is uncontained [24–26]. This can be used as a guide to surgeons.

Top Tip: Constrained implants and/or augmented components require enhanced fixation.

8.7   Practical Advantages of Sleeves

Sleeves simplify the operative procedure; preparation for a sleeve is through a broaching philosophy akin to preparing for a cementless hip stem. The broach matches the final sleeve, we get appropriate level of press-fit on both sides. They provide a robust intramedullary stability even with trial instrumentation offering an absolutely stable tibial platform upon which joint reconstruction can be built in a flexion-first balanced approach as previously outlined. Therefore, the instrumentation adds to the benefits of using sleeves in addition to their role in fixation. On the tibial side, we broach until we get axial and rotational stability and are able to lift the leg off the operating table with the broach handle attached. A refreshing tibial cut is then made off the trial sleeve and a tibial tray can be attached and secured efficiently thus completing the tibial preparation step of the surgery (Figs. 8.1, 8.2, 8.3, 8.4, 8.5 and 8.6).

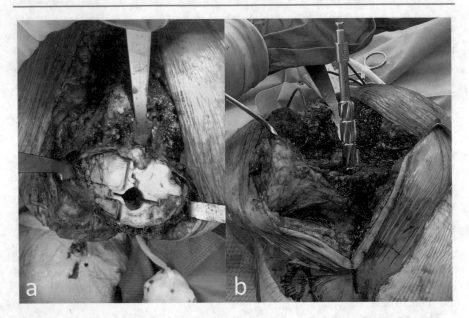

Fig. 8.1 a Following exposure and removal of components, surface cement is removed in the standard fashion; **b** an intramedullary tibial reamer is first used ensuring appropriate alignment

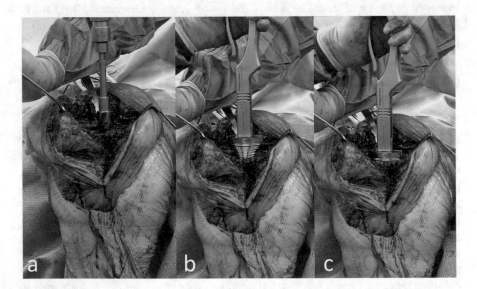

Fig. 8.2 a a cone reamer is used first; **b** sleeve broaches are used sequentially; **c** advanced to be flush on the proximal tibia

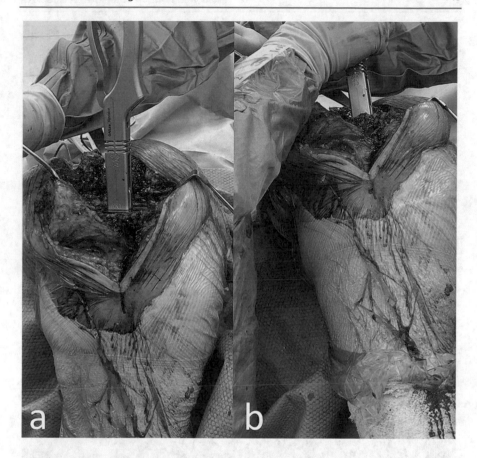

Fig. 8.3 a Rotational stability is ensured with a press-fit broach; **b** lift-off test *(lifting the leg off the operating table through the broach handle)* as a secondary check to ensure axial stability with the broach trial

Bone Contact: the minimum circumferential bone contact is 60–70% [27–29]. On the femoral side we almost always get >90%, considering any anterior bone loss, as the femoral sleeve is above the box of the component. On the tibial side, the more challenging cases are those with a large medial defect, here we ensure that tibial tubercle is still intact and the MCL bony insertion is still intact as a practical guide that we have enough posteromedial contact. Laterally, however, there is always enough contact.

Partial- or Fully-coated Sleeves? In our experience, > 90% of cases are adequately dealt with using partially-coated sleeves. These are the workhorse of sleeves with the benefits of getting fixation closer to the joint line on both sides, allow more bone loading near the joint line, are easier to revise, and have lower risk of intraoperative fracture during final impaction.

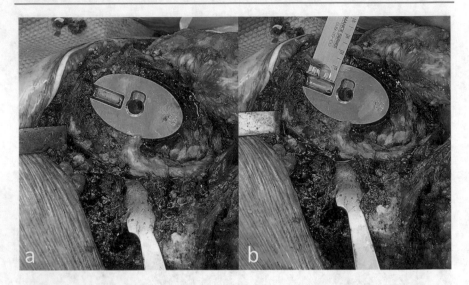

Fig. 8.4 **a** A stable broach trial is left in situ; **b** a refreshing tibial cut is made using the broach trial as a cutting guide

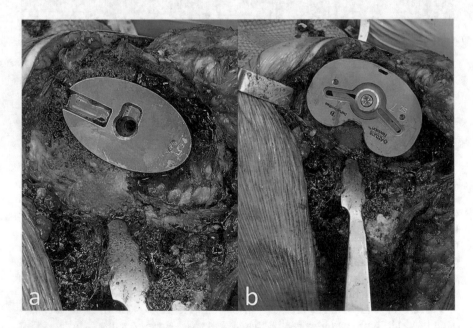

Fig. 8.5 **a** Once the cut is completed; **b** a trial tibial tray is attached to the broach handle bringing the tibial preparation to an end with a stable tibial platform

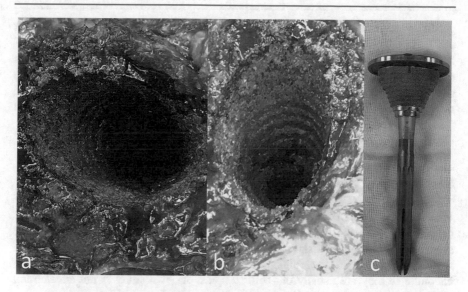

Fig. 8.6 **a–b** Final views of the metaphyseal bed before definitive implants are placed (**c**). Note the impacted stepped circular rings in the cancellous metaphyseal bone which ensure adequate bone contact with the coated sleeve for bone ingrowth

We use fully-coated sleeves, on the femoral side, when we have poor quality bone and we want to get a better press-fit across a bigger surface area. On the tibial side, we use fully coated sleeves for cases with big medial defects to ensure enough contact with the coated surface. Alternatively, in those cases we could downsize and distalise the sleeve and to get better coverage, remaining of course above the tibial tubercle, and then use a build-up tray which has chamfered sides recreating the native proximal tibial geometry. This latter is a preferred option to using a thicker poly insert in those cases.

8.8 Cemented Sleeves

Cemented sleeves have a different philosophy and act more as a void filler with the added advantage of being an integral part of the construct. A cemented sleeve reconstruction is a composite-beam construct and any failure will therefore occur at the cement bone interface. Using a rotating platform helps to dissipate some of the torsional torque on the tibial side while on the femoral side a longer cemented construct is needed to protect the fixation. In our practice, they are useful adjuncts and only used sparingly in selected cases particularly with hinged reconstructions. So, for low demand elderly frail patients undergoing hinged reconstructions, cemented sleeves can be used. Similarly, in selected salvage cases with massive metaphyseal bone loss where a sleeved-reconstruction is used with concerns about getting a cementless press-fit, cemented sleeves can be used reducing the amount of cement needed. Further, with their stepped geometry they provide excellent rotational stability. The other indication is where, in certain ethnic groups, the metaphyseal-diaphyseal junction is quite short and the bones are small even for the smallest of available press-fit sleeves. Here, cemented sleeves could be of help occupying the space without the risk of iatrogenic fracture. Finally, cemented sleeves are cheaper and reduce the overall cost of the reconstruction.

8.9 Complications

When faced with sclerotic bone from removed loose components, which can make broaching hard, we would advocate the use of a burr or a curette to clear the sclerotic bone and avoid risk of iatrogenic fracture during broaching. Intraoperative fractures adjacent to the joint line, while broaching, are rare. However, if encountered they are usually uni-cortical splits. Axial stability is not affected but slight torsional weakness is incurred.

Over the years, we have seen small splits near the joint line on the tibial side which required no adjunctive fixation. However, if the fracture is extending distally beyond the sleeve then adjunctive fixation of the fracture will be needed based on the individual case.

On the femoral side, as broaching progresses to get a press-fit we have rarely seen small splits on the anterior cortex and which seldom required a cerclage wire.

Top Tip: When broaching for a sleeve, regularly clean the broaches' cutting teeth and remove any central sclerotic or neocortical bone to prevent fractures or under-sizing.

8.10 Our Series of Sleeves in rTKA

In our single-surgeon series *(Peter James)*, we reported on the outcomes of metaphyseal sleeves of 319 rTKA over 10-year period (2006–2016) with a minimum 2-year follow up [9]. We used the DePuy Synthes revision TKA system which consists of different levels of constraint. The PFC Sigma Posterior Stabilized is the least constrained, but allows the attachment of stems and sleeves if required. Next is the TC3-RP which is a varus-valgus constrained device with a more constrained cam and post mechanism and a highly conforming mobile bearing. Finally, the S-ROM Noiles rotating hinge is used when there is ligamentous deficiency or a gross flexion–extension mismatch, and the Limb Preservation System (LPS) distal femoral replacement is reserved for large bony defects or periprosthetic fractures. All these femoral options are compatible with the mobile bearing tibia (MBT) rotating platform revision tibial component and the metaphyseal sleeve system. All 319 revisions had a tibial metaphyseal sleeve to address the central bone loss

(i)

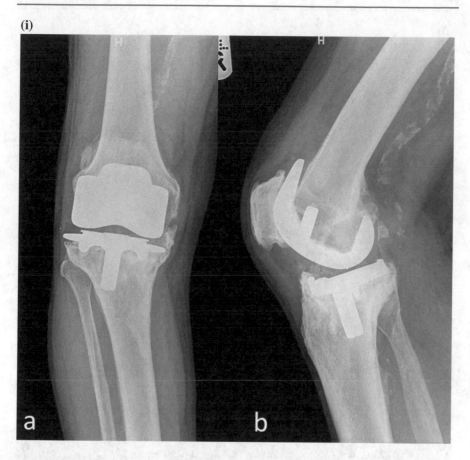

Fig. 8.7 **i** Anteroposterior and lateral weight-bearing radiographs of a 74-year-old woman with a failed cemented TKA and a collapsed tibial component with medial bone loss. **ii** Follow up radiographs at 8 years following reconstructing with a metaphyseal tibial sleeve and short cemented stemmed femoral component in a semi-constrained construct with a rotating platform. The femoral component and cemented stems are well-fixed with no evidence of loosening

associated with removal of the tibial component and 146 had femoral sleeves. Where there was significant bone loss on the femur, a femoral metaphyseal sleeve was used; but if the joint line could be adequately reconstructed with augments and there was sufficient condylar bone to support this, then either cementless or cemented stems without a sleeve were used.

(ii)

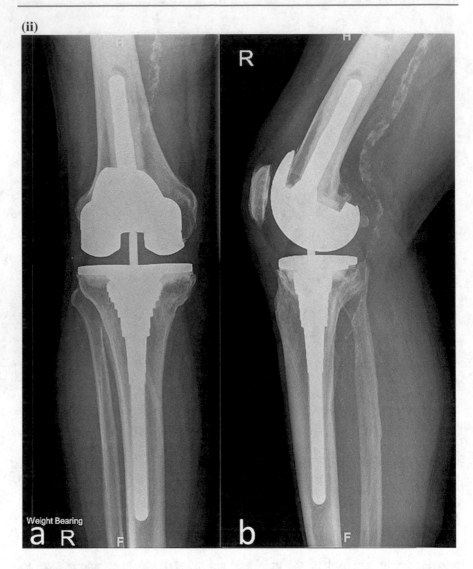

Fig. 8.7 (continued)

Five knees (1.57%) required re-revision surgery, at a mean of 35 months (median 18 months). Four of these were for infection; of which 3 required removal of the implants while the fourth was successfully treated with debridement, antibiotics, and implant retention (a DAIR procedure); 1 was revised for instability. No sleeve

(i)

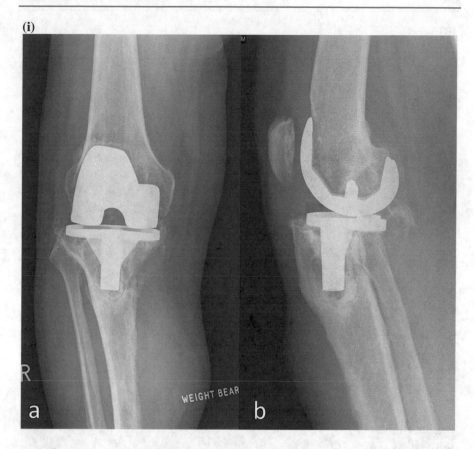

Fig. 8.8 **i** Anteroposterior and lateral weight-bearing radiographs of a 75-year-old man with a failed right TKA and catastrophic polyethylene failure and significant tibial lysis. Infection was ruled out. **ii** Anteroposterior and lateral radiographs at 4 years follow up following revision surgery with a hinged implant and metaphyseal sleeves fixation on both sides. **iii** Sequential radiographs at 2, 4 and 6 years of the femoral component with well-ingrown metaphyseal sleeve. **iv** Radiographs of the tibial reconstruction at 6 years follow up with well-ingrown tibial sleeve and tibial medial bone remodelling as it has been loaded through the ingrown sleeve

was revised for aseptic loosening. Twelve tibial sleeves (3.7%) showed radiographic subsidence >1 mm in subsequent radiographic follow up compared to immediate postoperative radiographs. All reached a position of stability without progressing further on subsequent radiographs and none required revision. Using re-revision as an endpoint, our implant survivorship was 99.1% at 3 years, 98.7% at 5 years and 97.8% at 10 years.

(ii)

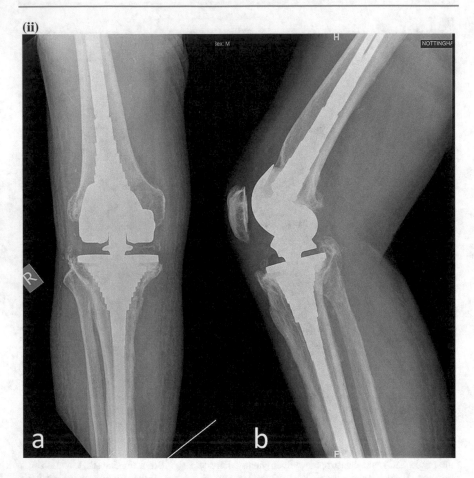

Fig. 8.8 (continued)

8.11 Overview of Metaphyseal Sleeves in the Literature

There is a growing body of evidence in the literature in support of using metaphyseal sleeves in rTKA. A number of recent systematic reviews have summarised
the available evidence and reached similar conclusions albeit with the inevitable
overlap of the studies included and the inherent limitations of level-IV evidence.
Zanirato et al. [30] reviewed 1,079 rTKA (13 studies) using 1,554 sleeves with
mean follow up of 4 years. They reported implant and sleeves aseptic survival rate
of 97.7 and 99.2%.

(iii)

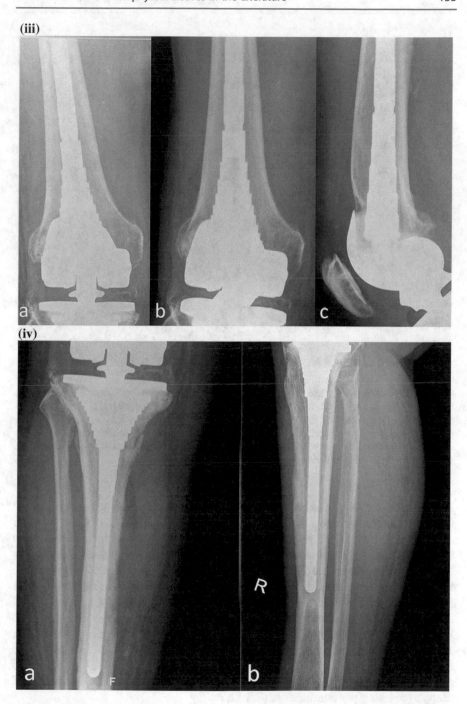

(iv)

Fig. 8.8 (continued)

(i)

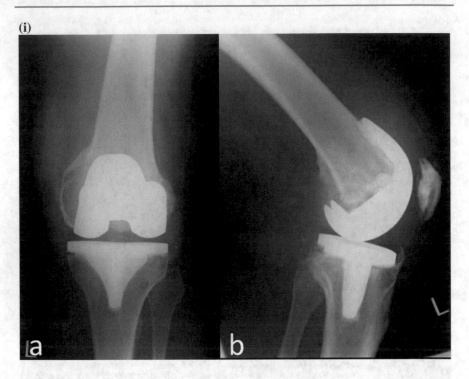

Fig. 8.9 **i** Anteroposterior and lateral weight-bearing radiographs of a 76-year-old man with a loose left TKA and a large osteolytic lesion in the medial femoral condyle. **ii** Coronal images demonstrating the extent of the lesion. **iii** Anteroposterior and lateral radiographs following reconstruction using a sleeved construct; on the femoral side the fixation achieved in the metaphysis bypassing the lesion with anterior/lateral/ posterior and proximal bone contact with the sleeve; the void is filled with cement

Bonanzinga et al. [18] reported on 928 revisions (10 studies) with mean follow up of 45 months with 888 tibial sleeves and 525 femoral sleeves. There were 36 septic re-revisions of the prosthetic components (4%), of which 5 sleeves were found loose during septic re-revision; rate of septic loosening of the sleeves was 0.35%. Further, there were 27 aspetic re-revisions (3%), of which 10 sleeves were found loose during aseptic re-revision; rate of aseptic loosening of the sleeves was 0.7%. They also reported overall intraoperative fracture rate (3.1%).

Roach et al. [11] reported on 27 studies of metaphyseal sleeves and cones (12 sleeves and 15 cones). In total, there were 1,617 sleeves implanted in 1,133 rTKA. The overall rate of reoperation was 110/1,133 (9.7%) and the total rate of aseptic loosening per sleeve was 13/1,617 (0.8%). They also reported on 701 cones in 620 rTKA with overall reoperation rate of 116/620 (18.7%), and the overall rate of aseptic loosening per cone was 12/701 (1.7%).

(ii)

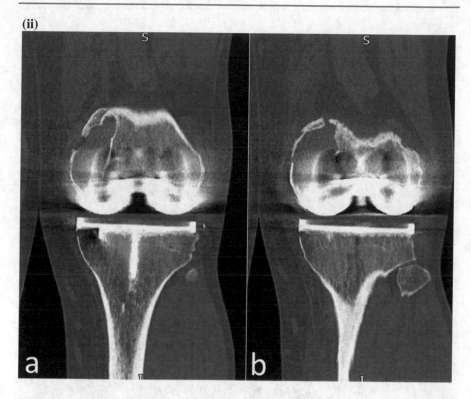

Fig. 8.9 (continued)

The studies included in these systematic reviews were of varying sizes and duration of follow ups. Our series [9] was not included in either of these reviews. Chalmers et al. [15] reported on their tertiary experience in the Mayo Clinic of 280 patients using 393 metaphyseal sleeves (144 femoral, 249 tibial) between 2006–2014 with mean follow up of 3 years. Their sleeves were commonly cemented (55% femoral, 72% tibial). Using re-revision as an end point, they reported 5-year survivorship for aseptic loosening at 96% and 99.5% for femoral and tibial sleeves respectively.

Despite the heterogeneity of the above studies in their indication for revisions, surgical techniques used and duration of follow up, there is clearly an emerging pattern with the success of metaphyseal sleeves in achieving osteointegration and excellent survivorship.

(iii)

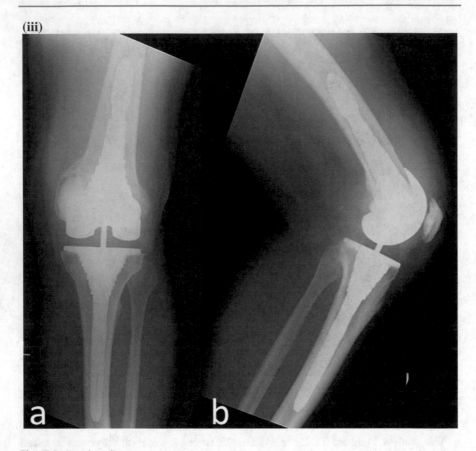

Fig. 8.9 (continued)

In conclusion, implant fixation is one of the main pillars of a durable revision knee construct. Adjunctive metaphyseal fixation is needed in cases of bone loss and compromised epiphysis where surface cementation is not enough to support the implants. Our preferred approach is to use metaphyseal sleeves to not only achieve durable fixation but also to help in joint reconstruction by the routine use of tibial sleeves to reliably establish a stable tibial platform with the *frame principle*. Short cemented-stem femoral construct, in a hybrid fixation technique, is preferred in cases of minimal metaphyseal femoral bone loss with femoral sleeves used when significant bone loss is encountered.

(i)

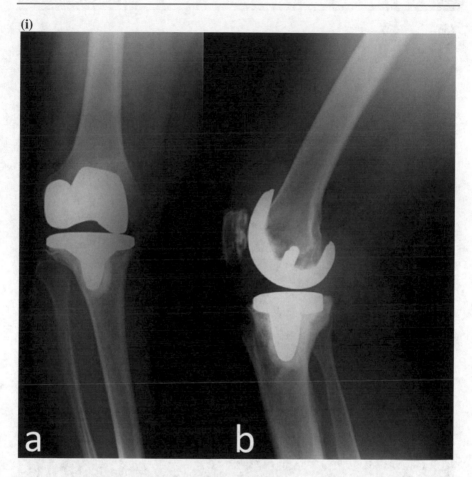

a   b

Fig. 8.10 **i** Anteroposterior and lateral weight-bearing radiographs of a 64 years old woman with a failed TKA; the patient is of short stature and small bones. **ii** Postoperative radiographs following reconstruction with a sleeve-augment combination on the tibial side; this feature is only possible with the smallest (29 mm) sleeve. **iii** Anteroposterior and lateral radiographs of the left side in the same patient with failed left TKA. **iv** Postoperative radiographs for a similar construct but without the tibial augment; cement filled in the space with the main fixation achieved through the sleeve in the metaphysis

(ii)

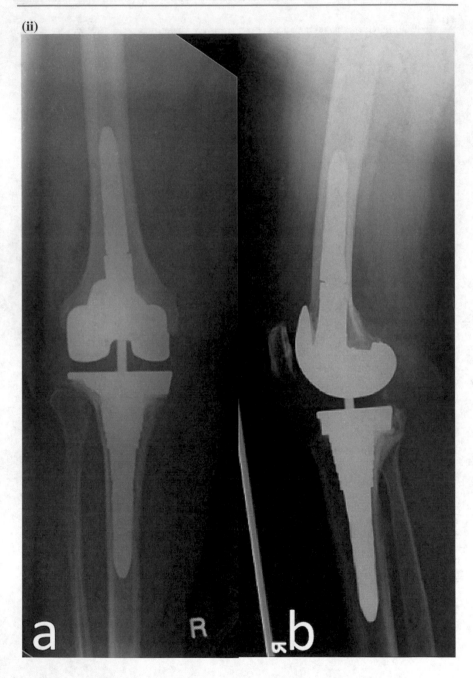

Fig. 8.10   (continued)

(iii)

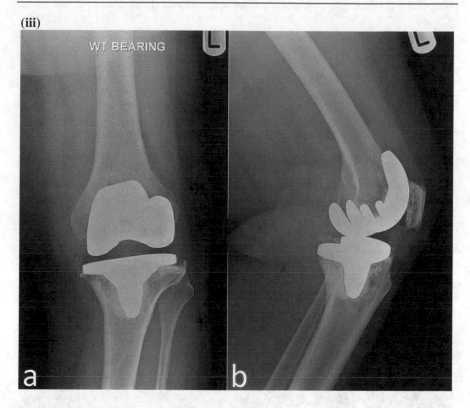

Fig. 8.10   (continued)

(iv)

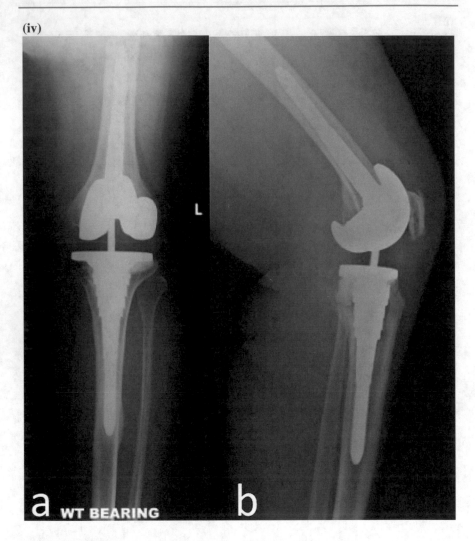

Fig. 8.10 (continued)

References

1. Ghomrawi HM, et al. Patterns of functional improvement after revision knee arthroplasty. J Bone Joint Surg Am. 2009;91(12):2838–45.
2. Fehring TK, et al. Stem fixation in revision total knee arthroplasty: a comparative analysis. Clin Orthop Relat Res. 2003;416:217–24.
3. Edwards PK, et al. Are cementless stems more durable than cemented stems in two-stage revisions of infected total knee arthroplasties? Clin Orthop Relat Res. 2014;472(1):206–11.
4. Elia EA, Lotke PA. Results of revision total knee arthroplasty associated with significant bone loss. Clin Orthop Relat Res. 1991;271:114–21.
5. Whaley AL, et al. Cemented long-stem revision total knee arthroplasty. J Arthroplasty. 2003;18(5):592–9.
6. Mabry TM, et al. Revision total knee arthroplasty with modular cemented stems: long-term follow-up. J Arthroplasty. 2007;22(6 Suppl 2):100–5.
7. Kang SG, Park CH, Song SJ. Stem Fixation in Revision Total Knee Arthroplasty: Indications, Stem Dimensions, and Fixation Methods. Knee Surg Relat Res. 2018;30(3):187–92.
8. Heesterbeek PJ, Wymenga AB, van Hellemondt GG. No Difference in Implant Micromotion Between Hybrid Fixation and Fully Cemented Revision Total Knee Arthroplasty: A Randomized Controlled Trial with Radiostereometric Analysis of Patients with Mild-to-Moderate Bone Loss. J Bone Joint Surg Am. 2016;98(16):1359–69.
9. Bloch BV, et al. Metaphyseal Sleeves in Revision Total Knee Arthroplasty Provide Reliable Fixation and Excellent Medium to Long-Term Implant Survivorship. J Arthroplasty. 2020;35 (2):495–9.
10. Matar HE, Bloch BV, James PJ. Role of metaphyseal sleeves in revision total knee arthroplasty: Rationale, indications and long-term outcomes. J Orthop. 2021;23:107–12.
11. Roach RP, et al. Aseptic loosening of porous metaphyseal sleeves and tantalum cones in revision total knee arthroplasty: a systematic review. J Knee Surg, 2020.
12. Barrack RL, et al. The use of a modular rotating hinge component in salvage revision total knee arthroplasty. J Arthroplasty. 2000;15(7):858–66.
13. Jones RE, et al. Total knee arthroplasty using the S-ROM mobile-bearing hinge prosthesis. J Arthroplasty. 2001;16(3):279–87.
14. Jones RE, Barrack RL, Skedros J. Modular, mobile-bearing hinge total knee arthroplasty. Clin Orthop Relat Res. 2001;392:306–14.
15. Chalmers BP, et al. Survivorship of Metaphyseal Sleeves in Revision Total Knee Arthroplasty. J Arthroplasty. 2017;32(5):1565–70.
16. Watters TS, et al. Porous-Coated Metaphyseal Sleeves for Severe Femoral and Tibial Bone Loss in Revision TKA. J Arthroplasty. 2017;32(11):3468–73.
17. Huang R, et al. Revision total knee arthroplasty using metaphyseal sleeves at short-term follow-up. Orthopedics. 2014;37(9):e804–9.
18. Bonanzinga T, et al. Are metaphyseal sleeves a viable option to treat bone defect during revision total knee arthroplasty? Syst Rev Joints. 2019;7(1):19–24.
19. Haidukewych GJ, Hanssen A, Jones RD. Metaphyseal fixation in revision total knee arthroplasty: indications and techniques. J Am Acad Orthop Surg. 2011;19(6):311–8.
20. Nadorf J, et al. Tibial revision knee arthroplasty with metaphyseal sleeves: The effect of stems on implant fixation and bone flexibility. PLoS One. 2017;12(5):e0177285.
21. Bobyn JD, et al. Characteristics of bone ingrowth and interface mechanics of a new porous tantalum biomaterial. J Bone Joint Surg Br. 1999;81(5):907–14.
22. Matar HE, Bloch BV, James PJ. High survivorship of short cemented femoral stems in condylar revision total knee arthroplasty without significant metaphyseal bone loss: minimum 5-year follow-up. J Arthroplasty. 2021;Online- ahead of print.
23. Engh GA, Ammeen DJ. Bone loss with revision total knee arthroplasty: defect classification and alternatives for reconstruction. Instr Course Lect. 1999;48:167–75.

24. Huff TW, Sculco TP. Management of bone loss in revision total knee arthroplasty. J Arthroplasty. 2007;22(7 Suppl 3):32–6.

25. Bush JL, Wilson JB, Vail TP. Management of bone loss in revision total knee arthroplasty. Clin Orthop Relat Res. 2006;452:186–92.

26. Backstein D, Safir O, Gross A. Management of bone loss: structural grafts in revision total knee arthroplasty. Clin Orthop Relat Res. 2006;446:104–12.

27. Awadalla M, et al. Influence of varying stem and metaphyseal sleeve size on the primary stability of cementless revision tibial trays used to reconstruct AORI IIA defects: a simulation study J Orthop Res. 2018;36(7):1876–86.

28. Awadalla M, et al. Influence of stems and metaphyseal sleeve on primary stability of cementless revision tibial trays used to reconstruct AORI IIB defects. J Orthop Res. 2019;37 (5):1033–41.

29. Fonseca F, Sousa A, Completo A. Femoral revision knee Arthroplasty with Metaphyseal sleeves: the use of a stem is not mandatory of a structural point of view. J Exp Orthop. 2020;7 (1):24.

30. Zanirato A, et al. Metaphyseal sleeves in total knee arthroplasty revision: complications, clinical and radiological results: a systematic review of the literature. Arch Orthop Trauma Surg. 2018;138(7):993–1001.

Kinematics of Constrained Condylar Revision Implants: A Practical Perspective

There is no greater evil for men than the constraint of fortune.

Sophocles

9.1 Introduction

Instability is a common cause of revision surgery following aseptic loosening and infection. True mechanical instability may result from loosening, bone loss, prosthetic breakage, component size or position, fracture, wear, or collateral ligament failure with only the latter typically requiring a fully-constrained implant [1]. Further, some implant designs and surgical techniques used in soft tissue balancing may potentially predispose to development of mid-flexion instability where the ligaments appear balanced at 0° and 90° of flexion but become lax in the mid-range with subsequent instability symptoms particularly when patients climb stairs or rise from a seated position [2]. Constrained implants are then used without necessarily addressing the underlying cause of instability leading to suboptimal clinical outcomes [3]. In this chapter we will focus on the practical implications of constraint in rTKA in the context of instability, particularly the kinematics of condylar revision implants.

H. E. Matar et al., *Revision Total Knee Arthroplasty*,
https://doi.org/10.1007/978-3-030-81285-0_9

9.2   What is Constraint?

Constraint is defined as the effect of the elements of knee implant design that provide the stability needed in the presence of a deficient soft-tissue envelope [4]. It is well-established that knee implants can be categorised based on the intrinsic degree of constraint from the least to the most constraint:

(a) PCL-retaining or cruciate-retaining (CR)
(b) PCL-substituting/cruciate-substituting (CS) or posterior-stabilised (PS)
(c) Unlinked constrained/semi-constrained or varus-valgus constrained (VVC)
(d) Rotating-hinge implants
(e) Fixed-hinge implants

It is also well-established from the early work of *Hugh Cameron* in 1980s [5] and others [6] that as the amount of constraint is increased, the stress transmitted to the implant-bone interface is also increased which leads to eventual implant loosening and failure. Therefore, it is always recommended to use the least amount of constraint necessary for a satisfactory outcome.

9.3   Constraint and Kinematics

In revision cases, the aim is to deliver near-normal knee kinematics in the presence of a compromised bone stock and a compromised soft tissue envelope as a result of either the original failure or repeated operations. Therefore, we require a revision system that allows an element of bone restoration with different fixation options on both femoral and tibial sides. Bone stock at the surface/epiphyseal area is often compromised to a varying degree, and metaphyseal or even segmental bone loss is also encountered. Thus, a degree of modularity is also essential to any revision system in order to augment and achieve enhanced fixation.

On the femoral side, this means the ability to attach a stem which in turn connects to the femoral component; it is very difficult to attach the stem anywhere else but centrally. So, we need a robust connection between the intramedullary part of the construct and the femoral component. Most revision systems do so by taking a fixed boss with an adaptor bolt or similar mechanisms at the back of a stabilised implant. There are no cruciate-retaining revision femoral components that we can attach stems to reliably. Therefore, we are immediately into the territory of a boxed femoral component to be able to attach stems. So, kinematically we are driven to at least a PS articulation.

From a kinematic point of view, the articulating geometry of a revision femoral component should be the same as that of a PS primary TKA in that portfolio. The kinematic pattern in terms of articulation design on the femoral side should be compatible with PS articulation on the tibial side. The next level of constraint then is a VVC insert, which again in terms of its condylar pattern should match the PS insert. The only difference between a PS insert and a VVC insert is the height and the size of the post. The box therefore would be deeper to accommodate that height but should also be able to deliver the same kinematics with a PS insert. In other words, the VVC femur should be compatible with both a VVC and a PS insert. Condylar kinematics with a cam-post engagement and post-contact kinematics should be the same between PS and VVC constraint. It is worth noting here that a deficient or incompetent MCL is an absolute contraindication for a VVC articulation [7].

In most contemporary revision systems, the initial kinematic pattern of the knee is delivered by the condylar geometry and its interaction with the tibial insert. The articular geometry is the initial driver of stability and it also drives the rollback to give clearance and to then slowly engage and control the transition point between condylar control and cam-post control. In deeper flexion, the kinematics is controlled by the cam-post mechanism, rather than by condylar control. It is important to avoid any conflict between condylar control and cam-post control once the latter is engaged. With this principle in mind, when designing a revision knee implant this kinematic pattern should be predictable and reproducible.

Top Tip: A desired feature of a revision knee implant is that condylar control should transition to cam-post control with no conflict.

9.4   In First Principles, Why Have a Cam-Post Mechanism and Why in Revision Surgery?

The problem we have in revision surgery is in getting well-balanced flexion/extension gaps in addition to the required fixation parameters. Even in a PS articulation, we get better control of flexion as it gives a physical barrier to paradoxical anterior slide. The cam-post gives control of rollback, so we are not dependent on condylar control as much. Here, we can cope with small fluctuations at the joint line but maintain better flexion stability with this approach.

9.5   What About Fixed-Bearings in Revision Surgery?

First principles in a fixed-bearing rTKA is to minimise the amount of rotational constraint. The downside of a VVC implant is that with better varus-valgus stability comes a degree of rotational constraint as well. Therefore, it is recommended to use the least amount of constraint that you can in a fixed-bearing rTKA, so beware of relying on a VVC articulation to compensate for a lack of stability that should be first addressed surgically in terms of joint line positioning and soft tissue balancing. A VVC articulation would sort the problem out short-term but in the longer-term you will see early loosening and failure.

Ideally, what we need is a physiological varus-valgus constraint to support the ligamentous structures but without rotational constraint as the knee rotates in the physiological flexion–extension arc. This often leads to eccentric post wear and edge-loading in addition to the issues of eventual loosening.

Top Tip: In fixed-bearing VVC articulation, it is important to consider the implications on rotational constraint and on the fixation interfaces.

9.6   What About Mobile-Bearing VVC Articulation?

One solution to the dilemma of having rotational constraint with a fixed-bearing VVC is a rotating platform insert. Early fixed hinges had significant failure rates and loosening which had been substantially improved by the introduction of rotating hinge designs. Kinematically, a mobile-bearing or rotating platform VVC insert offers the advantages of coronal constraint without the downside of rotational constraint and its potential impact on aseptic loosening and failure. National joint registries have reported 80–85% survivorship of fixed-bearing VVC condylar revisions. While aseptic failure is a multifactorial process with complex interactions between implant characteristics, fixation methods, surgical technique, and patients' factors, there is emerging evidence indicating improved longevity with a mobile-bearing philosophy. Certainly, our experience with condylar revisions and mobile-bearing VVCs indicate that excellent long-term survivorship can be expected with increased protection of fixation interfaces; >95% at 10 years [8]. The Mayo clinic and others have also reported similar results [9, 10].

9.7   Impact of Constraint on Patellofemoral Joint (PFJ)

The downside of having a deeper box on the femoral component is its impact on patellofemoral mechanics with less protection of the PFJ. The angle of the box is governed by the exit point of the stem which has to be attached to the box at a given angle to achieve a central position in the canal. This depth means that the box in revision implants is involved earlier in the PFJ during flexion range compared to a primary PS component, where the box can be angled and is shallower with the ability to keep the trochlear groove intact deeper into flexion.

Optimising PFJ mechanics, restoring the joint line, and managing the soft tissues around the patella (clearing and excising scar tissue which could impinge on the box) are all important surgical steps that would help to improve patients' outcomes. We believe that revisions should have a resurfaced patella. The aim from resurfacing here is to really optimise the position of the patella button in relation to the joint line.

(i)

(ii)

(iii)

(iv)

(v)

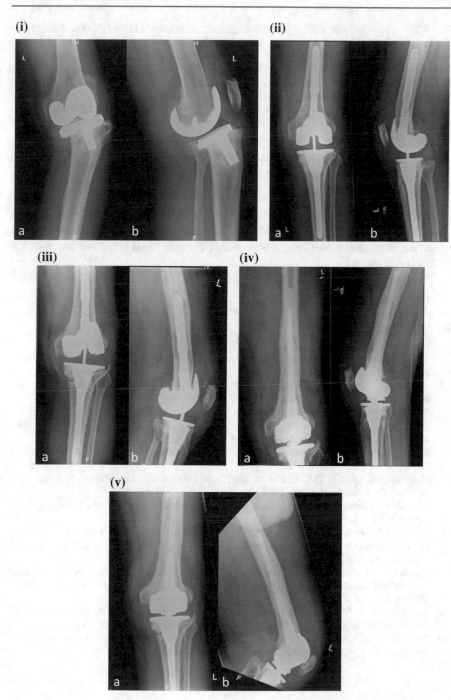

◄ **Fig. 9.1** **i** Anteroposterior and lateral radiographs of a catastrophic failure 7 years post primary CR knee. **ii** Anteroposterior and lateral radiographs post revision surgery with a VVC implant using a tibial sleeve and an offset press-fit femoral stem. Intraoperatively, the MCL was intact. **iii** Anteroposterior and lateral radiographs 12 months post revision surgery following a fall with a ruptured MCL and rotated VVC insert. **iv** Anteroposterior and lateral radiographs following re-revision; the tibial sleeve was well-ingrown, single component femoral revision was performed using a cemented S-ROM femur with a bridging bearing. **v** Anteroposterior and lateral radiographs following re-revision at 3 months

> **Top Tip: With revision implants, the PFJ is interacting with the box much earlier. Understanding this point helps to further highlight the importance of restoring the joint line to as near native as possible for better PFJ mechanics.**

In conclusion, the use of constraint in revision knee surgery is necessary in most cases. Understanding the implications of constraint on fixation interfaces and the construct durability is essential in the decision making and choice of implants for individual cases.

This case demonstrates the limitation of a VVC implant (Fig. 9.1):

References

1. Vince KG, Abdeen A, Sugimori T. The unstable total knee arthroplasty: causes and cures. J Arthroplasty. 2006;21(4):44–9.
2. Athwal KK, et al. Clinical biomechanics of instability related to total knee arthroplasty. Clin Biomech (Bristol, Avon). 2014;29(2):119–28.
3. Wilson CJ, et al. Knee instability as the primary cause of failure following Total Knee Arthroplasty (TKA): A systematic review on the patient, surgical and implant characteristics of revised TKA patients. Knee. 2017;24(6):1271–81.
4. Morgan H, Battista V, Leopold SS. Constraint in primary total knee arthroplasty. J Am Acad Orthop Surg. 2005;13(8):515–24.
5. Cameron HU, Hunter GA. Failure in total knee arthroplasty: mechanisms, revisions, and results. Clin Orthop Relat Res. 1982;170:141–6.
6. McAuley JP, Engh GA. Constraint in total knee arthroplasty: when and what? J Arthroplasty. 2003;18(3):51–4.
7. Athwal KK, et al. An in vitro analysis of medial structures and a medial soft tissue reconstruction in a constrained condylar total knee arthroplasty. Knee Surg Sports Traumatol Arthrosc. 2017;25(8):2646–55.
8. Bloch BV, et al. Metaphyseal Sleeves in revision total knee arthroplasty provide reliable fixation and excellent medium to long-term implant survivorship. J Arthroplasty. 2020;35(2):495–9.
9. Reina N, et al. Varus-Valgus Constrained Implants With a Mobile-Bearing Articulation: Results of 367 Revision Total Knee Arthroplasties. J Arthroplasty. 2020;35(4):1060–3.
10. Gurel R et al. Good clinical and radiological outcomes of the varus-valgus constrained mobile-bearing implant in revision total knee arthroplasty. Int Orthop, 2021.

Rotating-Hinge Implants

10

A moving door hinge never corrodes, flowing water never grows stagnant.

Ming-Dao Deng

10.1 Introduction

In rTKA practice, the indications to use a rotating-hinge implant include ligament attenuation or deficiency particularly of the medial collateral ligament, bone loss that compromises ligament attachments, gross flexion–extension mismatch, recurvatum and gross multidirectional instability [1]. Early hinged designs were highly constrained, only allowing for flexion–extension, and had high failure and complication rates [2–4]. Second generation designs saw the introduction of varus-valgus motion and axial rotation reducing the level of prosthetic constraint and subsequently the torque stresses on the implant-cement and implant-bone interfaces [5–7]. The contemporary, third generation, implants saw the introduction of an improved rotating-hinge mechanism, improved patellofemoral biomechanics with a deepened femoral anterior flange to enhance patella tracking, increased component modularity and improved fixation techniques, all leading to significant improvements in survivorship and clinical outcomes [8–11]. In a systematic review of rotating-hinge implants in rTKA, survivorship ranged from 51 to 92.5% with complication rates ranging from 9.2 to 63%. Infection and aseptic loosening were the most common complications, although the majority of included studies were or short- to medium-term outcomes [12]. In this chapter, we will focus on the practical aspects of hinge implants and their kinematics to avoid common hinge-related complications.

© The Author(s), under exclusive license to Springer Nature Switzerland AG 2021   169
H. E. Matar et al., *Revision Total Knee Arthroplasty*,
https://doi.org/10.1007/978-3-030-81285-0_10

10.2 When to Use Hinges?

The common indications in our practice are soft tissue failure; posterior capsule, MCL and significant complex bone loss. They are also part of segmental bone replacing prostheses, either as a distal femoral replacement (DFR) or using massive augments to fill in major bone defects. They also play a role in complex primary situations with significant deformities, particularly in elderly patients (Fig. 10.1).

10.3 What About Fixed-Hinges?

True fixed hinges are incredibly constrained, and are therefore used very sparingly in our practice, for example a gross ligamentous laxity such as *Ehlers-Danlos* syndrome with a failed rotating-hinge (Fig. 10.2). The downside is expected loosening within 10 years or so. The other indication is for cases with extensor mechanism failure undergoing allograft reconstruction. Rotating-hinges in this

(i)

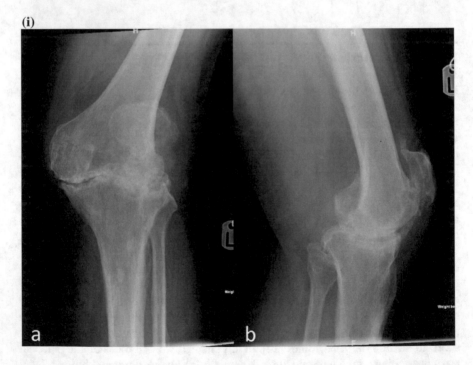

a   b

Fig. 10.1 i Anteroposterior and lateral radiographs of left knee in an elderly patient with significant fixed valgus deformity and end stage OA. **ii** Anteroposterior and lateral postoperative radiographs following a complex primary TKA using a rotating hinge implant (S-ROM) with press-fit metaphyseal sleeves

(ii)

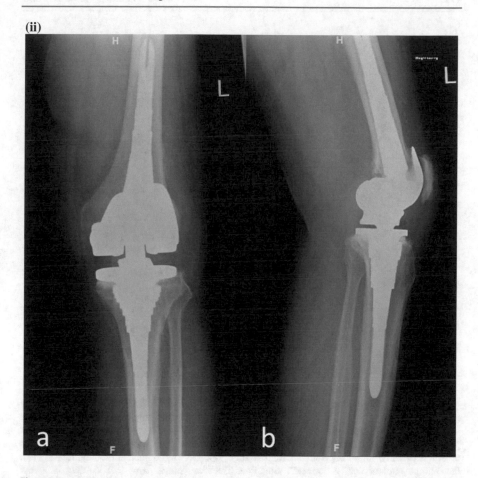

Fig. 10.1 (continued)

scenario are at risk of dissociation should the allograft fail. Similarly, we used fixed
hinge reconstructions in cases of DFRs with extensor mechanism failure and lack of
capsular support. The other indication is in cases of chronically dislocated patellae
where femoral rotation needs to be fixed in a more favourable position in addition
to soft tissue reconstruction procedures to centralise the patella (see Chap. 14).

10.4   Where Should the Hinge Mechanism Be?

Posterior: older designs have the hinge mechanism posterior, theoretically mim-
icking femoral rollback in flexion, but this opens like a clamshell creating pressure
on the extensor mechanism in flexion. From experience, if we leave the extension
gap too tight (a 'tight hinge'), particularly in older patients with compromised soft

(i)

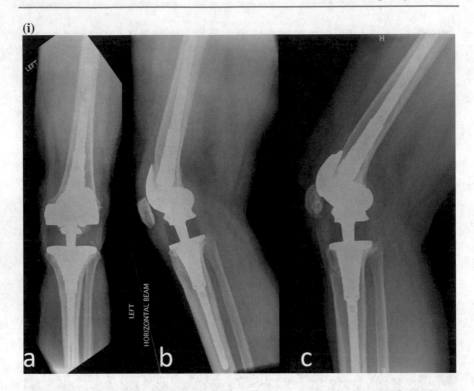

Fig. 10.2 **i** Anteroposterior and lateral radiographs of an unstable left knee in 53 years old tertiary referral patient with Ehlers-Danlos Syndrome and multiple previous surgeries. She had undergone a revision of her hinge with poly exchange due to instability. Now referred with a complex presentation of pain and instability. Radiographically, she had joint line elevation and iatrogenic patella baja with a subluxing patella in flexion. **ii** Postoperative radiographs following revision to a fixed-hinge implant with a corrected joint line. The fixed hinge helps PFJ stability in a rare indication of a fixed-hinge. Further, in this rare syndrome the soft tissues where stretching out leading to hyperextension instability which is addressed by having a fixed-hinge

tissue envelope or valgus deformities, this leads to significant load on the extensor mechanism. With a posterior axis of rotation, as the patient goes into flexion around the posterior axis, the lever arm or distance from the centre of rotation to the extensor mechanism gets bigger. This puts increased load on the extensor mechanism and we see a number of predictable complications. Either you will get escape of the extensor mechanism with a dislocated patella, or extensor mechanism failure manifesting in either quadriceps rupture, patella fracture or patella tendon rupture; all of which are debilitating complications.

Top Tip: When using a posterior hinge design, de-tension the extension gap (a 'slack gap') and ensure the extensor mechanism is tracking centrally.

(ii)

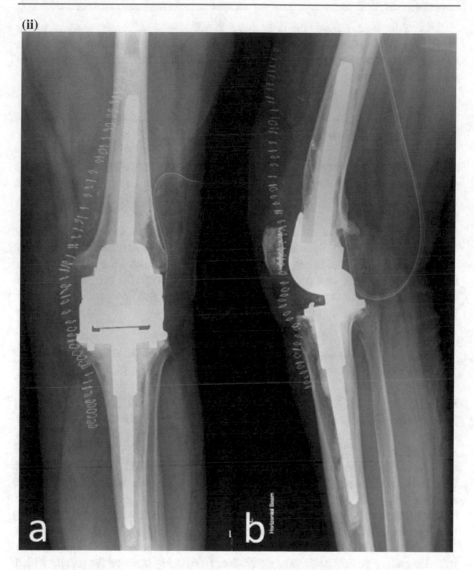

Fig. 10.2 (continued)

Central: the other design is a central hinge mechanism, with the axis of rotation closer to the anterior flange. This design is more PFJ friendly although it decreases the quads lever arm with potential weakness of the extensor mechanism. Further, it decreases range of motion with early impingement.

Surgeons have their preference in what type of hinge or philosophy they believe in or whether it is based on the portfolio of the system that they use. We are not aware of high-quality evidence to demonstrate that one design philosophy in terms of hinge position is better than the other; it is always a trade-off.

Top Tip: understand the practical implications of your chosen hinge implant and minimise the impact on outcomes; potential extensor mechanism failure with posterior hinges or quads weakness and reduced range of motion with central hinges.

10.5 Patellofemoral Issues with Hinges

This is a complex area with a lot of factors at play; tibiofemoral rotation, quads tension, position of the hinge mechanism with the resulting stress on the soft tissue envelope anteriorly, trochlea groove design, whether it is part of megaprostheses (DFR) among others.

As surgeons, we need to ensure we restore the joint line, with the appropriate soft tissue tension in extension, and understand the design used and its features in terms of the rotating mechanism. Here, different designs also have variations with the rotation occurring on top of the tibial tray or underneath the tray, how much of the hinge mechanism is delivered through the bushings and how much is condylar bearing i.e. understanding the hinge kinematics.

10.6 Practical Perspective on Hinge Kinematics

In older hinges, all of the load goes through an axle and bushings, these are posterior hinges, they have some rotational mechanism within the hinge but all of the load is delivered from a femoral component to a tibial component through a small surface area; like a *Stanmore Smiles Hinge* (Fig. 10.3). In this design, there is some rotational control built in the under-surface of the tibial component, so as it rotates it rides up slightly. It is not a constrained rotation but rather a resisted rotation. So, with that in mind, by meticulously setting tibiofemoral rotation intraoperatively, we can optimise positioning the extensor mechanism more centrally particularly in resting extension. The proposed benefit of that is if the patella starts in the correct position, as we go into flexion, the patella will engage in the trochlea groove getting a secondary stabiliser from the implant on the patella which helps in maintaining patella stability.

Top Tip: Ensure that the patella is central in resting extension to minimise risk of instability once the knee goes into flexion.

In contrast, hinges such as the *S-ROM Noiles hinge* (Fig. 10.4), have evolved over the years but remain theoretically *load-sharing* with an axle and bushings mechanism which shares load with the condylar geometry. Logically, however, it cannot be both, but as the bushings wear, which is inevitable being a low contact area with high stresses, perhaps then we may get more condylar contact and a degree of load sharing. Condylar contact is desirable as it gives more stability which

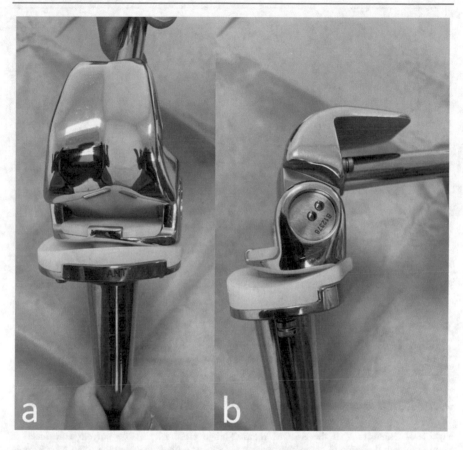

Fig. 10.3 a-b Photograph of the SMILES rotating-hinge prosthesis; the polyethylene insert is beveled against the tibial plate and limits rotational motion to ±5°

is derived from the geometry of the femoral and tibial components in extension, though this lessens as we get into flexion with a preponderance of load now passing through the axle and the bushings. The advantage of this locking mechanism is, theoretically at least, better alignment of the knee in extension with the caveat of having a totally unconstrained rotating bearing.

In the S-ROM design, for example, the insert is simply a polyethylene insert with a peg on a flat metal surface with no inherent resistance to rotation; delivering complete rotational freedom which is advantageous in protecting the fixation interface. But there are potential negative impacts on tibiofemoral and especially patellofemoral kinematics which are more pronounced with increased bone resection/loss such as a DFR construct. Here, for example, we lose the soft tissue envelope/capsule that connects the femur to the tibia thus losing the soft tissue restraint or stabilisers connecting the native femur and tibia which would resist excessive rotation.

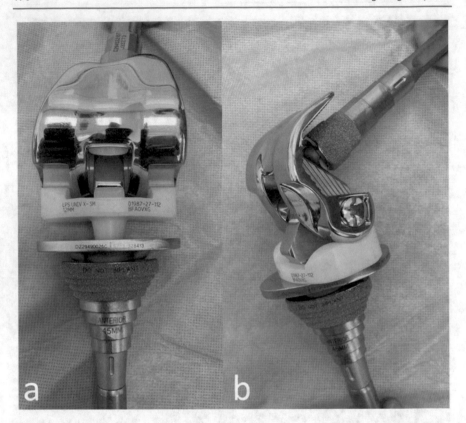

Fig. 10.4 Photograph of the S-ROM rotating-hinge prosthesis; **a**) the polyethylene insert is congruent with the femoral component with a flat-on-flat articulation with the tibial tray; **b**) note that there is no inherent resistance to rotation at the insert-tibial tray interface

Therefore, we have to be very careful in these unconstrained rotating platform hinge designs in terms of its implications on PFJ mechanism. If the patella starts to track slightly more laterally, the tibial tubercle will externally rotate because the extensor mechanism is pulling it and there is no rotational constraint. Here, the patella will drift more laterally and in rotating hinge knees once the patella starts to escape there is no coming back as the external rotation accelerates. This is less of an issue in a standard hinge case with enough capsular attachment, as there is enough soft issue constraint, unlike in a DFR scenario where there is little soft tissue connection between the femur and tibia.

Top Tip: Rotating-hinge designs with no rotational constraint have higher propensity for PFJ instability if the patella is not tracking centrally.

Other implant designs with modern linked hinges have some of the rotation occurring above the tibial tray, so the plastic is a fixed-bearing to the tray with the rotating mechanism attached to the femur sitting on top. In such a design, some condylar control is possible in extension which can block or limit excessive rotation near full extension. However, this contact is quickly lost in flexion with relative rotational freedom. The condylar geometry in these designs is useful in optimising kinematics in relation to the PFJ. Therefore, it is essential to get the rotational alignment of the components correct, and to get the patella resting position correct in extension and ensure that it is centralised on the component so at least it starts off at the right point.

Top Tip: The axle and bushings type designs are robust to failure although we tend to get bushing wear which can be changed without catastrophic failure.

10.7   What is An Ideal Hinge Design?

The ideal hinge from a kinematic point of view is a sliding-hinge, that is a condylar hinge that can piston slightly to keep condylar control but also with a hinge mechanism that can slide so the point of rotation is not fixed. The point of rotation would be driven by both the condyles and the hinge mechanism. It would need to last 15–20 years and preserve bone.

In other words, a sloppy hinge that does not fix the centre of rotation, pistons a little bit, blocks hyperextension, and gives guaranteed varus-valgus stability for revision surgery for instability issues and ligamentous laxity. Sadly, such an implant is not currently available but this is indeed an area in revision knee surgery that requires great engineering minds to explore further.

10.8   Hinges in Megaprostheses

We must have hinges on these implants as by definition there are no collateral ligaments. The load goes through the fixation quite significantly; the larger the segmental replacement we have, the longer the lever arm before reaching the fixation. This is why megaprostheses have a higher failure rate particularly in older patients. The standard tumour implants do well in good young bone. Most have coated collars where the periosteum can be attached to giving a secondary point of fixation with an element of biological fixation. In salvage revision knee cases in elderly patients, however, we can only really rely on implant-bone interface fixation whether cemented or cementless, and long-term longevity remains an issue (Fig. 10.5).

(i)

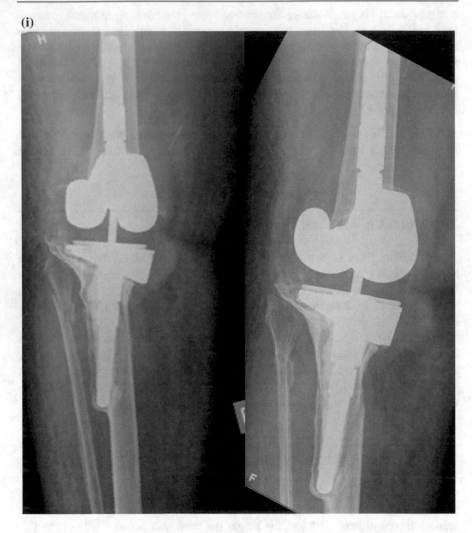

Fig. 10.5 **i** Preoperative radiographs of an 81 year old female with gross aseptic loosening of right revision total knee arthroplasty. **ii** Radiographs at 3 years follow up following reconstruction with SMILES fixed-hinge and METS proximal tibial replacement with well-fixed stems on both sides

(ii)

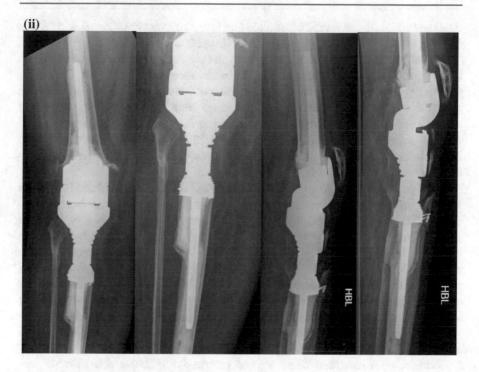

Fig. 10.5 (continued)

10.9   Our Series of Rotating Hinges

We evaluated our medium- to long-term survivorship, complications and outcomes of rTKA using two contemporary rotating-hinge prostheses (fully cemented vs. cementless systems) in a consecutive series between 2005–2018. The choice of fixation method, and subsequently type of implant used, is dictated by patient factors, the degree of osteopenia or osteoporosis, and whether adjunctive fixation is required. Fixation technique is one of the differences between the two implants used with the cemented system requiring fully cemented fixation, and the cementless system allowing for metaphyseal sleeve fixation. Both groups in this study achieved comparable outcomes although there were some differences in the demographics of both groups.

Implants: we use two rotating-hinge implants; the Stanmore Modular Individualized Lower Extremity System SMILES® Knee System (Stanmore Implants Worldwide Ltd) and the S-ROM® NOILES™ Rotating Hinge Knee System (DePuy, Warsaw, IN).

SMILES® Knee System (Fig. 10.3): is a third-generation fully cemented hinged knee, introduced in 1992. It is made from a cast cobalt-chromium-molybdenum and titanium alloy. The rotating-hinge knee articulation includes a beveled polyethylene bearing surface placed on the tibial plate and limits rotational motion to $\pm\ 5°$ while hyperextension is constrained by a bumper that acts as a secondary bearing surface. This system has three tibial options in two sizes; a rotating-hinge all-polyethylene tibia, a rotating-hinge metal cased tibia with short (140 mm) and long stem (180 mm) options, and a fixed hinge tibia with short and long stems. In our practice, we use the rotating-hinge metal cased tibia. The femoral component is either small or standard size with 140 mm long femoral curved titanium stem of 13 mm diameter for standard components and 12 mm for small components. The hinge is assembled with a cobalt-chromium-molybdenum axle, a pair of poly-ethylene bushes and a titanium circlip.

S-ROM® Rotating Hinge Knee System (**Fig. 10.4**): is also a third-generation modular mobile-bearing implant that has evolved from the original Noiles pros-thesis. The components of this condylar design are made of highly polished cobalt-chromium with a mobile-bearing polyethylene which is highly congruent with the femoral component and linked via a yoke and axle assembly hinge mechanism. The femoral component is available in three sizes (Extra-Small, Small and Medium). This system is compatible with the MBT revision tibial tray and has modular titanium metaphyseal sleeves (cemented or cementless), that can be added as part of the construct through a Morse taper junction, to enhance fixation. In our practice, we routinely use cementless metaphyseal sleeves on the tibial side and in selected patients on the femoral side [13].

Patients were identified using a local prospective database and linkable data obtained from the NJR for rTKA. We excluded patients that required endopros-theses with distal femoral replacements and patients with periprosthetic fractures.

Operative Technique: utilizing the old midline incision and extending as far proximally as needed to expose the distal femur, knees were approached through a standard medial parapatellar arthrotomy with subluxation of the patella following complete synovectomy. Components are then removed in the standard fashion with minimal bone loss. The tibia is then prepared and the canal is reamed to accept an appropriate diameter stem for either cemented or cementless systems. Attention is then turned to the femur and the canal is similarly prepared. In cases where the cementless system was used, we prepared for a press-fit cementless stem with a femoral metaphyseal sleeve. A trial is then assembled and articulated with the tibial component. The joint line level is restored in flexion and extension and checked using a combination of anatomical markers, soft tissue tension (particularly the extensor mechanism), and length measurements including patellofemoral articula-tion [14]. Once satisfactory trial positioning is obtained, definitive implants are assembled to match the trials. For cemented implants, we use Palacos R + G (Hereaus Medical GmbH, Germany). Additional antibiotics can be added to the cement as required [15]. Routine closure is then performed in layers over a drain which is removed in 24 h. Full weight-bearing is commenced as tolerated with routine physiotherapy. Follow-up was performed regularly at 6 weeks, 3 months and 12 monthly thereafter.

There were 158 consecutive patients (158 knees) during the study period and were all included in the analysis. These included 93 females (59.5%) and 64 males (40.5%) with mean age 73.9 (range 38–95). Mean BMI was 30.9 (range 19–51) with a median of 30 kg/m^2. The majority of patients (92.4%) had ASA score II/III. The main indications were infection (37.3%) with most patients managed through a two-stage approach (46/59), aseptic loosening with instability (36%), and instability (18.3%). Eighty-nine patients (56.3%) received the cementless sleeved system (Figs. 10.6, 10.7 and 10.8) and 69 (43.7%) received a fully cemented hinge knee prosthesis (Figs. 10.9). There were no statistically significant differences in baseline patients' characteristics between the two groups. Although the cementless system group were marginally younger with more males than females and higher number of patients with ASA-II reflecting a healthier cohort.

(i)

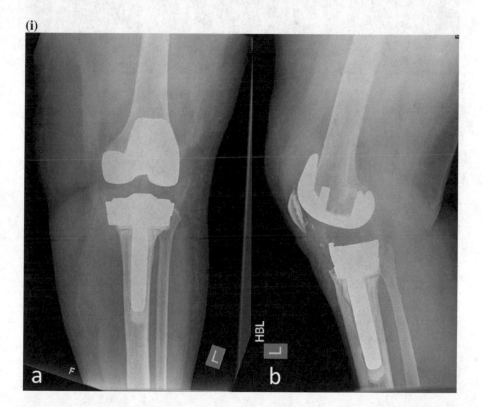

Fig. 10.6   i Anteroposterior and lateral weight-bearing radiographs of a 67 year old woman with a failed revised left TKA with aseptic loosening and instability. **ii** Postoperative radiographs following revision surgery and reconstruction with a sleeved rotating hinge implant and built-up tibial tray. Follow up radiographs at 7 years with satisfactory clinical outcomes and well-ingrown sleeves with no evidence of loosening. **iii** The tibial component and sleeve had subsided few millimetres to stability with a pedestal in the canal with well-ingrown sleeve. Both stems have non-progressive radiolucent lines

(ii)

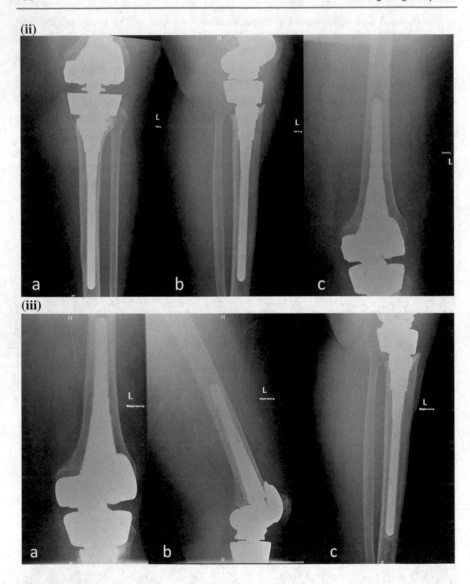

(iii)

Fig. 10.6 (continued)

(i)

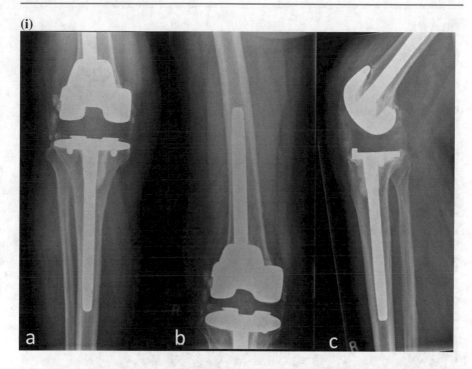

Fig. 10.7 **i** Anteroposterior and lateral radiographs of a failed right revised knee in a 56 year old man with previous patellectomy and flexion instability symptoms. **ii** Postoperative radiographs following rotating hinge reconstruction with press-fit sleeves both sides. **iii** Follow up radiographs at 8.5 years follow up with well-fixed components and a satisfactory functional outcome

In the SROM group, the mean follow-up was 7.4 years with a median 7 years (range 2–17). The overall rate of re-operation, for any cause, was 10.1% with rate of implant revision of 6.7%; there were three reoperations and 6 component revisions. Kaplan Meier implant-survivorship analysis, using "revision for any cause" as an end point, was 93.3% at 10 years. In the SMILES group, the mean follow-up was 7.9 years (range 2–17), overall complication rate was 7.24%; all with patellofemoral complications. Failure rate with 'any cause revision' was 4.34%. There were

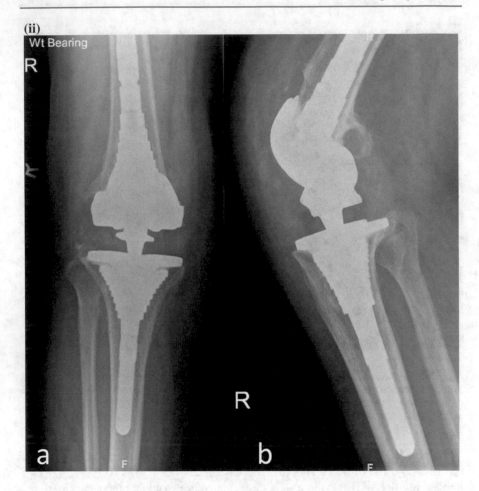

Fig. 10.7 (continued)

no cases of mechanical failure. At 10 years, 17/69 (24.63%) patients had died. Implant-survivorship was 94.2% at 10 years. There was no statistically significant difference in 10-years survivorship between the two groups (P = 0.821).

A number of studies on contemporary rotating-hinge implants in rTKA have been published although most with short- to medium-term outcomes [10, 16–20] (Table 10.1).

(iii)

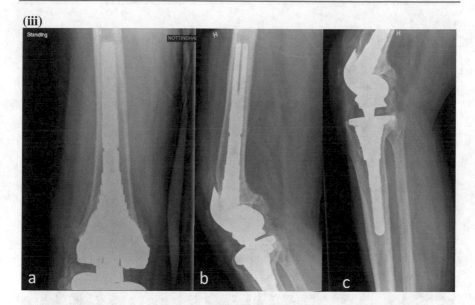

Fig. 10.7 (continued)

Top Tip: In our series, both systems were comparable in terms of fixation technique (cemented or sleeved cementless), restoring joint line and component rotation were more important in preventing kinematic complications particularly PFJ's.

In summary, hinged components in rTKA are an important tool within our armamentarium. However, they must be approached with caution and care must be taken to adequately reconstruct the joint line and re-establish the correct component rotation in order to avoid complications that will compromise the functional outcome. Where possible we would always advocate a rotating hinge design in order to avoid the transmission of stresses to the implant-bone or fixation interfaces, potentially leading to early loosening.

(i)

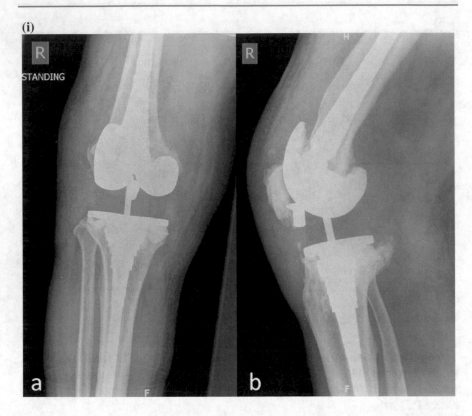

Fig. 10.8 i Anteroposterior and lateral radiographs of a 76 year old man with a varus valgus constrained revision right knee presenting with instability and inability to walk. Both radiographs demonstrate a broken bolt between the femoral component and the well-fixed sleeve adaptor. **ii** Postoperative radiographs following single-component revision to a rotating hinge component

(ii)

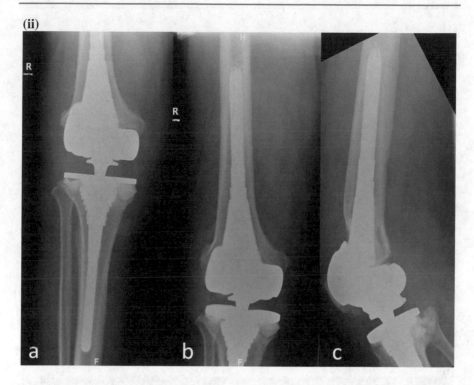

Fig. 10.8 (continued)

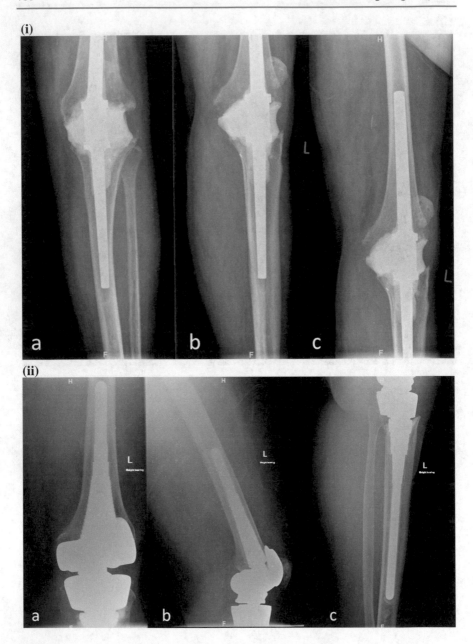

Fig. 10.9 i Anteroposterior and lateral radiographs of a left knee in a 71 year old woman following 1st stage revision for infection using a fusion nail as a static stabiliser. **ii** Anteroposterior and lateral radiographs **a–b** at 2 years and **c–d** 4 years follow up with well-fixed implant following 2nd stage reconstruction with a cemented fixed-hinge implant

(i)

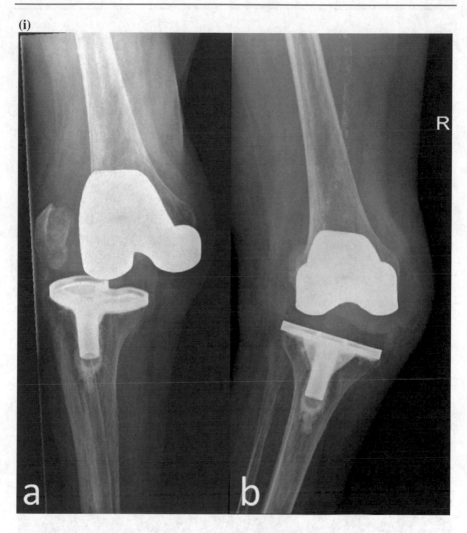

Fig. 10.10 **i** Preoperative anteroposterior and lateral radiographs of right knee in 89 years old female with gross rotatory instability and a failed MCL. **ii** Anteroposterior and lateral radiographs at 3 years follow-up using following revision to a cemented fixed-hinge with no loosening and satisfactory clinical outcomes

(ii)

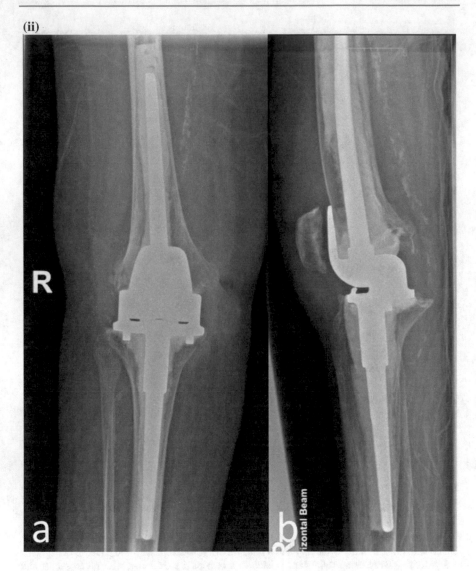

Fig. 10.10 (continued)

Table 10.1 Summary of published studies on contemporary rotating hinge implants in revision knee arthroplasty

Study	Indication	No Patients /Knees	Implants	Mean FU (yrs)	Complications	Revision rate	Survivorship
Joshi 2008 [19]	Aseptic loosening (60%), instability (31%), periprosthetic fracture (5%), extensor mechanism failure (4%)	78 rTKA	Waldemar Endo-Model Rotational Knee Prosthesis	7.8	Instability (5%), aseptic loosening (5%), infection (3%)	8 (12.8%): septic 2 (2.6%), aseptic 8 (10.3%)	73% at 7.8 years
Baier 2013 [16]	Aseptic loosening (45%), component malrotation (23%), instability (18%), stiffness (9%)	78 rTKA	TC3, DePuy, Warsaw, IN	6.7	Arthrofibrosis (7%), aseptic loosening (6%), deep infection (4%), patellar complication (3%)	7 (8.9%): septic 3 (4%), aseptic 4 (6%)	reoperation rate 26% at 6.7 years, no survivorship data
Smith 2013 [20]	Infection (46%), instability (34%), aseptic loosening (24%)	59 rTKA/ 111	Stryker Kinematic 1&2, Stryker Duracon Modular Rotating Hinge, SROM, Biomet Finn Rotating Hinged	5	Infection (24%), soft tissue failure (12%), aseptic loosening (7%), periprosthetic fracture (5%)	28 (47.5%): septic 14 (23.7%), aseptic 13 (22.0%)	77% at 1 year 52% at 5 years
Guirea 2014 [21]	Osteoarthritis (56%), infection (13%), aseptic loosening (13%), instability (15%)	62 rTKA/ 152	Aesculap EnduRo rotating hinge	2	Deep infection (3%), aseptic loosening (1%), periprosthetic fracture (1%), extensor dysfunction (1%)	14 (9.2%): septic 5 (3.3%), aseptic 9 (5.9%)	85.4% at 2 years
Farid 2015 [17]	Infection (43%), arthrofibrosis (11%), aseptic loosening (11%), instability	131 rTKA / 142	Biomet Orthopedic Salvage System	4.7	Aseptic loosening (16%), deep infection (15%), periprosthetic fracture	49 (34.5%): septic 21 (14.8%), aseptic 28 (19.7%)	51% at 10 years

(continued)

Table 10.1 (continued)

Study	Indication	No Patients /Knees	Implants	Mean FU (yrs)	Complications	Revision rate	Survivorship
	(11%), periprosthetic fracture (5%)				(7%), quad/patellar tendon rupture (4%)		
Cottino 2017 [10]	Infection (35%) Aseptic loosening (13%) Periprosthetic fractures (13%) Non-union (5%) Primary TKA (18%)	334 rTKA / 408	Howmedica (59%) NexGen RH Knee (31%) S-ROM (9%), Biomet Finn (0.5%)	4	Deep infection (11%), delayed wound healing (3%), stiffness (2.5%), aseptic loosening (2.5%), superficial infection (1.2%)	22.5% at 10 years	71.3% at 10 years
Our series	Infection (37.3%) Aseptic loosening (36%) Instability (18.3%) Dislocation (5.7%) Others (2.7%)	158 rTKA	S-ROM (56.3%) SMILES (43.7%)	7.6	13 (8.2%)	SROM implant revision of 6.7% at 10-years. SMILES implant revision of 4.34% at 10-years	70.9% at 10 years

References

1. Rodríguez-Merchán EC. Total knee arthroplasty using hinge joints: Indications and results. EFORT Open Rev. 2019;4(4):121–32.
2. Jones EC, et al. GUEPAR knee arthroplasty results and late complications. Clin Orthop Relat Res. 1979;140:145–52.
3. Jones GB. Total knee replacement-the Walldius hinge. Clin Orthop Relat Res. 1973;94:50–7.
4. Lettin AW et al. The Stanmore hinged knee arthroplasty. J Bone Joint Surg Br. 1978; 60-b (3):327–32.
5. Murray DG, et al. Herbert total knee prosthesis: combined laboratory and clinical assessment. J Bone Joint Surg Am. 1977;59(8):1026–32.
6. Shaw JA, Balcom W, Greer RB 3rd. Total knee arthroplasty using the kinematic rotating hinge prosthesis. Orthopedics. 1989;12(5):647–54.
7. Walker PS, et al. The kinematic rotating hinge: biomechanics and clinical application. Orthop Clin North Am. 1982;13(1):187–99.
8. Jones RE, Barrack RL, Skedros J. Modular, mobile-bearing hinge total knee arthroplasty. Clin Orthop Relat Res. 2001;392:306–14.
9. Barrack RL. Evolution of the rotating hinge for complex total knee arthroplasty. Clin Orthop Relat Res. 2001;392:292–9.
10. Cottino U, et al. Long-term results after total knee arthroplasty with contemporary rotating-hinge prostheses. J Bone Joint Surg Am. 2017;99(4):324–30.
11. Myers GJ, et al. Endoprosthetic replacement of the distal femur for bone tumours: long-term results. J Bone Joint Surg Br. 2007;89(4):521–6.
12. Kouk S, et al. Rotating hinge prosthesis for complex revision total knee arthroplasty: a review of the literature. J Clin Orthop Trauma. 2018;9(1):29–33.
13. Bloch BV, et al. Metaphyseal sleeves in revision total knee arthroplasty provide reliable fixation and excellent medium to long-term implant survivorship. J Arthroplasty. 2020;35 (2):495–9.
14. Bellemans J. 52 joint line restoration in revision total knee replacement. In: Hirschmann MT, Becker R, editors. The unhappy total knee replacement: a comprehensive review and management guide. Cham: Springer International Publishing; 2015. p. 631–8.
15. Frew NM et al. Comparison of the elution properties of commercially available gentamicin and bone cement containing vancomycin with 'home-made' preparations. Bone Joint J. 2017; 99-b(1):73–7.
16. Baier C, et al. Assessing patient-oriented results after revision total knee arthroplasty. J Orthop Sci. 2013;18(6):955–61.
17. Farid YR, Thakral R, Finn HA. Intermediate-term results of 142 single-design, rotating-hinge implants: frequent complications may not preclude salvage of severely affected knees. J Arthroplasty. 2015;30(12):2173–80.
18. Hossain F, Patel S, Haddad FS. Midterm assessment of causes and results of revision total knee arthroplasty. Clin Orthop Relat Res. 2010;468(5):1221–8.
19. Joshi N, Navarro-Quilis A. Is there a place for rotating-hinge arthroplasty in knee revision surgery for aseptic loosening? J Arthroplasty. 2008;23(8):1204–11.
20. Smith TH, et al. Comparison of mechanical and nonmechanical failure rates associated with rotating hinged total knee arthroplasty in nontumor patients. J Arthroplasty. 2013;28(1):62-7. e1.
21. Giurea A et al. Early results of a new rotating hinge knee implant. Biomed Res Int. 2014; 2014:948520.

Salvage Revision Total Knee Arthroplasty

11

A sound man is good at salvage, at seeing nothing is lost.

Laozi

11.1 Introduction

Salvage revision TKA is a complex and challenging surgery with unpredictable results and requires significant resources. The demand for salvage surgery is increasing, with more and more patients coming to their third or fourth revision in a situation with increasing bone loss.

The UK National Joint Registry reported re-revision rates of 3.52% at 1 year, rising to 16.77% at 7 years and 19.38% at 10 years following first rTKA, with aseptic loosening, infection and instability accounting for the majority of re-revisions [1]. The overall risk of failure and complications of further sequential re-revisions is much higher than those of first revisions [2, 3].

Most of the problems that we are facing are currently on the femoral side, partly due to periprosthetic fractures but also due to segmental or massive bone loss. However, increasingly we will start to see more issues on the tibial side with the need for salvage endoprostheses on the tibial side becoming more common. This chapter focuses on the practical aspects of salvage endoprostheses and presents our tertiary experience with case demonstrations.

© The Author(s), under exclusive license to Springer Nature Switzerland AG 2021
H. E. Matar et al., *Revision Total Knee Arthroplasty*,
https://doi.org/10.1007/978-3-030-81285-0_11

11.2   Options for Salvage

The Anderson Orthopaedic Research Institute (AORI) classification system, developed by *Engh*, is widely used to classify bone loss both pre- and intra-operatively [4]. AORI-III are large defects with deficient metaphyseal bone or uncontained defects [5–7]. In cases of massive segmental AORI-III defects, limb-sparing options are limited. Here, the salvage options are:

(a) Allograft-prosthetic composite techniques
(b) Massive Endoprostheses
(c) Arthrodesis techniques
(d) Amputation

High failure rates have been reported with allograft-prosthetic composites with fractures, collapse, and high risk of infection [8–10]; our experience in this technique is limited. Implant-arthrodeses are preserved for low demand patients with chronic pain, infections, and deficient extensor mechanisms with relatively poor functional outcomes [11, 12]. While above knee amputation remains an option for treating recurrent infections; better functional and ambulatory status has been demonstrated with knee arthrodesis [13].

11.3   Massive Endoprostheses

Endoprostheses include condylar replacing distal femoral replacement (DFR) and the less commonly used proximal tibial replacement prosthesis (PTR). Rarely, sub-total or total femoral replacement prostheses are required. The modular endoprostheses with rotating-hinge mechanisms provide a viable limb-salvage alternative in rTKA practice with the ability to restore some function and immediate mobilisation in this complex cohort of patients [14–16].

Evidence from the orthopaedic oncological literature, where PTR prostheses are used more frequently in the management of bone tumours, indicate that PTRs have an increased risk of complications, infection, and failure compared to DFRs [17–19]. This is in part due to anatomical factors with the subcutaneous location of the proximal tibia, tenuous soft-tissue coverage, poor supportive bone for fixation, and extensor mechanism complications [20].

11.4   Issues Related to Massive Endoprostheses

In rTKA practice, massive endoprostheses are mainly used in the form of a DFR with a hinge mechanism. There are specific issues with endoprostheses that relate to the hinge mechanism and the constraint in the implant, with the resultant transmission of that constraint to the fixation interfaces.

On the tibial side: most of the time we can use augments or build up trays as most of the bone loss we see is above the tibial tubercle and extensor mechanism attachment. The bone here is loaded through the extensor attachment, as long as the quads are working, so the bone here is usually strong. Thus, in our experience, most cases can be managed with metaphyseal fixation with either sleeves or cones to restore joint height with a good fixation for a revision tibial component. However, in cases of DFR or certain hinge implants such as Stanmore where sleeves or cones cannot be used, long cemented stems are an alternative. Provided we then couple the tibial component with a rotating-hinge mechanism, even in a megaprosthesis situation, the tibial construct fixation remains protected and functions in a similar manner to a standard rotating-hinge implant.

Top Tip: On the tibial side, unless it is a PTR case, there is very little difference in the mechanics of massive endoprostheses compared to standard hinge implants.

On the femoral side: the hinge mechanism attaches to the distal femur with a similar loading and kinematic pattern at the joint surface to a standard rotating hinge as discussed in the previous chapter. There is however a significant impact on the stresses at the fixation interface due to the increased lever arm which is an effect of the separation between the implant-bone interface and the articulation.

The axial load is well-tolerated on both tibial and femoral sides. However, the challenge is in resisting torsional loading. In the coronal plane, the varus-valgus constraint coupled with a long lever arm from the articulation to the fixation interface will have an impact in addition to the rotational constraint. Just like a rotating-hinge, the torque from rotational constraint is partially dissipated by the rotating bearing on the tibial side. On the femoral side, any load that is generated with the knee slightly flexed will create a turning moment, which in turn is transmitted over a long lever arm before reaching the fixation interface. So, in loading the knee in standing position from sitting, we are applying a load asymmetrically to the distal femur creating a turning moment on it. We have a very long segment and that load is going to be amplified. Here, lies our problem in massive endoprostheses which is resisting that load on the proximal femur which eventually leads to loosening and failure.

Top Tip: The long lever arm of a massive endoprosthesis amplifies the stresses on the fixation interface in the proximal femur.

11.5   Fixation of Massive Endoprostheses

Our experience in uncemented stems on the femoral side in these DFRs is limited because of early failure. This is because the torque being put on that interface very early, even if we get a good press-fit, is very high and seems to affect ingrowth. Cemented fixation is therefore outperforming cementless fixation because at least with cement we can get good interdigitation, rotational stability between the implant and cement which resists that rotation, with better early and midterm survivorship. Long term fixation remains an issue with repeated loading and high stresses on the fixation interface with progressive failure.

In tumour prostheses, having a secondary fixation is a good solution by using hydroxyapatite- or porous metal-coated collars with younger patients than those seen in salvage arthroplasty population. Here, the periosteum is sutured to the collar with potential for bony ingrowth onto the collars. So, there will be a primary fixation with cement and a secondary biological fixation. In rTKA practice however, with elderly patients with osteoporotic bone this is not practically possible with almost non-existent periosteum. The challenge remains in how to optimise fixation of these salvage endoprostheses so that we can have a hybrid fixation with either cemented stem and some form of secondary biological fixation or have a primary biological cementless fixation with a secondary fixation to give us better rotation stability while we get the ingrowth.

Practical Technique for Secondary Fixation: this involves the creation of a sleeve of bone with any remaining periosteal attachment or muscle. Once we decide on the resection level, we keep some bone distal to that, then osteotomise the tube, leaving as much attachment to it as possible and then bring that tube around the collar for a secondary fixation point which has the potential for healing and ingrowth of the coated collar (Fig. 11.1).

Top Tip: All attempts should be made to obtain a secondary fixation of massive endoprostheses such as the use of coated collars, whether the primary fixation is cemented or cementless.

11.6   Extensor Mechanism and Massive Endoprostheses

The challenge on the tibial side is attachment of the extensor mechanism. Our preferred approach is to create a long tibial crest osteotomy early on during initial exposure. The crest includes the tibial tubercle with the intact extensor attachment and a broad bed of anterior tibial bone. We then resect the proximal tibia as planned and once trials are satisfactory and the definitive prosthesis is implanted, we wire the osteotomy back to the front of the prosthesis. We use, and advocate, a prosthesis that has some ingrowth surface to attach the crest osteotomy with the extensors attached (Fig. 11.2).

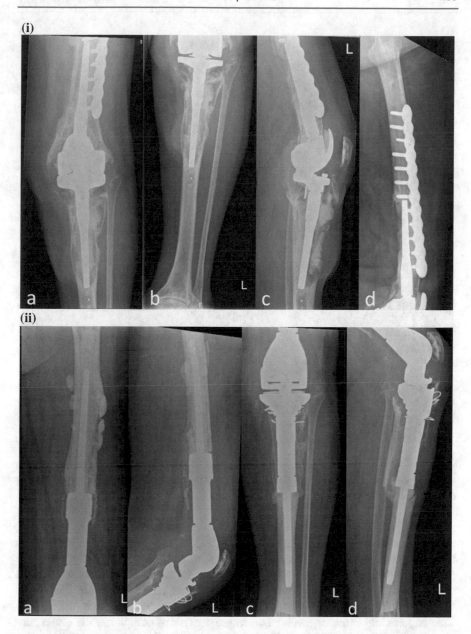

Fig. 11.1   i Preoperative radiographs of left knee in 80 years old females with catastrophic failure of re-revised knee with ipsilateral femoral plating for previous femur periprosthetic fracture. **ii** Postoperative radiographs following salvage reconstruction with DFR and PTR with satisfactory outcome at 3 years follow up

(i)

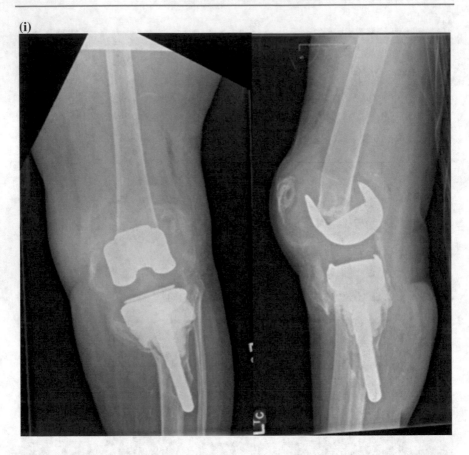

Fig. 11.2 **i** Preoperative anteroposterior and lateral radiograph of left knee with catastrophic failure of revision components in 82 years old lady. **ii** Postoperative radiographs with DFR and PTR at 2 years follow up

The other important point here is getting the joint line correct. Ensuring that we have appropriate extensor mechanism tension and rotation is of paramount importance because in these salvage cases there is no soft tissue connection between femur and tibia; they are completely independent of each other. Therefore, we have much less rotational control and rotational stability for the articulation. This exposes the extensor mechanism to greater risk of complications; either rupture, patella fracture or failure with dislocation/subluxation. If we over-tension the extensor mechanism it will inevitably escape laterally. Further, because there is no

(ii)

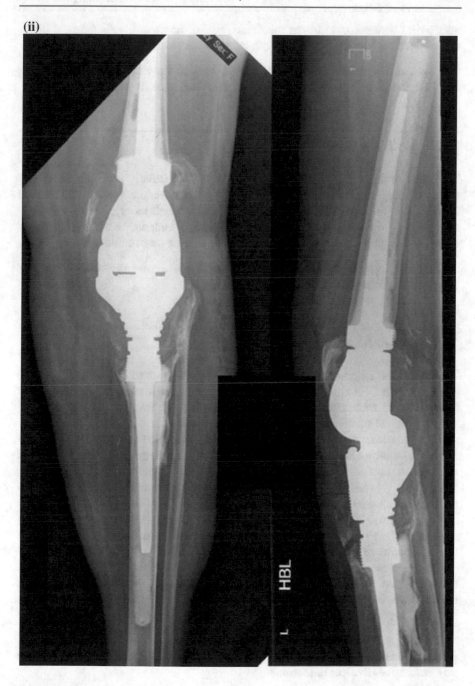

Fig. 11.2 (continued)

attachment between the tibia or the femur, risk of implant dissociation and dislo-cation becomes significantly high with extensor mechanism escape.

Top Tip: Do not overstuff the PFJ, over-tension the extensor mechanism, or distalise the joint line otherwise the extensor mechanism will escape.

11.7 Soft Tissue Coverage

The other problem with salvage endoprostheses, particularly on the tibia, is soft tissue coverage. In most cases we can get good coverage around the femoral implant with the extensors. On the tibial side, it is much more exposed with only skin covering the proximal tibia. An infected salvage endoprosthesis is a disastrous complication with a very high likelihood of above knee amputation as the next step.

Top Tip: Respect the soft tissues, ensure adequate coverage, and get plastics support for local or free flaps when needed.

11.8 What About Ipsilateral THA?

That can cause significant problems, for most cases there will be enough room to get a stem in a DFR case. The decision is then on how to protect the junction which has a potential stress riser with the risk of interprosthetic fracture. Do you protect it with a plate, adjunctive fixation, or custom implants?

Each manufacturer's engineers have different strategies to deal with these sce-narios on case-by-case basis. Our preferred technique is to get primary fixation with a cemented stem using an implant with supplementary plate to span the weak area. These are usually CT-based custom implants manufactured with a hydroxyapatite-coated plate as an integral part of the prosthesis. The fixation points on the plate are either cables or screws driven by the individual case depending on what accessibility we have. The plate can also help to position the implant on the femur in terms of rotation (Fig. 11.3).

Other techniques of custom implants is to use a cement-linked DFR prosthesis to the well-fixed and functioning THA where a hollow cylindrical component is inserted over the retained femoral stem to provide a solid diaphyseal reconstruction and it allows immediate weight bearing (Fig. 11.4) [21].

Top Tip: The use of custom implants demands meticulous technique, patience, and precise execution; there is little salvage choice left to deal with any intraoperative complications.

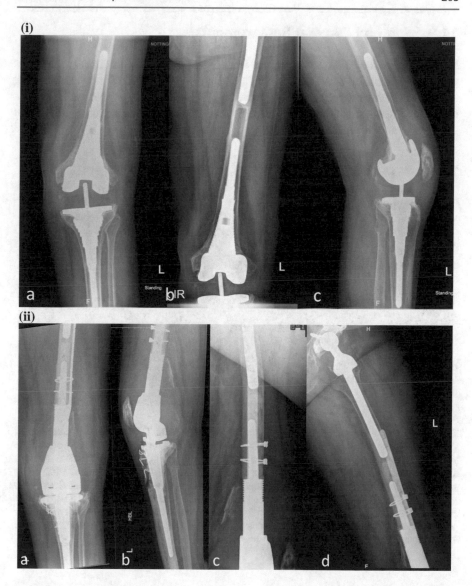

Fig. 11.3 **i** Example of a challenging case with instability and deficient MCL with an ipsilateral THA. **ii** Follow up radiographs at 2 years following salvage reconstruction using custom-implant DFR with a lateral plate to span the interprosthetic area to reduce risk of fracture

11.9 Subtotal Femoral Replacements

In our experience, the need for these massive prostheses is fortunately rare and often in low demand patients. The mechanics are similar to a DFR implant with the same challenge of durability of the fixation interfaces with the potential for early aseptic failure. In most cases, a subtotal femoral replacement is a staging procedure to a total femoral replacement.

(i)

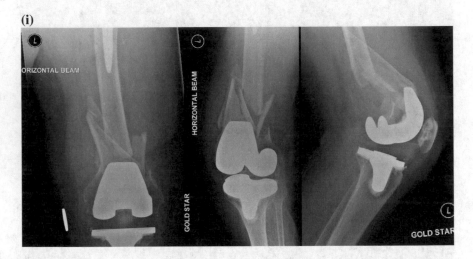

Fig. 11.4 **i** Another example on how to deal with an ipsilateral THA in an acute comminuted periprosthetic fracture case distal to a well-fixed cementless hip stem in a 71 years old woman. The remaining length of intact femur distal to the stem is inadequate to support a DFR stem. Further, fracture fixation is likely to fail due to the significant comminution. **ii** Anteroposterior pelvic radiograph at initial presentation demonstrating well-fixed, well-aligned uncemented total hip replacement. **iii** Template as provided by the manufacturer of a custom-made implant with a DFR and a proximal cement-linked integral attachment to the pre-existing hip stem. **iv** Anteroposterior and lateral radiographs of a custom-made cement-linked DFR at 5-year follow up with satisfactory clinical outcomes

(ii)

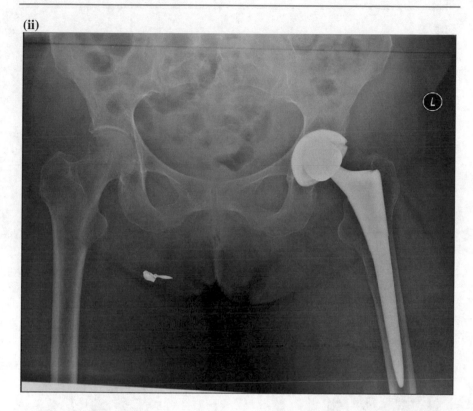

Fig. 11.4   (continued)

11.10   Total Femoral Replacements

The use of TFRs for non-oncological indications is extremely rare. There are layers of complexities around the use of this salvage option; inherent mechanical limitations, surgical technique, and perioperative care in generally elderly patients with poor soft tissues and numerous previous surgeries. Nonetheless, TFRs do provide the ability to ambulate in appropriately selected patients at short- to medium-term accepting that there is a high risk of complications [22–25].

In our practice, we position the patient laterally and use a long lateral incision over the hip curving it more anteriorly over the knee. The remining femur is resected which usually is associated with significant intraoperative blood loss. Tibial preparation of the knee is performed in the standard fashion, adequate view can be achieved even though the patient is in lateral position once the femur is

(iii)

Implant type:	Distal Femoral Replacement
Type of fixation:	Cemented Tibial Component – Cement Fill Bore
Joint type:	Standard METS (To be decided during operation)
Material:	CoCrMo – Ti – HA
Side:	Left

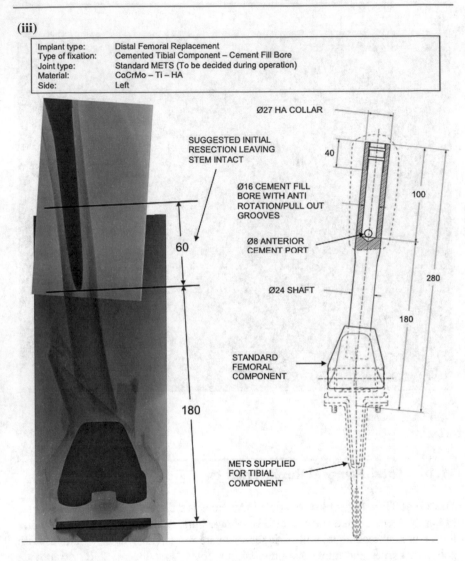

Fig. 11.4 (continued)

resected. We use a fixed-hinge mechanism to better control the extensors, protecting the fixation interfaces is less of a concern here. We also use captive liners to reduce the risk of hip dislocation. Mechanically, all the stresses and torque generated go through the acetabulum. (Fig. 11.5).

(iv)

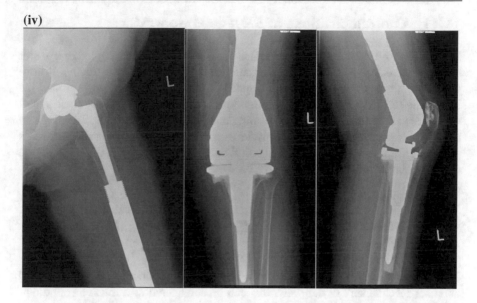

Fig. 11.4 (continued)

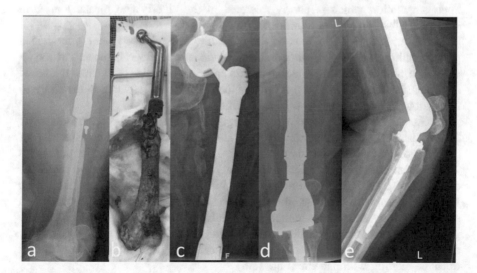

Fig. 11.5 Example of a total femoral replacement performed as a second stage procedure salvage for chronic proximal femoral replacement infection and distal femoral osteomyelitis

11.11 Contraindications of Salvage Endoprostheses

In addition to the generic cardiovascular fitness of the patients to undergo major reconstructive surgery, the main contraindications from a reconstructive arthroplasty point of view are related to the status of the soft tissue envelope around the knee. The soft tissue envelope is of paramount importance and robust anterior soft tissues are needed to ensure wound healing and protect the prosthesis. The aim is to re-establish the retinaculum and capsule over the prosthesis. A plastic surgeon's input is often needed to get a healthy soft tissue envelope in a staged fashion before definitive implantation.

11.12 What About Concurrent Extensor Mechanism Failure?

The question here is there any merit in salvage massive endoprosthesis with a failed extensor mechanism? In our view, this can be considered as a relative contraindication. If the soft tissues are poor in a frail elderly host, then embarking on major reconstructive surgery is not advised. Conservative measures such as a brace and a wheelchair may suffice. Other options here, include ablative surgery with above knee amputation which is poorly tolerated in the elderly and means long-term wheelchair use, or salvage arthrodesis.

However, if the soft tissue envelope is healthy in a relatively young, motivated patient with a sensate foot, then extensor mechanism allograft reconstruction as well as a massive salvage endoprostheses may be considered. In this combined approach, implant failure is a medium- to long-term concern, while in the short- to medium-term it is extensor mechanism failure.

Technically, we would use a fixed-hinge in those cases of combined salvage. This is because if the extensor mechanism failed, a rotating hinge is at risk of dissociation and knee dislocation. Alternative options can be hinge endoprostheses where separation or dissociation is inherently blocked by distraction. In those circumstances, even if the extensor allograft fails, patients can still ambulate with a fixed-hinge implant with rehabilitation focused on back-knee gait for stability in stance, and they can achieve limited but meaningful function and activities of daily living. This sort of complex reconstructive surgery requires a specialist capability and MDT support with vascular and plastic surgical input and a shared decision-making with patients (Fig. 11.6).

Top Tip: Patients with a sensate foot and a stable limb in extension can ambulate; elderly frail patients with above knee amputation are often confined to a wheelchair.

(i)

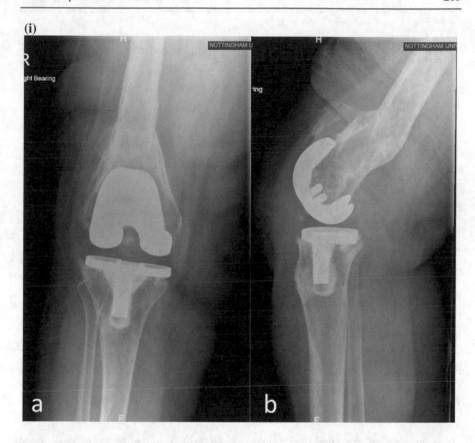

Fig. 11.6 i Example of a combined approach of salvage reconstruction and allograft extensor mechanism in a 64 years old man who was referred to us with (a-b) with an infected complex primary TKA with previous ipsilateral distal femur fracture and failed extensor mechanism. **ii** Radiographs following 1st stage revision for infection and temporary static spacer using arthrodesis nail. **iii** Radiographs at 3 years follow up following major combined reconstruction with a DFR/fixed hinge mechanism and allograft extensor mechanism reconstruction

11.13   Implant-Arthrodesis

Knee arthrodesis offers a salvage option for failed infected knee arthroplasties, chronic pain and instability. The aim is to provide patients with a stable, pain-free lower extremity that supports ambulation. Whilst above knee amputation (AKA) may be an option for some patients, it often renders elderly patients with failed knee arthroplasties wheelchair-bound due to the increased energy expenditure required for ambulation with an AKA prosthesis [26, 27]. However, knee arthrodesis requires 25% less energy expenditure compared with AKA [28] and has better functional results [29].

(ii)

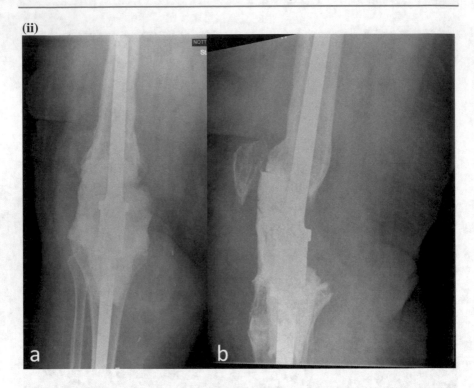

Fig. 11.6 (continued)

A number of classical techniques are described in order to achieve knee arthrodesis using both intra- or extra-medullary options such as nailing, compression plating and external fixation, as well as the use of vascularised bone grafts to achieve osseous union. However, patients with failed rTKA, who have undergone multiple previous surgeries, have significant segmental bone loss where osseous fusion is unachievable. In those cases, implant-arthrodesis is used with modular intramedullary endoprostheses.

Standard arthrodesis nails such as the LINK® Endo-Model® Arthrodesis Nail (Waldemar Link GmbH & Co Hamburg, Germany) can be used (Fig. 11.7). We routinely use this as part of our two-stage approach for infection as a static spacer in cases with significant bone loss *(see infection chapter)*. However, when faced with segmental bone loss, a custom-made knee arthrodesis prosthesis (Fig. 11.8) can be used. These implants are made from cobalt-chrome with dimensions determined from preoperative imaging (plain radiographs and CT). Most of these implants are also cemented and consist of tapered femoral and tibial

(iii)

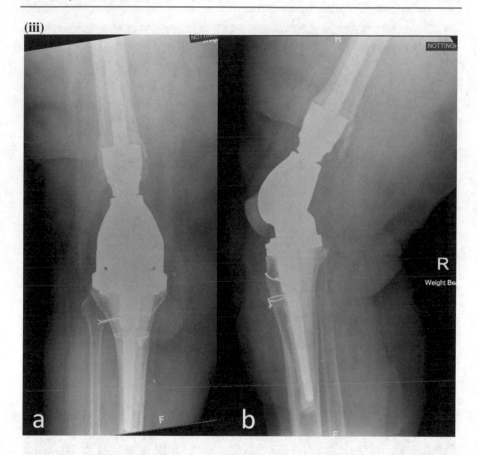

Fig. 11.6 (continued)

stems that couple with a cam and post mechanism and are locked using an axle and circlip. Silver coated options are also available. The prosthesis allows full tibio-femoral extension and incorporates a 6° valgus angle. A number of case-series have reported reasonable outcomes at short- to medium-term using implant-arthrodesis as an alternative to ablative surgery [12].

Top Tip: When using Implant-arthrodesis as a definitive salvage, we still need to eradicate infection first.

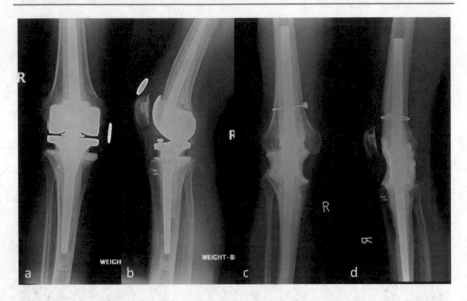

Fig. 11.7 a–b Anteroposterior and lateral preoperative radiographs of right failed knee arthroplasty following multiple revision surgeries with chronic debilitating pain and dysfunction; **c–d** Anteroposterior and lateral radiograph of implant arthrodesis using LINK cemented modular nail at 5-year follow up

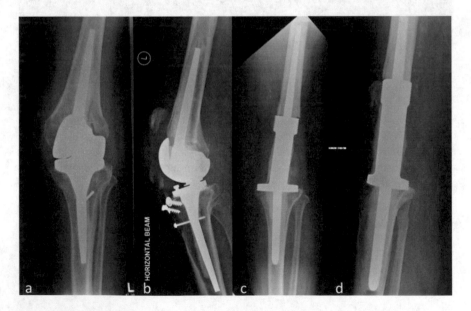

Fig. 11.8 a–b Anteroposterior and lateral preoperative radiograph with chronically infected left knee arthroplasty following repeated failed 2-stage revision surgery for infection with deficient extensor mechanism; **c–d** Anteroposterior and lateral radiograph of implant-arthrodesis using custom made implant at 7-year follow up

11.14   Amputation

One of the main challenges when reconstructive surgery is no longer an option for patients is whether the outcomes of above knee amputation are better than arthrodesis. Things to consider in the shared-decision making with the patients are that arthrodesis allow patients to keep their leg and with a sensate foot they can ambulate. However, the difficulty here is in a sitting position with the leg sticking out. Low demand elderly patients do spend a lot of their time sitting. So, amputation does have a role for those patients who would find it difficult to ambulate with an arthrodesis but would prefer to sit more comfortably.

11.15   Our Recent Experience in Salvage Endoprostheses (Fig. 11.9, 11.10, 11.11 and 11.12)

We recently reviewed our consecutive series of patients who underwent a salvage DFR with minimum 2-year follow up between 2005–2018. Patients who had acute DFR for periprosthetic fractures were excluded [30].

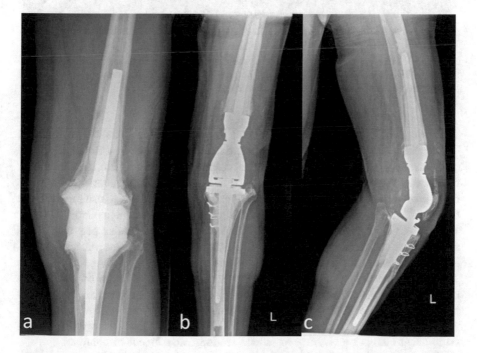

Fig. 11.9 a Preoperative anteroposterior and lateral radiograph of left knee following 1st stage revision for infection in 78 years old man. **b–c** Postoperative radiographs following reconstruction with DFR at 4 years follow up

(i)

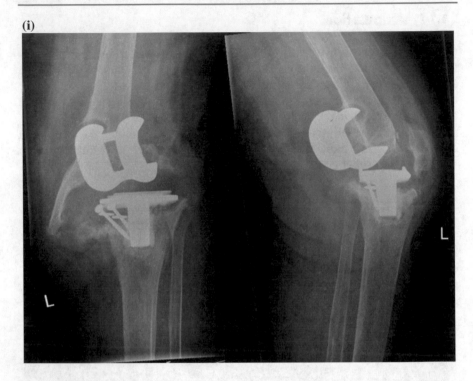

Fig. 11.10 i Preoperative anteroposterior and lateral radiograph of left knee with catastrophic failure with multiple previous surgeries in 77 years old female. **ii** Anteroposterior and lateral radiographs at 3 years follow up with satisfactory outcome

Implants: The METS® SMILES Total Knee Replacement (Stanmore Implants Worldwide Ltd) which is a modular system consisting of a SMILES distal femoral component, a range of shafts in 15 mm increments to suit differing lengths of resections, options of hydroxyapatite (HA) coated or uncoated collars, and a range of cemented stems to fit the intramedullary canal. Our practice is to use this with the SMILES knee rotating hinge metal casing tibia with cemented stems (140 or 180 mm). This system also offers the option of METS modular proximal tibial replacement for cases with concurrent massive bone loss of the proximal tibia. Similarly, this system consists of a proximal tibial component, range of shafts in 15 mm increments to suit differing lengths of resection, a range of HA coated collars of different diameters to match the size of the resected bone and a range of cemented stems to fit the intramedullary canal. The individual components of the tibial shaft are connected using interlocking taper junctions. The proximal tibial component also has a HA-coated patella tendon reattachment mechanism.

We also use the LPS™ Limb Preservation System (DePuy, Warsaw, IN) with cemented or cementless stems, porous-coated metaphyseal sleeves and mobile-bearing hinge. The minimum distal femoral resection for LPS™ is 70 mm

(ii)

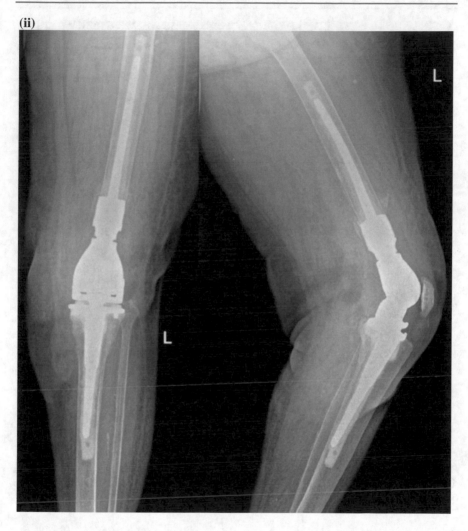

Fig. 11.10 (continued)

when using extra-small DFR component. Choice of implant is dictated by the degree of bone loss and need for adjunctive fixation, patient factors, and the soft tissue envelope.

Operative Technique: Utilising the old midline incision and extending as far proximally as needed to expose the distal femur, knees were approached through a standard medial parapatellar arthrotomy with subluxation of the patella following complete synovectomy. Components were then removed in the standard fashion with minimal bone loss. The level of femoral resection was then determined as per preoperative planning and a transverse osteotomy performed perpendicular to the

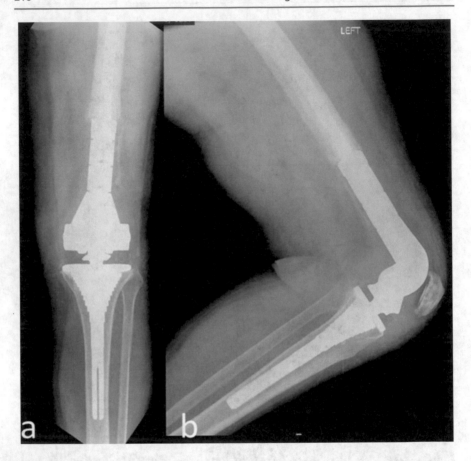

Fig. 11.11 Anteroposterior and lateral radiographs at 7 years follow up with satisfactory outcome in 65 years old male patient using hybrid fixation with cemented DFR and cementless tibial stem with metaphyseal sleeve (LPS system)

anatomical axis of the distal femur. *Hey Groves* bone holding forceps are then applied just proximal to the osteotomy.

The capsule and soft tissues are then dissected off the bone, using a femoral peel approach, in a proximal to distal direction allowing removal of the resected distal femur. Care is taken to avoid injury to the popliteal vessels or posterior tibial and peroneal nerves. The femoral canal is then prepared with reamers to accept an appropriate diameter cemented stem. Attention is then turned to the tibia which is prepared in the standard fashion, removing the component with minimal bone loss. The canal is reamed to accept an appropriate diameter cemented stem. In cases where the LPS system is used with metaphyseal sleeves, we use a press-fit cementless stem. A trial is then assembled and articulated with the tibial component. The joint line level is restored and checked using a combination of anatomical markers, soft tissue tension and length measurements including patellofemoral

(i)

(ii)

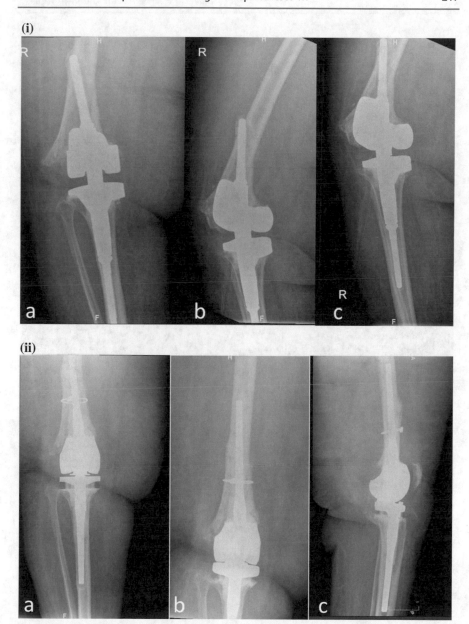

Fig. 11.12 i This is an example of a tertiary referral case that had failed multiple revisions and illustrates the importance of MDT approach and specialist centres for salvage revision surgery; (i–a–c) anteroposterior and lateral radiographs of a failed revision TKA with compromised distal femoral bone and perforated anterolateral femoral cortex in a 65 years old lady with significantly high BMI at 47. **ii** Radiographs following revision surgery in a different centre using cemented DFR implant with predictable mode of failure with a short segment of femoral fixation. **iii** 2-years follow up radiographs with catastrophic yet predictable failure of fixation. **iv** 3-years following salvage revision with a DFR and segmental collars with a long-cemented stem and cemented sleeved tibial component with a build-up tray to restore joint line

(iii)

(iv)

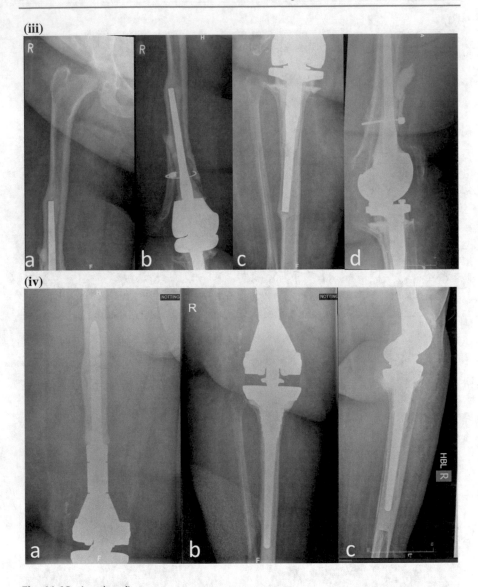

Fig. 11.12 (continued)

articulation. Achieving correct rotation of the components is crucial to ensure patellofemoral tracking, and this can be challenging with the loss of traditional landmarks such as the trans-epicondylar axis. Once satisfactory trial positioning is obtained, a mark is placed on the femur using diathermy to identify the position of the definitive implants which are assembled to match the trials and cemented in place, using Palacos R + G (Hereaus Medical GmbH, Germany). Additional antibiotics can be added to the cement as required.

In cases where PTR is planned, one of the main challenges is the reconstruction of the extensor mechanism. The METS® SMILES system with proximal tibial replacement provided with HA-coated metal tubercle attachment allowing the patella tendon to be reattached. We preserve the bony attachment of the patella tendon for reconstruction. Similar to the technique used in the distal femur, the level of resection is determined and a transverse osteotomy is performed with the remaining metaphyseal and diaphyseal bone removed to accommodate the proximal tibial replacement. In contrast to oncological applications of PTR where clear margins of resections are needed, in revision knee practice remnants of the posterior cortex of the proximal tibia can be left in situ protecting the posterior neurovascular structures. Routine closure is then performed in layers over a drain which is removed in 24 h. Full weight-bearing is commenced as tolerated with routine physiotherapy. Follow-up was performed regularly at 6 weeks, 3 months and 12 monthly thereafter.

Outcome Measures: clinical outcomes, surgical complications, reoperations, revision for any cause, loosening and mortality data were collected. Knee Society Score (KSS) at final follow up was used as patient' reported outcome measure.

Results: there were 33 consecutive patients with average age 79.6 years (range 58–89); 15 males and 18 females. All patients had multiple previous surgeries (median 4; range 3–8) and AORI-III massive bone defects in the distal femur and received DFRs. Six patients had concurrent AORI-III massive bone defects in the proximal tibia and also received PTRs. The indication for this salvage re-revision was infection in 16/33 (48.5%) patients following 2-stage procedures and aseptic loosening in the remining 17 patients (51.5%). One patient required pre-planned soft tissue coverage with gastrocnemius flap. In 21 patients (63.6%), we used METS® SMILES Total Knee Replacement (Stanmore Implants Worldwide Ltd) system including 6 PTR. The remining 12 (36.4%) patients had LPS™ Limb Preservation System (DePuy, Warsaw, IN).

Four patients had postoperative complications (12.1%). Two patients had a significant extensor lag; one patient with previous infected hinged knee who underwent 2-stage revision for infection and DFR reconstruction had a 20° extensor lag at 3 years follow up which limited his mobility. One patient with previous loose revision knee and catastrophic wear underwent DFR & PTR with a 25° extensor lag at 4 years follow up with subsequent limitation on her mobility and function. One patient with a previous infected hinged knee who underwent 2-stage revision procedures with DFR reconstruction developed patella dislocation 7 months post-operatively but maintained reasonable function and opted for conservative management. Finally, one patient who underwent 2-stage revision for infection with DFR reconstruction had recurrent infection and developed a sinus and was treated with suppressive lifelong antibiotic treatment having refused amputation.

The median follow-up was 5 years (range 2–15). At final follow up, median arc of flexion–extension was 100° (range 60–120). KSS was available for 29/33 patients with an average of 73.2 (range 51–86). However, patients with "infection" (n = 14) as their indication for limb-salvage had poorer scores with average 66.1 (range 51–81) vs. 81.6 (range 61–86) for "aseptic loosening" (n = 15). This difference was statistically significant (P < 0.0001). There was no difference in functional scores in relation to the implant used or patients' gender. Only one patient (3%) developed aseptic loosening of the femoral stem at 3 year follow up but remains asymptomatic and under close monitoring.

Survivorship analysis: None of the components have been revised to date. Eleven patients have died at median 4 years postoperatively (range 2–7) for unrelated causes. There was no difference in patients' survivorship between the two indications for salvage: infection vs. aseptic loosening. The overall patients' survivorship at 5-year was 80%.

In conclusion, salvage revision knee surgery is complex and challenging and requires significant resources and should only be undertaken within a multidisciplinary team approach.

References

1. *17th Annual Report of the National Joint Registry for England, Wales, Northern Ireland, the Isle of Man and the States of Guernsey*. [cited 2020 23rd Oct]; Available from https://reports.njrcentre.org.uk/Portals/0/PDFdownloads/NJR%2017th%20Annual%20Report%202020.pdf.
2. Hamilton DF et al. Dealing with the predicted increase in demand for revision total knee arthroplasty: challenges, risks and opportunities. Bone Joint J. 2015; 97-b(6):723–8.
3. Geary MB et al. Why Do Revision Total Knee Arthroplasties Fail? A Single-Center Review of 1632 Revision Total Knees Comparing Historic and Modern Cohorts. J Arthroplasty; 2020.
4. Engh GA, Ammeen DJ. Bone loss with revision total knee arthroplasty: defect classification and alternatives for reconstruction. Instr Course Lect. 1999;48:167–75.
5. Huff TW, Sculco TP. Management of bone loss in revision total knee arthroplasty. J Arthroplasty. 2007;22(7 Suppl 3):32–6.
6. Bush JL, Wilson JB, Vail TP. Management of bone loss in revision total knee arthroplasty. Clin Orthop Relat Res. 2006;452:186–92.
7. Backstein D, Safir O, Gross A. Management of bone loss: structural grafts in revision total knee arthroplasty. Clin Orthop Relat Res. 2006;446:104–12.
8. Clatworthy MG et al. The use of structural allograft for uncontained defects in revision total knee arthroplasty. A minimum five-year review. J Bone Joint Surg Am. 2001;83(3):404–11.
9. Dennis DA. The structural allograft composite in revision total knee arthroplasty. J Arthroplasty. 2002;17(4 Suppl 1):90–3.
10. Panegrossi G, et al. Bone loss management in total knee revision surgery. Int Orthop. 2014;38 (2):419–27.
11. Wilding CP, et al. Can a silver-coated arthrodesis implant provide a viable alternative to above knee amputation in the unsalvageable, infected total knee arthroplasty? J Arthroplasty. 2016;31(11):2542–7.
12. Matar HE, Stritch P, Emms N. Outcomes of implant-arthrodesis as limb salvage for failed total knee arthroplasties with significant bone loss: case series. J Long Term Eff Med Implants. 2018;28(4):347–53.
13. Chen AF, et al. Better function for fusions versus above-the-knee amputations for recurrent periprosthetic knee infection. Clin Orthop Relat Res. 2012;470(10):2737–45.
14. Pala E, et al. Megaprosthesis of the knee in tumor and revision surgery. Acta Biomed. 2017;88(2s):129–38.
15. Höll S, et al. Distal femur and proximal tibia replacement with megaprosthesis in revision knee arthroplasty: a limb-saving procedure. Knee Surg Sports Traumatol Arthrosc. 2012;20 (12):2513–8.

16. Korim MT, et al. A systematic review of endoprosthetic replacement for non-tumour indications around the knee joint. Knee. 2013;20(6):367–75.
17. Biau D, et al. Survival of total knee replacement with a megaprosthesis after bone tumor resection. J Bone Joint Surg Am. 2006;88(6):1285–93.
18. Albergo JI, et al. Proximal tibia reconstruction after bone Tumor resection: are survivorship and outcomes of Endoprosthetic replacement and Osteoarticular allograft similar? Clin Orthop Relat Res. 2017;475(3):676–82.
19. Bus MP, et al. What are the long-term results of MUTARS(®) modular endoprostheses for reconstruction of tumor resection of the distal femur and proximal Tibia? Clin Orthop Relat Res. 2017;475(3):708–18.
20. Henderson ER, et al. Failure mode classification for tumor endoprostheses: retrospective review of five institutions and a literature review. J Bone Joint Surg Am. 2011;93(5):418–29.
21. Engh CA, Bobyn JD, Glassman AH, Porous-coated hip replacement. The factors governing bone ingrowth, stress shielding, and clinical results. J Bone Joint Surg Br. 1987;69(1):45–55.
22. Amanatullah DF, et al. Non-oncologic total femoral arthroplasty: retrospective review. J Arthroplasty. 2014;29(10):2013–5.
23. Fonseca F, Sousa A, Completo A. Femoral revision knee Arthroplasty with Metaphyseal sleeves: the use of a stem is not mandatory of a structural point of view. J Exp Orthop. 2020;7 (1):24.
24. Lombardi AV, Jr, Berend KR, The shattered femur: radical solution options. J Arthrop. 2006;21(4 Suppl 1):107–11.
25. Berend KR, et al. Total femoral arthroplasty for salvage of end-stage prosthetic disease. Clin Orthop Relat Res. 2004;427:162–70.
26. Sierra RJ, Trousdale RT, Pagnano MW, Above-the-knee amputation after a total knee replacement: prevalence, etiology, and functional outcome. J Bone Joint Surg Am. 2003;85-a (6):1000–4.
27. Fedorka CJ, et al. Functional ability after above-the-knee amputation for infected total knee arthroplasty. Clin Orthop Relat Res. 2011;469(4):1024–32.
28. Pring DJ, Marks L, Angel JC. Mobility after amputation for failed knee replacement. J Bone Joint Surg Br. 1988;70(5):770–1.
29. Rodriguez-Merchan EC. Knee fusion or above-the-knee amputation after failed two-stage Reimplantation total knee arthroplasty. Arch Bone Jt Surg. 2015;3(4):241–3.
30. Matar HE, Bloch BV, James PJ. Outcomes of salvage Endoprostheses in revision total knee arthroplasty for infection and aseptic loosening: experience of a specialist centre. Knee. 2021;29:547–56.

Managing Infection in Revision Total Knee Arthroplasty: A Practical Perspective

12

> *Wise and humane management of the patient is the best safeguard against infection.*
>
> Florence Nightingale

12.1 Introduction

Periprosthetic joint infection (PJI) is a devastating complication with significant implications on patient-reported outcomes and mortality [1, 2]. Estimates of the incidence of PJI after primary TKA ranges between 0.85% in Germany, 1.0% in the UK, 1.4% in Finland and 2.2% in the USA [3–6]. PJI is associated with increased costs to healthcare systems with a significant economic burden [7].

The principles and concepts of managing PJI in rTKA are well-established. The International Consensus Meeting on musculoskeletal infections and PJIs provided a framework for treatment and a comprehensive review of PJI literature [8]. The worldwide gold standard for managing chronic infections in TKA has traditionally been a two-stage revision approach, with success rates of 70 to 90% being reported [9–11]. High success rates have also been achieved with a single-stage revision approach, with a growing body of evidence demonstrating both its effectiveness and improved outcomes in appropriately selected patients [12, 13]. In this chapter, we will focus on the practical aspects of PJI management and present our recent tertiary experience.

© The Author(s), under exclusive license to Springer Nature Switzerland AG 2021   223
H. E. Matar et al., *Revision Total Knee Arthroplasty*,
https://doi.org/10.1007/978-3-030-81285-0_12

12.2   PJI Classifications

A number of risk factors for failure to eradicate PJI have been identified including longer duration of symptoms, *Staphylococcus aureus* infections especially with methicillin-resistant strains, culture-negative infections, prior revisions, and the integrity of the surrounding soft tissues [14–19]. Several classification systems which take account of these risk factors are used for the diagnosis of PJI, with the most recent coming from the Musculoskeletal Infection Society (MSIS) [8].

Practically, however, what we found most useful in our decision-making process is that of duration of symptoms; acute versus chronic:

Acute infections either occur within 4–6 weeks of surgery, usually caused by *Staphylococcus aureus,* or are acute haematogenous infections that can happen years after surgery. The latter is very often caused by *streptococci* infections or other bacteraemia that can seed deposits around the implants. Patients with acute infections present unwell with fever, leucocytosis, an inflamed swollen joint, and with significantly raised inflammatory markers. Here, the diagnosis is often easy to make. Early joint aspiration is advised before systemic antibiotics are given, the fluid should be sent for urgent gram stain, microscopy and culture analyses. In the majority of cases, urgent gram stain will reveal *gram-positive cocci* with numerous white cells on microscopy examination.

Chronic infections tend to be of low virulence. Here, the presentation is more disparate ranging from chronic PJI presenting with sinuses, usually with a history of the knee being very unhappy, to a knee that has never been satisfactory and grumbling along since the time of implantation. In the latter, while there are a lot of aseptic causes for pain, infection must always be ruled out. Radiographically, we occasionally see changes around the implant but very often radiographs look relatively normal in the early stages. Chronic changes include scalloping around the component, particularly under the tibial tray or behind the femoral component. Further, unhealthy looking bone with periosteal reactions or elevations are seen in neglected cases.

Top Tip: Acute PJI has a clear presentation with 4–6 weeks of duration of symptoms, chronic PJI are more disparate from a grumbling unhappy knee to chronically infected knees with discharging sinuses.

12.3   Practical Approach to Diagnosing PJI

Acute PJI: relatively straightforward, unwell septic patient with hot swollen joint, raised inflammatory markers. Aspiration is mandatory before systemic antibiotics are given and operative strategy is planned.

Chronic PJI: diagnosing chronic PJI is more challenging. By far, the most important factor is clinical suspicion which is then supported by confirmatory investigations. In our practice, we rely on the history and traditional inflammatory markers early in the process; white cell counts, C-reactive protein (CRP) and Erythrocyte sedimentation rate (ESR).

If the inflammatory markers are completely normal and we have a low index of suspicion clinically, then the chances of infection are very low although not completely excluded.

If the CRP is persistently elevated with mildly raised ESR and no other explanation or systemic issues with a painful TKA, the chances of infection are much higher. Here, we have to hunt for it and get a definite microbiological diagnosis before embarking on revision surgery.

The next easy step is joint aspiration for culture and microscopy which are readily available. The presence of numerous white cells in the aspirate are usually consistent with infection even if the organism could not be identified. In 75–80% of cases, a culture yields an organism [20]. In approximately 1/5 cases where there is high index of suspicion of infection, we fail to culture an organism. Here, a repeat aspiration might be useful. Newer technologies such as polymerase chain reaction (PCR) can be helpful if available. Alternatively, a synovial or bone biopsy done arthroscopically might aid the diagnosis.

12.4 How Would Identifying an Organism Change the Management of Chronic PJI?

(a) Knowing the infecting organism in advance facilitate choice of antibiotics based on the sensitivities, both to be added to the cement intraoperatively and for tailored postoperative antibiotic therapy.

(b) Allows discussion with microbiology specialists on the susceptibility of the organism to antibiotic treatment i.e., a *'friendly bug'* or *'unfriendly bug'*.

(c) Helps with the decision making of whether a single- or two-stage approach is appropriate. For example, if we have a *coagulase-negative staphylococcus (CNS)* that is fully sensitive in a chronic PJI case with preservation of bone stock and good soft tissues in an immunocompetent host, then a single-stage approach is appropriate. If, on the other hand, we have a *gram-negative organism, Enterococcus, or Staphylococcus lugdunensis* i.e. an 'unfriendly bug', then a two-stage approach is more appropriate. This is despite the fact that *Staphylococcus lugdunensis* is a low-grade infection but it is characteristically difficult to eradicate and a two-stage approach would have better chance of success.

In modern arthroplasty practice, as we strive to improve patients' outcomes, gaining all the necessary information about the profile and characteristics of the infecting organism facilitates an informed discussion in a multidisciplinary team meeting with microbiology specialists to decide duration of antibiotic treatment, route of administration, antibiotics usage in cement, etc. This will help improve outcomes and success rate, and so the entire journey of a PJI case should be provisionally planned preoperatively.

Top Tip: Identifying the infecting organism preoperatively helps the decision-making and operative strategy of a single- versus two-stage approach.

12.5   Culture Negative PJIs

There will always be a group of patients where the above investigations will not yield a positive result. If we clinically suspect infection and we have raised inflammatory markers but no organism, we will still treat it as infection.

This is likely because the current commonly used technologies in most hospitals worldwide are insufficient to detect the indolent low-grade organisms that exist in the biofilm especially because we do not sample the biofilm preoperatively. Sonification of the implant is therefore useful in giving a retrospective identification. Interestingly, in an old study, we have demonstrated that in all revision cases (septic and aseptic) organisms can be identified through prolonged cultures and ultra-sonification. Implant colonisation at time of implantation was the main theory behind this, which may not be clinically significant, but in some patients when the balance tips in favour of the organism, symptoms can ultimately develop [21].

Traditionally, CN-PJIs are treated with a two-stage approach. Although, logically these are low-grade infections and with an immunocompetent host and good soft tissues, a single-stage technique might be considered within an MDT approach using wide-spectrum antibiotics (Teicoplanin or equivalent) until operative samples are cultured as we have successfully done in a number of cases [22].

Top Tip: Culture negative PJI is where infection is clinically suspected with raised inflammatory markers but no identifiable organism (approximately 20% of PJI cases). It is important to decide your operative strategy within an MDT framework and in conjunction with a microbiology specialist.

12.6   Operative Strategies

Acute Infections: with certain prerequisites in place, a DAIR procedure should always be attempted first in the acute settings to decrease the septic load and prevent overwhelming systemic sepsis. If a DAIR fails to cure the infection ($\sim 20\%$), then by definition the infection becomes chronic.

Chronic Infections: although a two-stage approach is the worldwide gold standard and remains the preferred strategy in specific scenarios, a single-stage approach has also been proven to be as effective in appropriately selected patients.

12.7 When to Do a DAIR?

Debridement, antibiotics and implant retention is indicated when the following criteria are met:

(a) Well-fixed implants with no radiographic changes suggestive of loosening
(b) History of a well-functioning knee until recently or immediate postoperative infection (<4–6 weeks)
(c) Must be performed by an experienced arthroplasty surgeon.

DAIR is not simply an arthrotomy and washout, it is a radical debridement of all infected tissues with synovectomy, clearing the interfaces, and clearing out the posterior space as much as possible. This is the most difficult part of the operation and mandates the removal of the modular polyethylene insert. We then physically scrub the implant with a brush to disrupt the biofilm, copiously wash the knee with mechanical lavage (pulsatile lavage) and finally exchange the polyethylene. Closure is performed over a 24-h drain.

12.8 DAIR and Revision Implants

Exposure is harder here with a varus valgus constraint implant, but easier with hinged implants with no collaterals and where the hinge mechanism can be disassembled. VVC implants are more difficult, as we have to be patient to get sufficient access, clear the gutters, and sublux the tibia far enough forward to extract the polyethylene insert. The principles of DAIR are the same as those for a primary implant.

If, however, the infected revision knee is very stiff precluding adequate access, then one should question the rationale behind salvaging the implant with a DAIR, and a formal revision strategy for infection is needed through either a single- or two-stage approach based on the individual case. If the previous revision was performed for infection, we would routinely consider a two-stage approach.

What About Arthroscopic Washout? This is only indicated in emergency cases (out of hours) as a life-saving procedure to reduce the septic load, decompress the joint, obtain microbiological samples, and start intravenous antibiotics in view of a formal DAIR within 24–48 h.

Top Tip: DAIR is not simply an arthrotomy and washout, it is a radical debridement of all infected tissues with synovectomy, posterior space clearance, physical disruption of the biofilm, mechanical lavage and a modular polyethylene exchange.

12.9 Duration of Antibiotics Following DAIR

This is guided by microbiology support, the infecting organism profile and host factors. However, typically three months of antibiotics are required. Historically, this used to be 3 months intravenous followed by 3 months oral antibiotics. However, in our practice we now use intravenous antibiotics for a maximum of 6 weeks followed by oral therapy for the remining 6 weeks. This is supported by the recent multi-centre OVIVA randomised controlled trial *(Oral versus Intravenous Antibiotics for Bone and Joint Infection)* which demonstrated that oral antibiotic therapy was non-inferior to intravenous antibiotic therapy when used during the first 6 weeks for complex orthopaedic infections, as assessed by treatment failure at 1 year [23]. This has encouraged us to further shorten the period of intravenous administration with earlier transition to an oral alternative.

12.10 Outcomes of DAIR for Acute PJI

The literature suggests that a well-done DAIR has 70–80% chance of success in salvaging the implant [24–27], and our experience is also in keeping with this. A successful DAIR is certainly a better outcome for the patient than a full revision surgery through either a single- or two-stage approach. Those who fail a DAIR would become a chronic PJI and are usually managed through a two-stage approach.

Top Tip: We would caution against deploying a single-stage strategy to treat acutely septic patients.

12.11 Chronic PJIs—Single or Two-Stage?

Historically, our standard practice in treating chronic PJIs has been a two-stage approach. Since the mid-2000s, we have also routinely used a single-stage approach in selected patients with a single infecting organism and known sensitivities in immunocompetent patients without soft tissue compromise and in the absence of systemic sepsis or a draining sinus [28]. We adopt a shared decision-making process with patients within an MDT framework including a specialist microbiologist (Table 12.1). A recent systematic review of observational studies using a meta-analytic approach (10 single-stage studies including 423 patients and 108 two-stage studies including 5,129 patients), reported re-infection rates within 2 years of 7.6% in single-stage versus 8.8% in two-stage approach [12]. However, indications for either approach differ significantly among institutions making direct comparisons difficult.

Table 12.1 factors that may influence the decision to use a two-stage revision approach

Patient factors	Microbiological factors	Surgical factors
Poor soft tissues	Culture-negative PJI	Previous failed DAIR or revision for infection
Chronic immunosuppression	Antibiotic resistant organism	Extensor mechanism loss
Sinus tract	Fungal PJI	Soft tissue defect requiring plastic surgical cover

PJI: periprosthetic joint infection; DAIR: debridement, antibiotics and implant retention

The essence of surgery for infection in either single- or two-stage approach is debridement of all infected materials. The technique is simple and reproducible; a full synovectomy, full clearance of the gutters, getting to the posterior space once the implant is removed, mechanical debridement, copious washout, and multiple samples throughout taken with multiple scalpel blades and forceps to minimise cross contamination.

12.12   Operative Technique

(a) *Single-stage approach:* using a standard midline incision and medial parapatellar approach, a radical synovectomy is performed with debridement and removal of all components and cement. Multiple tissue samples are taken for microbiology before administration of antibiotics and thorough irrigation with pulsatile lavage. The wound is then soaked in aqueous Chlorhexidine (0.5%) and the wound edges are approximated, wrapped with sterile crepe bandage and the tourniquet is deflated. The patient is then re-draped, the surgical team rescrubs, and new instruments are used. Further lavage is undertaken, and implantation of a new prosthesis is performed using antibiotic-loaded cement according to known sensitivities. Postoperatively, patients continue antibiotic therapy for 12 weeks (6 weeks intravenous followed by 6 weeks of oral preparations whenever possible based on patients' tolerance and organisms' sensitivities), with regular monitoring of the clinical response and inflammatory markers. This is supervised and closely monitored by a specialist microbiologist both as an inpatient and in Outpatient Parenteral Antibiotic Therapy clinic (OPAT clinic) settings.

(b) *Stage-1 of two-stage approach:* as above, this involves a thorough debridement with radical synovectomy and removal of all components, cement and infected tissue. We aim to use an articulating spacer whenever possible; our preference is a standard TKA prosthesis with an all-poly tibia component (Figs. 12.1, 12.2). If there is not enough bone to support a temporary spacer, or there is ligamentous disruption, then a static spacer spanning the knee joint is utilised. Our routine practice in these cases is to use a temporary fusion nail as a static

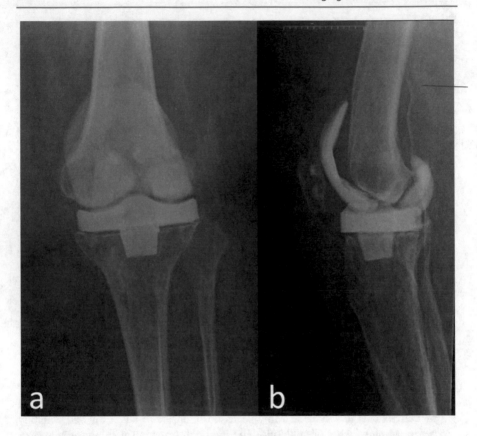

Fig. 12.1 Example of a fractured cement mould articulating spacer

spacer (Fig. 12.2). These spacers are implanted with antibiotic-loaded bone cement and the antibiotics are tailored to the infecting organism. Our standard practice is to add 1 g of Vancomycin per 40 g mix cement, unless advised otherwise by our microbiologist based on the microbiological profile of the infecting organism when identified.

Antibiotic therapy is continued for 6 weeks, with regular monitoring of the clinical response and inflammatory markers in OPAT clinic. In those rare cases where little progress is made, this stage can be repeated with further debridement and change of spacer. Once the infection is controlled and eradicated (relying on clinical assessment of patients' symptoms, status of their soft tissue envelope around the knee, and normalisation of inflammatory markers), we procced to stage-2 with joint reconstruction within 6–9 months. However, if patients with 'articulating spacers' achieve good functional outcomes with their all-poly TKA prosthesis, no further surgery is undertaken and revision is only considered for future aseptic loosening.

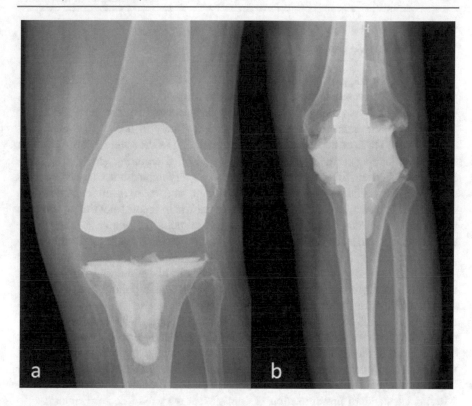

Fig. 12.2 Examples of **a** articulating spacer using a definitive knee prosthesis (all-poly tibial component); **b** example of intramedullary fusion nail used as a static spacer following stage 1/two stage-revision with significant bone loss and ligamentous instability

(c) ***Stage-2 of two-stage approach:*** following appropriate preoperative planning for joint reconstruction including normalised inflammatory markers and a negative aspiration for infection, the joint is exposed using the old scar, and a radical synovectomy is once again performed with further debridement of scar tissue recreating the medial and lateral gutters. The spacer is explanted, and multiple samples are taken for microbiological analysis. An assessment is then made of the bone loss and ligamentous integrity. In our practice, we routinely use implants with metaphyseal sleeves for biological fixation on the tibial side and in selected cases on the femoral side with both cemented and cementless options available with varying degrees of constrained implants based on individual factors such as bone loss, joint line restoration and ligamentous insufficiency. We routinely continue antibiotics until all the intraoperative culture results are available and stop antibiotics if samples are culture negative.

12.13   Why Do We Use a Definitive Prosthesis as an Articulating Spacer?

The interval management between stages is challenging. As outlined, in our practice, we use an articulating spacer whenever possible, using a TKA prosthesis (PFC Sigma, all-poly tibia). We developed this approach in the early 2000s, to replace the static cement spacers which were routinely in use at that time. Our experience of static cement spacers was disappointing as they were poorly tolerated by patients leaving them with poor function and often requiring an external brace for support. Further, 2nd stage reconstruction was very unpleasant with oedematous tissues, spacers that would move and dislodge, and as a result exposure was unnecessarily difficult. We realised that going back in to reconstruct the joint within 6–8 weeks was not ideal from a soft tissue point of view as they were non-compliant and very oedematous which made exposure much more difficult to achieve safely.

We then moved to cement articulating moulds to allow the knee to move but these were also problematic as they creaked, broke, were painful and offered no robust stability for mobilisation (Fig. 12.1). We then elected to use a knee prosthesis, with an all-poly tibia which is the cheapest option with numerous advantages. First, it offers patients stability to mobilise, and additional tailored antibiotics can be added to the cement. We must have adequate bone to support it, as it will not work with significant bone loss. We also require intact collateral ligaments in order to get a stable construct with it. We cement it well enough so that it is well-fixed but without the standard pressurisation of cement that we would do for primaries.

Secondly, it keeps the patients mobile, comfortable, and therefore as there was not such a compelling rush for a 2nd stage revision within 6–8 weeks, we started going back in for the second stage much later, at 6–9 months. In this prolonged interval, we are able to monitor inflammatory markers ensuring that infection remains eradicated long after the antibiotics had stopped, and we gained more confidence in achieving a successful outcome. As patients were mobilising, the soft tissues improved and it became easier to identify anatomical planes, so we realised that 2nd stage reconstruction was a far more pleasant operation at 6 months compared with 6 weeks. Finally, a good proportion of those patients never required a 2nd stage revision and were functioning very well with their definitive knee prosthesis [22].

Top Tip: Using a definitive knee prosthesis as an articulating spacer offers numerous advantages: stability, mobility, function, a longer interval to 2nd stage, and in many cases it acts as a definitive prosthesis with no further surgery required.

12.14   Why Do We Use a Fusion Nail as a Static Spacer?

If we have significant bone loss or ligamentous instability, then we must use static spacers. Originally the only option was to use a manually fashioned 'hamburger-like' cement spacer. Again, these were unstable and they migrated, dislodged and fractured. Patients did not trust these spacers to mobilise and we were forced to go back and reconstruct with a 2nd stage earlier with suboptimal soft tissues.

We therefore use a temporary modular fusion nail (Figs. 12.3 and 12.4), locked inside the knee with two screws. This offers skeletal stability from the nail, and we can then pack the joint between the femur and tibia with antibiotic loaded cement. This technique ensures that we keep the right length and tissue tension, allows delivery of antibiotics, provides stability at the knee for mobilisation and weight bearing, and allow us to plan 2nd stage at a time of our choosing with better soft tissue status.

We do not cement the stems in the canals, but we do cement in the metaphysis to give us stability in the bone from the nail at the joint surface, and the cement wrapped around the nail into the metaphysis gives us excellent stability for mobilisation. We use long enough nails to give us adequate working length for stability and engage the diaphysis for axial loading. This is short term stability that we require in the interval period. This combination gives us 6–12 months interval before 2nd stage reconstruction.

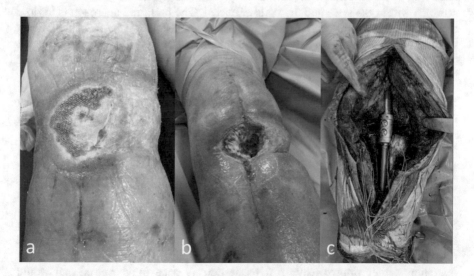

Fig. 12.3 (**a-b**) Example of a case with infected local flap; (**c**) intraoperative photograph at the end of the debridement of a 1st stage revision following crest osteotomy for exposure and trialling a static fusion nail spacer

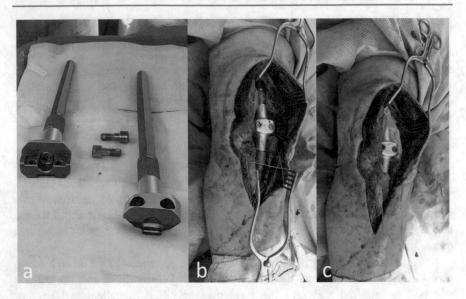

Fig. 12.4 **a** Example of a different modular fusion nail implant; **b** assembled intraoperatively following debridement with centrally locked bolts; **c** antibiotic-loaded cement is used to stabilise the nail

However, at the time of the 2nd stage, the knees are stiff, and the nail requires removing which is straightforward as they are centrally locked and can be disassembled within the knee and the nails extracted. The preferred approach is to do a crest osteotomy for exposure. Reconstruction is not prejudiced by this, and we can still use condylar revisions unless there is significant bone or ligamentous loss that would require a hinge reconstruction. After all, we have healthy compliant soft tissues in a sterile field to work with.

Top Tip: In cases with significant bone loss following 1st stage, a temporary fusion nail is our static spacer of choice. It offers stability, mobility, function, and allows a longer interval to 2nd stage with better soft tissues.

12.15 What to Do with Sinuses?

Sinuses are pathways of pus and infected fluids; they often form an epithelial tract and require full excision. If at the end of debridement, you have pliable tissues and no tension, they can be closed primarily. It is important not to compromise your operation; larger sinuses leave soft tissue defects once fully excised and would require local or regional flaps with plastic surgical input.

12.16   Why Do 1st Stages Fail?

If we do not appreciate the extent of the infected mass, particularly the posterior space into the condyles, we can leave infected tissue behind and compromise the outcome. Inadequate debridement is the biggest single cause of failure. Other causes, however, include a poor host, an unfriendly bug, lack of stability for the temporary reconstruction, or inadequate soft tissue cover.

While the same process can be repeated above, we should always be self-critical and ask whether we needed better soft tissue cover or plastic surgical input? Is it a different bug? Is there a fungus? Should we re-culture? Can we improve the host (e.g. nutritional status)? Etc.

12.17   Can We Use Press-Fit Metaphyseal Sleeves at Time of Reconstruction?

At single stage revision, the traditional teaching is to use antibiotic-loaded cemented fixation to get local antibiotic delivery, which is appropriate to the bacterial sensitivity. At 2nd stage reconstruction, here we have a sterile field with eradicated infection, hence our choice of implant is dictated by the amount of bone loss and ligamentous stability ranging from the use of condylar revision implants to hinged prosthesis and salvage endoprostheses. Our standard choice of adjunct fixation is metaphyseal sleeves particularly on the tibial side, with antibiotic-laden cement at the joint surface.

Press-fit sleeves can still be used as they are accompanied by surface-cementing of the component with antibiotic loaded cement. Secondly, PJI is a joint infection rather than a bone infection. We do often see how the infection is walled off from the intramedullary canals by a neocortex. We therefore maintain that if the joint infection is treated appropriately, joint reconstruction should not be compromised and if press-fit cementless sleeves or stems are needed for a durable fixation, they should be used once a bed of healthy bone for ingrowth is prepared.

Top Tip: Managing PJI is challenging and should be undertaken as part of an MDT framework with senior experienced colleagues, specialist microbiologists and plastic surgical input. Dual-consultant operating may be beneficial to help ensure a successful outcome.

12.18   Our Case Series on *Chronic* PJI

In a retrospective consecutive study, we reported on all patients who underwent rTKA for first-time *chronic* infection at our unit between 1st April 2003 and 31st Dec 2018 [22]. Patients with acute infections (<6 weeks duration of symptoms) were excluded.

Outcome measures: the primary outcome measure was failure to eradicate infection defined by any of the following outcomes [29]:

(a) Persistent or recurrent infection by either the same or a different organism
(b) Receipt of long-term antibiotics as suppressive treatment of infection
(c) Implant-arthrodesis as salvage for infection
(d) Limb amputation occurring at any point during follow-up
(e) Death within 90-day after a surgical procedure. We used 90-day mortality as this is a nationally collected NJR-linked data.

Reoperations and any further surgeries were recorded. Variables evaluated for failure were prospectively collected and included gender, age, BMI, ASA score and infecting organisms. Patients' survivorship data were also collected. Death was identified through both local hospital electronic databases and linked data from the National Joint Registry/NHS Personal Demographic Service.

Statistical Analysis: Differences in patient characteristics were assessed using the *chi-square test* for categorical variables and the *t-test* for continuous variables; differences were considered significant for *P*-value <0.05. A forward, stepwise, logistic regression model to identify independent predictors of failure was performed. The validity of the model was assessed by estimating the goodness-of-fit to the data with *Hosmer–Lemeshow* test. Statistical significance was defined as a two-tailed P <0.05. A priori, the following covariates were included in the model, known to be associated with PJI treatment outcome: age, the causative microorganism (categorised into *Staphylococcus aureus*, culture-negative PJI and other), presence of a sinus, BMI and ASA grade [9, 12, 14–17]. *Kaplan–Meier survival* curves were used to estimate time to failure and time to death. The *log-rank test* was used to test statistical significance. Statistical analyses were performed using SPSS 16.0 software (SPSS Inc., Chicago, IL).

Results: During the study period, 292 consecutive first-time knee revisions for chronic infection were performed on 288 patients. There were 82 single-stage (28.1%) and 210 (71.9%) two-stage revisions.

The average age was 71 years (range 27–90) with 165 females (57.4%) and average BMI of 30.9 (range 20–53) with no significant differences between the two groups in basic demographic characteristics (Table 12.2).

Thirty-six rTKA (17.14%) had tracking sinuses and hence were not deemed suitable for a single-stage approach. Significantly more patients had a known infecting organism in the single-stage group (93.9% vs. 80.47%; P = 0.0047), again reflecting the different indications for each approach. The overall number of cases per year has been increasing steadily during the study period; number of single-stage revisions has also been increasing annually particularly over the last 10 years which reflects the intended change in clinical practice (Fig. 12.5).

Microbiological data (Table 12.3): the infecting organism was identified pre-operatively in 246 cases (84.2%) with 46 (15.8%) CN-PJI. Only 5 CN-PJI cases were in the single stage group; these patients were immunocompetent with no soft tissue defects and opted for a single stage approach rather than our standard

Table 12.2 Demographic and surgical data

Demographics	TOTAL	Single-stage	Two-stage	P-value
Number of revisions	N = 292	N = 82	N = 210	–
Demographics:				
Patient Age (y) [Median (IQR)]	71 (65–78)	71 (65–79)	71 (64–78)	0.395
Female [N (%)]	165 (57.4)	47 (57.9)	118 (56.2)	0.792
BMI [Median (IQR)] Mean ± SD (range)	30 (27–34) 30.9 ± 6.0(20–53)	30 (27–33) 29.9 ± 5.6 (20–51)	30 (27–35) 31.3 ± 6.1(20–53)	0.07
Presence of sinus N (%)	36 (17.14)	–	36 (17.14)	**0.0001**
Known organism N (%)	246 (84.24)	77 (93.9)	169 (80.47)	**0.0047**
ASA: N (%) I	12 (4.10)	7 (8.53)	5 (2.38)	**0.0175**
II	150 (51.36)	41 (50.0)	109 (51.9)	0.7707
III	113 (38.69)	29 (35.36)	84 (40.0)	0.4652
IV	17 (5.85)	5 (6.11)	12 (5.72)	0.8985
Follow up (years) [Median (IQR)] Mean ± SD (range)	5.4 (4.4–8.7) 6.3 ± 3.88(2–17.6)	4.5 (3.9–6.8) 4.47 ± 2.92 (2–13.7)	5.9 (4.9–8.52) 7.42 ± 4.15 (2–17.6)	**0.0001**

two-stage approach in CN-PJI cases. *Coagulase negative Staphylococcus* species were the most common (28.1%) followed by *Staphylococcus aureus* (25.3%). Of those patients who had failed treatment (27/292), *Staphylococcus aureus* was the most common infecting organism in 12/27 rTKA (44.4%).

Failure rate: the average follow-up of the entire cohort was 6.3 years (range 2–17.6) with longer follow up in the two-stage group (4.47 vs. 7.42 years; P = 0.0001). In the single-stage group there were 5/82 (6.1%) failures; 2 (2.4%) patients died within 90-days and three (3.7%) had recurrent infections; two were treated successfully with a two-stage approach and one had further infections and a failed extensor mechanism and was treated with definitive arthrodesis (Fig. 12.6). All failures occurred in the first four years following their rTKA (Fig. 12.7).

In the two-stage group, there were 210 rTKA; 6 patients (2.9%) required a repeat 1st stage procedure and 3 patients (1.4%) died within 90 days following their 1st stage. Of the remaining 207 rTKA, 46 (22.2%) achieved satisfactory functional outcomes with their articulating spacer, as a definitive knee prosthesis, and did not require further reconstruction; 161 rTKA proceeded to a 2nd stage procedure with 11.8% failure rate (n = 19) with recurrent infections; all recurred within 4 years of

Table 12.3 Microbiological data and infecting organisms

Infecting organisms	Total N (%)	Single-stage N (%)	Two-stage N (%)	P-value
Number of revisions	N = 292	N = 82	N = 210	-
Coagulase negative Staphylococcus	82 (28.1)	25 (30.49)	57 (27.14)	0.5677
Staphylococcus aureus	74 (25.3)	20 (24.40)	54 (25.71)	0.8174
MRSA	3 (1)	–	3 (1.43)	0.2772
Enterococcus species	18 (6.2)	1 (1.22)	17 (8.10)	**0.0283***
Escherichia coli	15 (5.1)	5 (6.09)	10 (4.76)	0.6441
Streptococci species (*milleri, gordonii, oralis, dysgalactiae, Viridans*)	14 (4.8)	8 (9.76)	6 (2.86)	**0.0133***
B-haemolytic Streptococcus (B, C, G)	18 (6.2)	11 (13.41)	7 (3.34)	**0.0013***
Mixed growth	8 (2.7)	–	8 (3.80)	0.0740
Others:	14 (4.8)	7 (8.54)	7 (3.34)	0.0622
– *Diphtheroid bacilli*		–2	–	
– *Pasteurella multocida*		–	–1	
– *Propionibacterium*		–1	–	
– *Proteus mirabilis*		–1	–1	
– *Pseudomonas aeruginosa*		–2	–5	
– *Ureaplasma parvum*		–1	–	
Culture Negative-PJI	46 (15.8)	5 (6.09)	41 (19.52)	**0.0047**[a]
Infecting organisms for patients with septic failures and early deaths^:				
Total	27 (9.2)	5 (6.09)	22 (10.48)	0.2453
– *Staphylococcus aureus*	12 (44.4)	–3 (60)	–9 (41)	0.4489
– *E. coli*	1 (3.8)	–1 (20)	–	
– *Streptococci*	3 (11.1)	–1 (20)	–2 (9.05)	0.4895
– *CNS*	6 (22.2)	–	–6 (27.3)	
–*Enterococci*	3 (11.1)	–	–3 (13.6)	
– *CN-PJI*	2 (7.4)	–	–2 (9.05)	

[a]*Statistically significant; MRSA: methicillin-resistant Staphylococcus aureus;* ^*death within 90 days*

the rTKA (Fig. XX). Eighteen cases underwent a further two-stage rTKA with a successful outcome in 11/18 (61%), four had a definitive arthrodesis with extensor failure and poor soft tissue cover with repeated surgeries and one required above knee amputation.

Regression analysis: the cumulative probability of treatment failure in two-stage group was statistically significantly higher for patients who had a sinus (OR 4.97; CI 95% 1.593 to 15.505; P = 0.006) and were aged > 80 years (OR 5.962; CI 95%

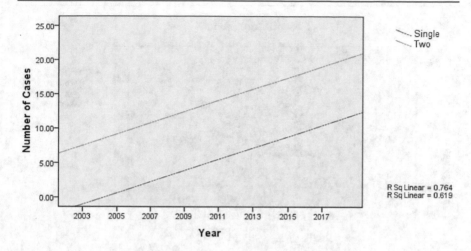

Fig. 12.5 Trend overtime of the use of single- versus two-stage approaches

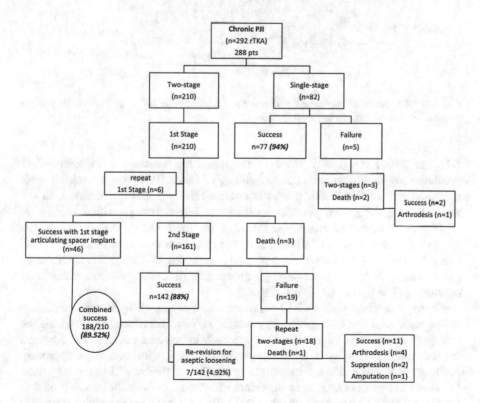

Fig. 12.6 Patients' flowchart and outcomes

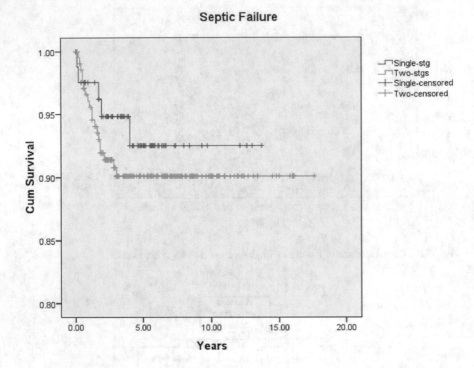

Fig. 12.7 Kaplan Meier survivorship curve with 'septic failure' as an end point; all failures occurred within the first 4 years postoperatively

1.156 to 30.73; P = 0.033). None of the remaining variables were independent predictors of failure in this cohort although higher BMI was associated with increased risk of failure but it was not statistically significant. Similarly, in the single-stage group no independent predictors of failure were identified.

10-year Patients' survivorship: At 10 years, there were 23/82 deaths in the single-stage group and 63/210 deaths in the two-stage group. Kaplan–Meier survivorship curves demonstrate 10-year survivorship rate of 72% in the single stage group versus 70.5% in the two-stage group; this difference was not statistically significant (P = 0.517, *Log-Rank test*).

During this study period of 17 years, our practice has changed with increasing deployment of a single-stage strategy which we have introduced in line with the emerging evidence in support of this approach in selected patients. We reported success rate of 94% with single stage versus 88% with two-stage approach. Although this is neither a randomised controlled trial, nor a direct comparison between the two cohorts due to important differences such as the absence of systemic sepsis or a communicating sinus and largely known single infecting organism in single-stage patients, a number of observations can be made from this data.

Firstly, a single-stage approach can achieve high rates of infection eradication in selected patients with meticulous surgical technique, aggressive debridement and removal of all cement, infected tissues and bone, judicious use of targeted antibiotic loaded cement and postoperative antibiotic protocol supported by a specialist microbiologist.

Secondly, a large group of the two-stage patients (46/210; 22%) who had their first of two-stage using a definitive knee prosthesis as a temporary spacer never required any further reconstruction. This subgroup is akin to a single-stage approach as we carry out our surgical debridement in the same fashion in both single-stage patients and stage one of two-stage patients. This adds to the validity of the results achieved using single-stage approach.

Thirdly, the standard practice in our unit in managing chronic PJI had been through the well-established two-stage approach for all patients. However, with the emerging evidence in the literature on the effectiveness and potential advantages [30, 31], we have cautiously introduced single-stage approach with strict selection criteria in the early stages. Our current contraindications are the presence of systemic sepsis, mixed bacterial infections, a tracking sinus or soft-tissue defects not amenable to primary closure, and failed previous revisions for infection or DAIR. Our experience with single stage revisions has increased over time and with good success rates our confidence has grown. We believe our data could serve as a model to units introducing a change to their practice whilst maintaining a high eradication rate and successful outcomes in treating chronic PJI.

In conclusion, managing PJI is challenging and a devastating complication both for the patient and the surgeon. Early intervention in acute infections with thorough debridement and modular exchange is preferred. Patient selection, meticulous surgical debridement, and targeted antibiotic treatment in conjunction with a specialist microbiologist are the most important factors to ensure success in managing chronic PJI in either single- or two-stage strategy.

References

1. Greidanus NV, et al. Quality of life outcomes in revision versus primary total knee arthroplasty. J Arthroplasty. 2011;26(4):615–20.
2. Zmistowski B, et al. Periprosthetic joint infection increases the risk of one-year mortality. J Bone Joint Surg Am. 2013;95(24):2177–84.
3. Blom AW, et al. Infection after total knee arthroplasty. J Bone Joint Surg Br. 2004;86(5):688–91.
4. Huotari K, Peltola M, Jämsen E. The incidence of late prosthetic joint infections: a registry-based study of 112,708 primary hip and knee replacements. Acta Orthop. 2015;86(3):321–5.
5. Kurtz SM, et al. Economic burden of periprosthetic joint infection in the United States. J Arthroplasty. 2012;27(8):61-5.e1.
6. Meyer E, et al. Impact of department volume on surgical site infections following arthroscopy, knee replacement or hip replacement. BMJ Qual Saf. 2011;20(12):1069–74.
7. Mathews JA et al. Top ten research priorities for problematic knee arthroplasty. Bone Joint J. 2020;102-b(9):1176–82.

8. Parvizi J, et al. The 2018 definition of periprosthetic hip and knee infection: an evidence-based and validated criteria. J Arthroplasty. 2018;33(5):1309-14.e2.
9. Kilgus DJ, Howe DJ, Strang A. Results of periprosthetic hip and knee infections caused by resistant bacteria. Clin Orthop Relat Res. 2002;404:116–24.
10. Romanò CL, et al. Two-stage revision of septic knee prosthesis with articulating knee spacers yields better infection eradication rate than one-stage or two-stage revision with static spacers. Knee Surg Sports Traumatol Arthrosc. 2012;20(12):2445–53.
11. Pangaud C, Ollivier M, Argenson JN. Outcome of single-stage versus two-stage exchange for revision knee arthroplasty for chronic periprosthetic infection. EFORT Open Rev. 2019;4 (8):495–502.
12. Kunutsor SK et al. Re-infection outcomes following one- and two-stage surgical revision of infected knee prosthesis: a systematic review and meta-analysis. PLoS One. 2016;11(3): e0151537.
13. Thakrar RR et al. Indications for a single-stage exchange arthroplasty for chronic prosthetic joint infection: a systematic review. Bone Joint J. 2019;101-b(1_Supple_A):19–24.
14. Kubista B, et al. Reinfection after two-stage revision for periprosthetic infection of total knee arthroplasty. Int Orthop. 2012;36(1):65–71.
15. Mortazavi SM, et al. Two-stage exchange arthroplasty for infected total knee arthroplasty: predictors of failure. Clin Orthop Relat Res. 2011;469(11):3049–54.
16. Massin P, et al. Infection recurrence factors in one- and two-stage total knee prosthesis exchanges. Knee Surg Sports Traumatol Arthrosc. 2016;24(10):3131–9.
17. Cunningham DJ, et al. Specific infectious organisms associated with poor outcomes in treatment for hip periprosthetic infection. J Arthroplasty. 2017;32(6):1984-90.e5.
18. Matar HE et al. Septic revision total knee arthroplasty is associated with significantly higher mortality than aseptic revisions: long-term single-center study (1254 Patients). J Arthroplasty. 2021.
19. Corona PS et al. Current actual success rate of the two-stage exchange arthroplasty strategy in chronic hip and knee periprosthetic joint infection. Bone Joint J. 2020;102-b(12):1682–88.
20. Tande AJ, Patel R. Prosthetic joint infection. Clin Microbiol Rev. 2014;27(2):302–45.
21. James PJ, et al. Methicillin-resistant Staphylococcus epidermidis in infection of hip arthroplasties. J Bone Joint Surg Br. 1994;76(5):725–7.
22. Matar HE et al. Long-term outcomes of single- and two-stage revision total knee arthroplasty for chronic periprosthetic joint infections: changing clinical practice in a specialist centre (292 Knees). Bone Joint J. 2021;Aug;103-B(8):1373–9.
23. Li HK, et al. Oral versus intravenous antibiotics for bone and joint infection. N Engl J Med. 2019;380(5):425–36.
24. Leta TH et al. Outcome of revision surgery for infection after total knee arthroplasty: results of 3 surgical strategies. JBJS Rev. 2019;7(6):e4.
25. Vahedi H, et al. Irrigation, débridement, and implant retention for recurrence of periprosthetic joint infection following two-stage revision total knee arthroplasty: a matched cohort study. J Arthroplasty. 2019;34(8):1772–5.
26. Barry JJ, et al. Irrigation and debridement with chronic antibiotic suppression is as effective as 2-stage exchange in revision total knee arthroplasty with extensive instrumentation. J Bone Joint Surg Am. 2021;103(1):53–63.
27. Weston JT et al. Irrigation and debridement with chronic antibiotic suppression for the management of infected total knee arthroplasty: a contemporary analysis. Bone Joint J. 2018;100-b(11):1471–6.
28. Freeman MA, et al. The management of infected total knee replacements. J Bone Joint Surg Br. 1985;67(5):764–8.

29. Fillingham YA et al. Definition of successful infection management and guidelines for reporting of outcomes after surgical treatment of periprosthetic joint infection: from the workgroup of the musculoskeletal infection society (MSIS). J Bone Joint Surg Am. 2019;101 (14):e69.

30. Gehrke T, Zahar A, Kendoff D. One-stage exchange: it all began here. Bone Joint J. 2013;95-b(11 Suppl A):77–83.

31. Nagra NS, et al. One-stage versus two-stage exchange arthroplasty for infected total knee arthroplasty: a systematic review. Knee Surg Sports Traumatol Arthrosc. 2016;24(10): 3106–14.

Orthoplastics and Revision Knee Arthroplasty

13

I'm not the smartest fellow in the world, but I can sure pick smart colleagues.

Franklin D. Roosevelt

13.1 Introduction

Compromised soft tissues around a TKA present significant challenges. There is a wide spectrum of scenarios ranging from a knee being considered for a primary TKA with a scarred soft tissue envelope to the multiply operated knee with a discharging sinus [1, 2]. In either case, the goal of soft tissue reconstruction is to ensure definitive coverage of the implant with pliable and durable tissue to facilitate joint function [3].

The concept of the 'reconstructive elevator' is used by plastic surgeons when planning to cover soft tissue defects around TKA. It allows ascension from the simplest to the most complex techniques, based on the specific characteristics of the wound and the soft tissue coverage needed. The focus is on early closure of the defect with stable soft tissue coverage over the implants, which would also allow for any future procedures to be undertaken. The options include primary closure, healing by secondary intention, skin grafts, local and free flaps [4].

This chapter will discuss some practical aspects of orthoplastic cases in rTKA within a multidisciplinary team approach.

© The Author(s), under exclusive license to Springer Nature Switzerland AG 2021
H. E. Matar et al., *Revision Total Knee Arthroplasty*,
https://doi.org/10.1007/978-3-030-81285-0_13

13.2   Why Do We Get Compromised Soft Tissues Around the Knee?

We usually see compromised soft tissues in the infrapatellar region at the distal end of the wound and more rarely in the suprapatellar region. This is due to a number of factors such as blood supply to this region, the relative subcutaneous location of the proximal tibia, skin fat necrosis, scarring with more adherent skin to the tissues underneath, previous trauma, skin grafting, the multiply operated knee, and infection (Figs. 13.1, 13.2, 13.3 and 13.4).

13.3   Managing Compromised Soft Tissues

To run a successful revision knee service, it is imperative to have strong links with plastic surgical colleagues within a multidisciplinary team approach. Such cases should be viewed as joint cases with early involvement and consultation as part of the preoperative assessment and surgical planning.

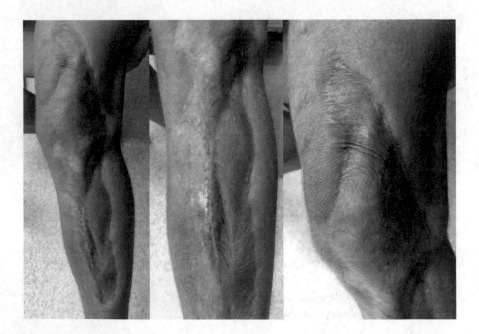

Fig. 13.1 Clinical photographs of a 56 years old man with post-traumatic osteoarthritis; previous polytrauma with flap reconstruction. Primary TKA was performed as a joint case with a plastic surgeon

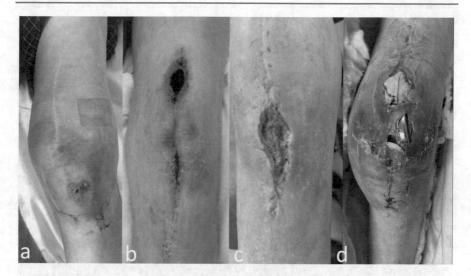

Fig. 13.2 a–d Example of compromised soft tissues around TKAs; **a** infrapatellar sinus; **b** suprapatellar wound defect; **c** example of infrapatellar defect over the patella tendon which require urgent coverage to salvage the patellar tendon; **d** catastrophic soft tissue compromise with an exposed infected implant

Fig. 13.3 Clinical photograph of a right knee following a two-stage reconstruction for infection with a medial head gastrocnemius flap which was performed at time of the 1st stage with a temporary fusion nail as a static spacer. Later at the time of the 2nd stage, the flap was raised, and the 2nd stage performed

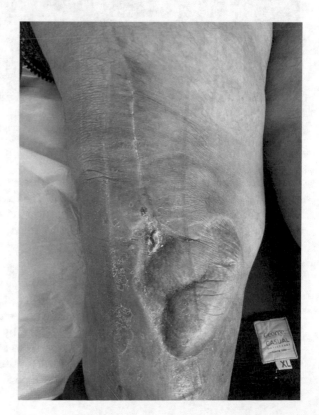

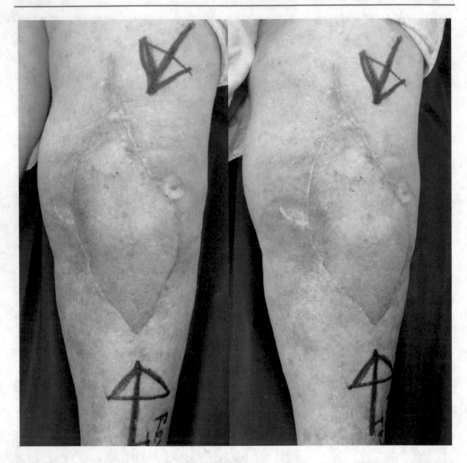

Fig. 13.4 Clinical photograph of a left knee following first-stage revision for infection with a well-healed free flap

Wounds around the knee joint are difficult to reconstruct effectively and this is especially the case in the presence of an implant. The technique used must allow for an easy access for a definitive implant and may need to be re-used in the case of a staged revision for infection. Here, we describe some of the common techniques used by colleagues in our unit:

(a) **Infrapatellar defects**

A defect over the patella tendon, or adjacent to it, is the most common defect encountered in practice. These defects are amenable to a pedicled *medial gastrocnemius flap* [3]. This is commonly done by transposing the flap, as a muscle-only flap, with a combined split-thickness skin graft. This flap is versatile because of its substantial size, mobility, ease of harvest, and minimal functional loss and donor-site morbidity. The medial head of the gastrocnemius is supplied by the medial sural artery and can be rotated. Flaps range from 5 to 9 cm in width and from 13 to 20 cm in length and it provides a vascular bed for the skin graft. Accurate planning that considers the arc of rotation and insetting must be integral to flap dissection. This will allow a tension free suturing of the distal part of the flap along the most superior aspect of the defect. A small skin paddle can also be incorporated with the muscle as a myocutaneous flap.

In cases of infection, the capsule of the joint is destroyed either by the infection or the surgical debridement. As such, the medial head of gastrocnemius fans out under the surrounding skin flaps during insetting creating a 'waterproof' effect.

(b) **Prepatellar defects**

The medial head of gastrocnemius will not reach this area without detaching the origin from the femoral condyle. The latter procedure may need to be coupled with the transverse scoring of the deep aspect of the muscle. Both of these procedures risk devascularising the flap. This will allow healing but it must be anticipated that further soft tissue reconstruction will need to be undertaken. A local *fasciocutaneous flap* may be planned as a random pattern flap [5].

(c) **Suprapatellar defects**

In the presence of PJI, these defects are exceptionally difficult to cover with vascularised tissue. Whereas the vastus muscles may seem attractive option due to their proximity, the morbidity from the harvest must be considered. The *distally-based gracilis flap* has been shown to be a reliable option in those cases especially when delayed [6].

(d) **Proximal incisional wounds**

A redeeming feature here is that this incision is over the quadriceps muscle group. Further, there is laxity of the skin and if primary closure cannot be undertaken, a Z-plasty may help to move the incision away from the defect in the knee extensors.

(e) **Posterior defects**

These are rare; usually from previous trauma with weakness in the posterior capsule. Nonetheless, small defects in the popliteal fossa can be excised and closed primarily with a Z-plasty. For larger defects *random pattern fasciocutaneous flaps* can be planned with a proximal back-cut.

13.4   When Do We Need *Free Flaps?*

Most of the reconstructive options rely on local tissue. This is both quick and effective when planned and executed well. There are however defects that are either located in hostile locations such as the lateral part of the knee or too large for local flaps. In these cases, free tissue transfer must be planned. Safe planning relies on having a good donor flap as well as good recipient vessels. The large popliteal vessels or the superficial femoral vessels seem obvious choices, but these will need vein grafts to allow realistic pedicle lengths. The genicular vessels, both medial and lateral, are consistent and are usually of a good calibre. The great saphenous vein must be used as the venous recipient. Free flap surgery has significant donor site morbidity and it is a much more prolonged surgery. Therefore, careful counselling of patients is paramount [1, 7].

13.5 When Should We Flap an Infected Knee with Tissue Defects?

Our short answer is to flap at time of 1st stage, however, very rarely in cases of gross infection we debride and VAC for a short period of time followed by a repeat 1st stage and a flap. The best chance of eradicating infection is at 1st stage revision with full debridement of all infected tissue and bone. The ability to close the knee should not compromise the debridement. A prerequisite to success is full debridement, stabilisation and good blood supply. In our practice, we stabilise with a temporary fusion nail and flap at time of the 1st stage.

Once the infection is cured, the soft tissues will become more pliable, the oedema will subside, and healthy tissues are much better to deal with at the time of the 2nd stage, making it easier to reconstruct the joint and leading to better outcomes. Our plastic surgical colleagues will be involved to safely raise the flap at the time of the 2nd stage and to close it again following definitive implantation.

In conclusion, orthopastic rTKA cases are challenging and should be managed closely with plastic reconstructive surgeons within a multidisciplinary team approach.

References

1. Louer CR, et al. Free flap reconstruction of the knee: an outcome study of 34 cases. Ann Plast Surg. 2015;74(1):57–63.
2. Nahabedian MY, et al. Salvage procedures for complex soft tissue defects of the knee. Clin Orthop Relat Res. 1998;356:119–24.
3. Ries MD, Bozic KJ. Medial gastrocnemius flap coverage for treatment of skin necrosis after total knee arthroplasty. Clin Orthop Relat Res. 2006;446:186–92.
4. Osei DA, Rebehn KA, Boyer MI. Soft-tissue Defects After Total Knee Arthroplasty: Management and Reconstruction. J Am Acad Orthop Surg. 2016;24(11):769–79.
5. Hallock GG. Salvage of total knee arthroplasty with local fasciocutaneous flaps. J Bone Joint Surg Am. 1990;72(8):1236–9.
6. Mitsala G, et al. The distally pedicled gracilis flap for salvage of complex knee wounds. Injury. 2014;45(11):1776–81.
7. Fang T, et al. Recipient vessels in the free flap reconstruction around the knee. Ann Plast Surg. 2013;71(4):429–33.

Managing Chronic Patella Dislocations in Revision Knee Arthroplasty: Surgical Technique

14

> *If you define the problem correctly, you almost have the solution*
>
> Steve Jobs.

14.1 Introduction

Patella dislocation after primary or revision TKA is a major challenge in revision surgery. A number of risk factors have been established for patella instability after TKA including internal rotation of the components, excessive valgus alignment, prosthetic design geometry, extensor mechanism contracture, medial capsular insufficiency, excessively tight lateral retinaculum, asymmetric patellar bone preparation, excessive patellar composite thickness, patella alta, and dynamic instability [1–5].

Historically, older knee designs, particularly those with short femoral flanges or a flat trochlea were associated with a higher incidence of patellofemoral instability; either tilting, subluxation or dislocation. Advances in prosthetic designs have reduced the incidence of patellofemoral instability [6]. However, in practice, the main reason for patella maltracking and instability following TKA is malrotation of the femoral and/or tibial components [7].

This chapter describes a novel surgical technique to manage chronic patella dislocations in revision TKA; originally developed by the distinguished *Dr Jeffrey Gollish* in Toronto and popularised by *Hosam Matar* [8] and adopted effectively in our unit as the *'Matar Procedure'*.

14.2 Historical Perspective

A number of procedures, once component malrotation is corrected, have been used to restore central patella tracking. These include quadricepsplasty, the proximal realignment procedure described by *Insall*, and distal patellar tendon realignment procedure using a tibial tubercle osteotomy described by *Whiteside* [5, 9–11]. These procedures were originally described for patellofemoral instability in patients with chondromalacia patellae. Madigan et al.described a *quadricepsplasty procedure* which included mobilisation of vastus medialis obliquus (VMO) laterally with a lateral retinacular release [12]. *Insall* later modified this procedure to a *proximal tube realignment procedure* which was a lateral and distal mobilisation of VMO as well as lateral retinacular release [13, 14]. Here, the lateral capsule was divided from tibial tubercle distally to vastus lateralis proximally. A medial flap consisting of the medial portion of the quadriceps tendon was then sutured overlapping the lateral half of the quadriceps mechanism [13]. Our technique relies on some of those principles but further developed and adapted to manage chronic dislocations in rTKA.

14.3 Rationale

In managing chronically dislocated patellae in rTKA settings, assuming the components are well-aligned and with the correct rotation, the aim is to change the vector of the extensor mechanism from a lateral to a more central position. This is achieved by performing extensive lateral release of vastus lateralis off the intermuscular septum and a partial release of the iliotibial band if required. This ensures that we relocate the patella to track more centrally. We further secure central tracking by advancing the VMO laterally to the lateral edge of the patella/vastus lateralis to act as a dynamic stabiliser. In most cases of chronic dislocation, the medial soft tissues are stretched and have adequate excursion to be advanced laterally. The degree of advancement needed will differ case by case based on the amount of the excursion of the VMO and the position of the dislocated patella in flexion (Fig. 14.1).

14.4 Surgical Technique

Position: patients are placed in the supine position and the leg prepped and draped in the usual fashion as per TKA (Fig 14.2).
Incision: the prior longitudinal skin incision is used. Dissection is then carried out to the prepatellar plane, elevating the soft tissues and exposing the extensor mechanism to the level of the tibial tubercle.

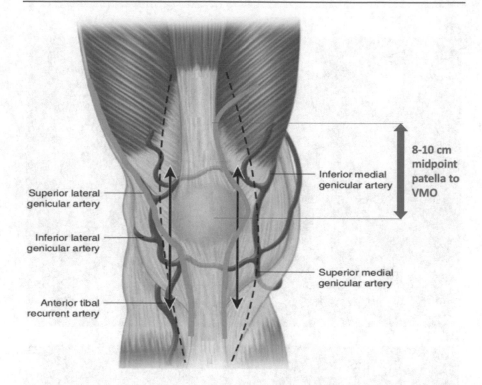

Fig. 14.1 Schematic demonstration of the procedure. Laterally, the release starts by defining the interval between lateral patella tendon and iliotibial band, developed more proximally lateral to vastus lateralis lifting it off the lateral intermuscular septum. Medially, medial parapatellar arthrotomy extending proximally to 8–10 cm from the midpoint of the patella obliquely into the VMO (short VMO split) to preserve its inferior blood supply and prepare it for advancement (adopted from Pawar et al. with permission from Copyright Clearance Centre)

Lateral releases: the lateral margin of the patellar tendon is then identified and the interval between the patellar tendon and the iliotibial (IT) band is opened. Here, the soft tissues are often tethered to the IT band requiring extensive elevation and separation of vastus lateralis. Then the aim here is to elevate vastus lateralis off the lateral intermuscular septum up to the mid-thigh. Significant tethering of the extensor mechanism can be seen laterally, particularly if previous surgeries such as lateral plating for fracture management or distal femoral osteotomies have been performed. The lateral release of the quadriceps is essential to allow it to mobilise medially and centralise. Partial release of the IT band may also be necessary. A number of perforators are to be expected. Ensure haemostasis is achieved to prevent haematoma collection in the lateral space.

VMO advancement: In chronically dislocated patellae, the medial soft tissues are often significantly attenuated. A medial arthrotomy is then performed; distally from the medial margin of the patella down to the tibial tubercle. Proximally; the

(i)

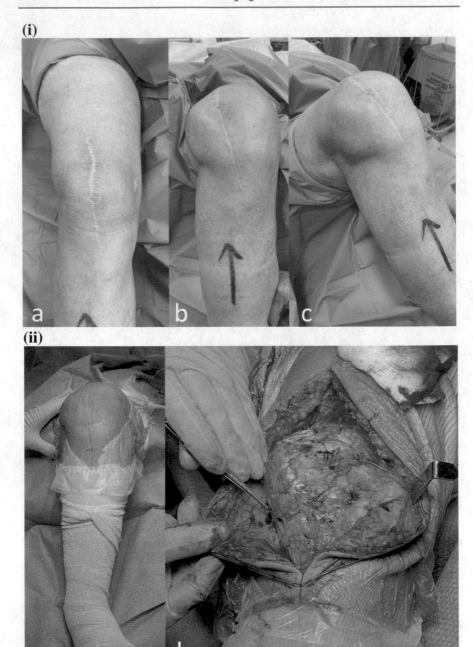

(ii)

◀ **Fig 14.2   i)** Case demonstration with clinical photographs of a 72 years old man with chronically dislocated patella in otherwise well-fixed and well-aligned knee with no femoral internal rotation. He underwent PS-TKA for a valgus knee 3 years earlier. He presents with chronic patella dislocation and difficulty mobilising following a fall a year ago; **a)** *in extension* the patella is subluxed laterally; **b–c)** *with flexion* the patella dislocates fully. **ii)** Intraoperative photographs; **a)** the knee is prepped and draped in the usual fashion; **b)** the old incision is used; full thickness skin flaps are raised and haemostasis achieved exposing the extensor mechanism. **iii) a)** The patella is dislocated laterally; lateral edge of vastus lateralis is identified. **b)** more distally, the interval between the iliotibial band and lateral edge of patella tendon is identified and developed. **iv) a)** Vastus lateralis is lifted off the intermuscular septum to allow the extensor mechanism to be mobilised more centrally; **b)** a number of perforators are usually encountered here, and haemostasis is achieved. **v) a)** The second part of the procedure (medial side) is then performed by **b)** identifying mid-point of the patella and marking 8–10 cm point proximally in the VMO where the medial arthrotomy extends obliquely to prepare VMO for advancement.**vi) a)** Medial parapatellar arthrotomy is performed; **b)** synovectomy and removing of all scar and granulation tissues; the patella is then inspected and patelloplasty is undertaken if necessary. **vii) a)** Scar tissue is removed leaving the VMO fascia intact; **b)** VMO is then prepared for lateral advancement. **viii) a)** VMO is advanced and temporarily held to check patella tracking in flexion; **b)** identifying any tight fibrous bands in vastus lateralis which can be released at this point. **ix) a)** Final preparations to ensure the extensor vector has been shifted more centrally; **b)** VMO is advanced and secured temporarily with sutures. In this case, there is abundant medial tissue with enough excursion of the VMO to be advanced laterally and sutured to the patella centrally and laterally. In other cases, the amount of advancement needed is dictated by VMO excursion and the lateral resting position of the patella. **x) a)** VMO advanced and secured with non-absorbable sutures; **b)** The remaining medial arthrotomy is then closed in the usual fashion.**xi) a–b)** At 90° flexion, the patella is central and tracks centrally throughout range of motion; in this case 0-100°; VMO advanced and secured with non-absorbable sutures. **xii) a)** The lateral space is closed over a 24 h drain; **b)** Subcutaneous tissues are closed in layers in the usual fashion. **xiv) a–b)** Postoperative radiographs at 10 weeks follow up with the patella tracking centrally and range of motion 0-100° and satisfactory outcome; **c)** skyline view

soft tissues are divided along the medial border of the rectus femoris and between rectus femoris and vastus medialis. The proximal dissection is carried out proximally over a distance of 8–10 cm from the midpoint of the patella, then a short mid-VMO split is performed in order to allow the later advancement of VMO whilst protecting its inferior blood supply. At this point, if the components are malrotated then a full revision is carried out in the usual fashion. The patella could then be inspected and patelloplasty and/or patella resurfacing undertaken where necessary, to improve its contact and tracking in the trochlea of the femoral component.

The next step is advancement of the VMO which has already been prepared; this can be done provisionally with towel clips or temporary sutures to ascertain the appropriate position of the advancement and test it throughout the range of movement. Then the medial edge of VMO is sutured, using absorbable interrupted sutures such as 1 *Vicryl*, to the lateral edge of the patella and the lateral edge of the proximal extensor mechanism. The repair is further reinforced with nonabsorbable 5 *Ethibond* sutures. Patellar tracking is then tested with the aim of achieving at least 90° flexion with the patella remaining central. In this position, the vastus lateralis is further inspected to identify any intramuscular fibrous bands which can be released.

(iii)

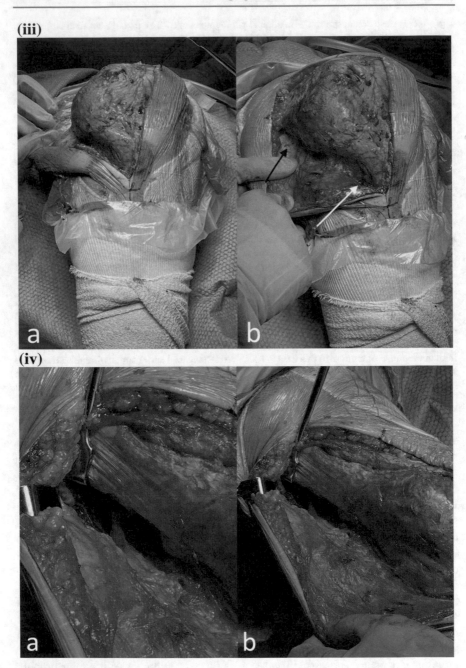

(iv)

Fig 14.2 (continued)

(v)

(vi)

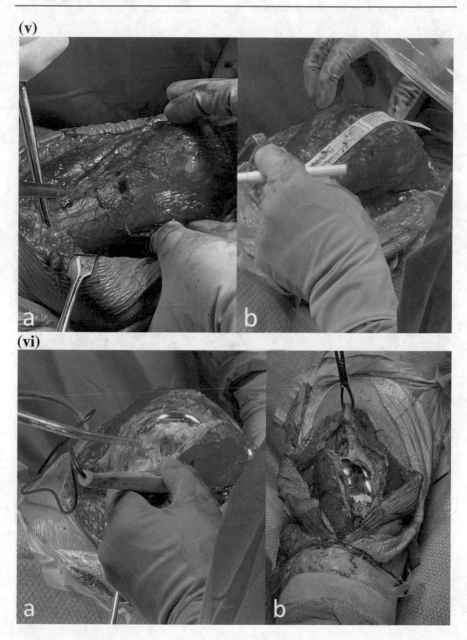

Fig 14.2 (continued)

(vii)

(viii)

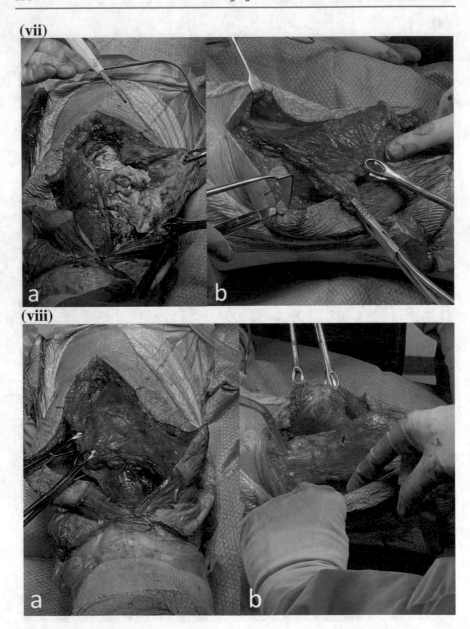

Fig 14.2 (continued)

(ix)

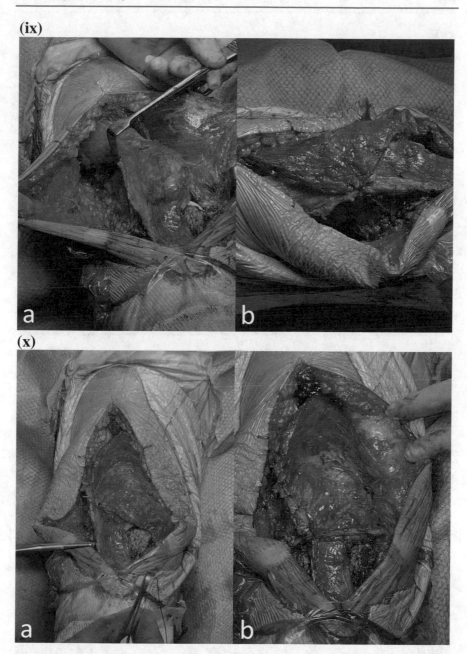

(x)

Fig 14.2 (continued)

(xi)

(xii)

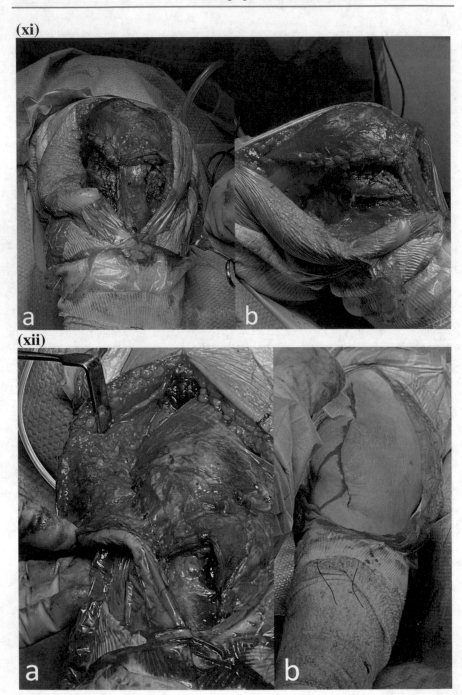

Fig 14.2 (continued)

(xiii)

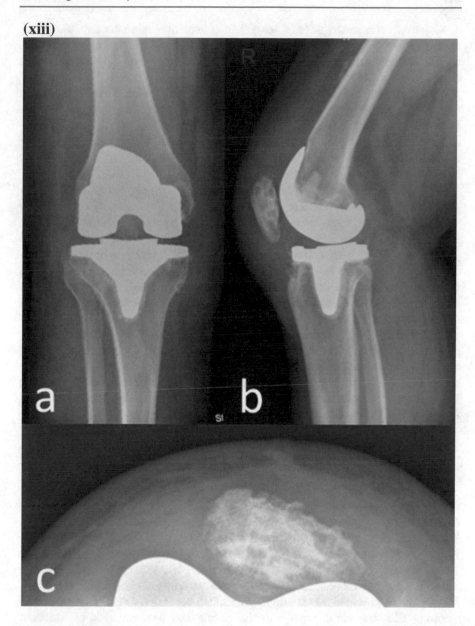

Fig 14.2 (continued)

Closure: the next step is to close the lateral interval eliminating any dead space by tacking the lateral soft tissues across the lateral margin of the extensor mechanism with interrupted absorbable sutures. The remainder of the wound is then closed in the usual fashion.

Postoperatively: A knee immobiliser is applied and the knee held in extension for 4 weeks whilst isometric quadriceps and hamstring exercises are encouraged. Full weight bearing as tolerated is allowed with assisted walking devices. A graduated physiotherapy protocol is then applied with the aim of maintaining knee extension whilst performing flexion exercises to 30°, 60° and 90° on two weekly basis. A hinged knee brace can also be used (Figs. 14.3 and 14.4).

Managing patellofemoral instability in TKA is challenging particularly in revision knee arthroplasty. The management is based on the aetiology of instability which in principle is related to surgical factors. Component malpositioning with internal rotation of the femoral and/or tibial components is one of the main culprits [15]. Nonsurgical measures such as strengthening the VMO and bracing are generally unsuccessful [6]. Revision arthroplasty is often needed to restore function and mobility. Whether the components are revised or retained, in the absence of component malpositioning, soft tissue reconstruction of the extensor mechanism is needed to restore function.

The technique we describe focuses on soft tissue reconstruction by performing an extensive lateral release of the vastus lateralis and VMO advancement. This allows the patella to sit more centrally. The VMO is advanced across to the midline of the extensor mechanism where the lateral margin of the VMO is advanced to the lateral edge of the patella and brought distally in order to provide dynamic stability for the patella during functional range of motion.

14.5   What About Blood Supply and Risk of Avascular Necrosis?

Maintaining blood supply to the VMO is crucial to the success of this technique. The mid-VMO split is designed to allow mobilisation of the VMO without disrupting its blood supply from the inferior medial genicular artery (Fig. 14.1). The lateral release is carried out by lifting the vastus lateralis off the intermuscular septum. Here, several perforators might be encountered and require ligation. However, the proximal blood supply to rectus and vastus lateralis remain intact ensuring adequate blood supply to the patella and negating risk of avascular necrosis. Pawar et al.assessed patella blood supply and viability in 36 primary TKAs requiring lateral release using Technetium-99 m methylene diphosphate (Tc-99 m MDP) scintigraphy. Fourteen knees with lateral release showed scintigraphic signs of hypovascularity in the early postoperative period that normalised by 8 weeks [16]. Further, Montserrat et al.reported on their long term follow up (43 patients with minimum 10 years) of Insall proximal realignment procedure and

(i)

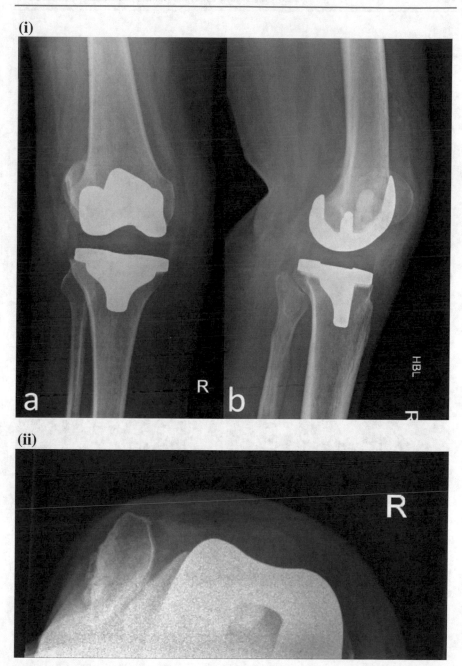

(ii)

Fig. 14.3 i) **a-b** Anteroposterior and lateral radiographs of a 68 years old woman with a failed right TKA, incompetent MCL and chronically irreducible dislocation patella. **ii)** Skyline view with the patella in the lateral gutter. **iii)** Anteroposterior and lateral radiographs at 1 year follow up following revision surgery to a hinged implant with extensor mechanism reconstruction and VMO advancement. The patella is tracking centrally with satisfactory clinical outcomes

(iii)

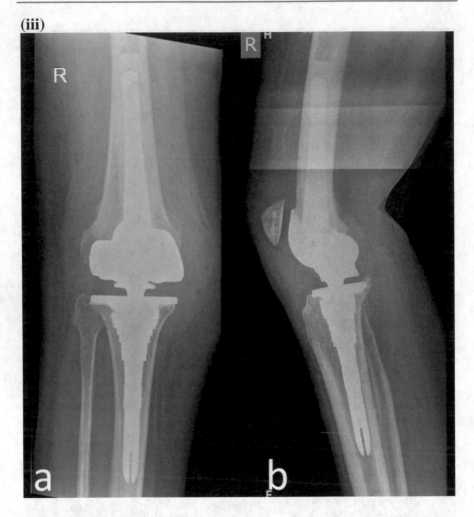

Fig. 14.3 (continued)

lateral facetectomy to treat patellofemoral arthritis with no reported cases of osteonecrosis [17].

14.6   Literature Overview

Very few studies have reported on any similar surgical techniques in the literature. *Insall* reported on 12 knees with patella dislocation following primary TKA which were treated with proximal realignment of the extensor mechanism in 10 knees, lateral retinacular release alone in one, and revision of the tibial and femoral

(i)

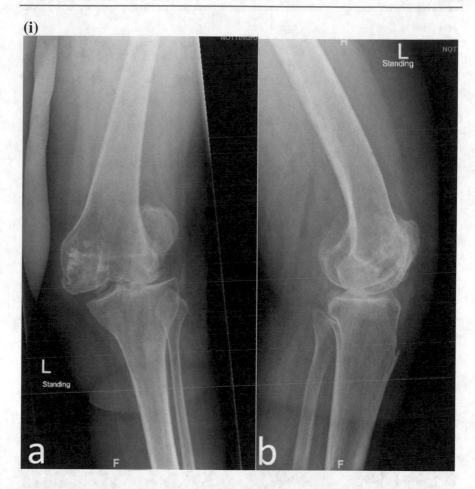

Fig. 14.4 i) a-b) Anteroposterior and lateral radiographs of a 73 years old woman with painful arthritic left valgus knee, incompetent MCL and chronically dislocated patella. **ii) a-b)** Postoperative radiographs at 9 months following complex primary TKA using a hinged implant. The patella is centrally tracking with successful outcomes

components combined with proximal realignment in one with no re-dislocations at average 34 months follow up [5]. Further, *Insall* reported similar results in 5 chronically dislocated irreducible patella dislocations using extensive proximal realignment procedure [18].

In conclusion, managing chronically dislocated patellae in rTKA is challenging. The 'Matar Procedure' described here has been developed based on the biomechanical principles of changing the vector force to centralise the patella and further reinforced by a viable dynamic VMO stabiliser to ensure durability and a sustained outcome.

(ii)

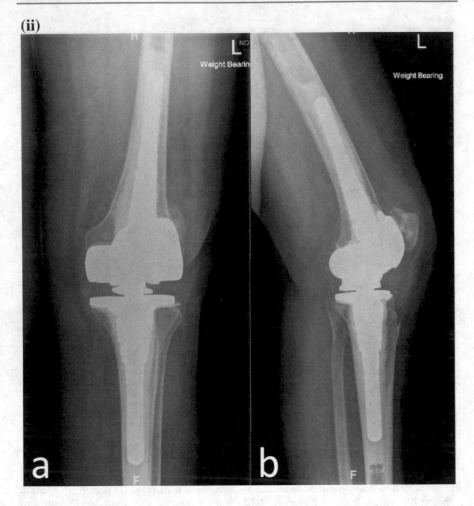

Fig. 14.4 (continued)

References

1. Cameron HU, Fedorkow DM. The patella in total knee arthroplasty. Clin Orthop Relat Res. 1982;165:197–9.
2. Grace JN, Rand JA. Patellar instability after total knee arthroplasty. Clin Orthop Relat Res. 1988;237:184–9.
3. Kirk P, et al. Management of recurrent dislocation of the patella following total knee arthroplasty. J Arthroplasty. 1992;7(3):229–33.
4. Lynch AF, Rorabeck CH, Bourne RB. Extensor mechanism complications following total knee arthroplasty. J Arthroplasty. 1987;2(2):135–40.
5. Merkow RL, Soudry M, Insall JN. Patellar dislocation following total knee replacement. J Bone Joint Surg Am. 1985;67(9):1321–7.

6. Malo M, Vince KG. The unstable patella after total knee arthroplasty: etiology, prevention, and management. J Am Acad Orthop Surg. 2003;11(5):364–71.
7. Donell S. Patellar tracking in primary total knee arthroplasty. EFORT Open Rev. 2018;3 (4):106–13.
8. Matar HE, Illanes FL, Gollish JD. Extensive Proximal Extensor Mechanism Realignment for Chronic Patella Dislocations in Revision Knee Arthroplasty: Surgical Technique. Knee. 2020;27(6):1821–32.
9. Whiteside LA. Distal realignment of the patellar tendon to correct abnormal patellar tracking. Clin Orthop Relat Res. 1997;344:284–9.
10. Brassard MF, et al. Complication of total knee arthroplasty. In: Insall JN, Scott WN, editors. Surgery of the knee. Churchill Livingstone: Philadelphia; 2006. p. 1753.
11. Dao Q, Chen DB, Scott RD. Proximal patellar quadricepsplasty realignment during total knee arthroplasty for irreducible congenital dislocation of the patella: a report of two cases. J Bone Joint Surg Am. 2010;92(14):2457–61.
12. Madigan R, Wissinger HA, Donaldson WF. Preliminary experience with a method of quadricepsplasty in recurrent subluxation of the patella. J Bone Joint Surg Am. 1975;57 (5):600–7.
13. Insall J, Falvo KA, Wise DW. Chondromalacia patellae: a prospective study. J Bone Joint Surg Am. 1976; 58(1): 1–8.
14. Insall J, Bullough PG, Burstein AH. Proximal "tube" realignment of the patella for chondromalacia patellae. Clin Orthop Relat Res. 1979;144:63–9.
15. Chin KR, et al. Revision surgery for patellar dislocation after primary total knee arthroplasty. J Arthroplasty. 2004;19(8):956–61.
16. Pawar U, et al. Scintigraphic assessment of patellar viability in total knee arthroplasty after lateral release. J Arthroplasty. 2009;24(4):636–40.
17. Montserrat F, et al. Treatment of isolated patellofemoral osteoarthritis with lateral facetectomy plus Insall's realignment procedure: long-term follow-up. Knee Surg Sports Traumatol Arthrosc. 2013;21(11):2572–7.
18. Bullek DD, Scuderi GR, Insall JN. Management of the chronic irreducible patellar dislocation in total knee arthroplasty. J Arthroplasty. 1996;11(3):339–45.

Extensor Mechanism Failure and Allograft Reconstruction

15

If you can't fly then run, if you can't run then walk, if you can't walk then crawl, but whatever you do you have to keep moving forward.

Martin Luther King Jr

15.1 Introduction

Extensor mechanism failure was traditionally considered a catastrophic failure with the only salvage option being arthrodesis to maintain some function. However, although it remains a catastrophic complication, there are a number of contemporary techniques with reasonable outcomes that restore function. Several graft options are available for reconstruction, but there is no consensus in the literature regarding optimal treatment. In a recent review of 28 reports on managing extensor mechanism disruption after TKA, the complication rate after direct repair of patellar tendon (63.16%) was higher than the complication rate after repair of quadriceps tendon (25.37%). However, the complication rate for patellar and quadriceps tendon tears after autograft, allograft, or mesh reconstruction was similar (18.8% vs. 19.2%, respectively). The most common complication after extensor mechanism repair or reconstruction was an extension lag of $\geq 30°$ (45.33%). This was followed by re-rupture (25.33%) and infection (22.67%). Early ruptures had a higher overall complication rate than late injuries [1].

In this chapter, we will describe our surgical technique in allograft extensor mechanism reconstruction with case demonstrations.

15.2   Why Do Extensor Mechanisms Fail After TKA?

In a native knee, we see either patella tendon failure, patella fracture or quads tendon failure. There are different pathophysiological causes for these failures ranging from traumatic to degenerative. In TKA population, these processes persist and can be further accentuated by TKA-related risk factures including patella resurfacing, multiple surgeries, or disruption to the extensor mechanism blood supply [2].

Patella tendon failure: if this occurs in the early postoperative period following a TKA, it may be iatrogenic—caused either during exposure of a stiff knee with tendon avulsion from the tibial tubercle, or by inadvertent injury during tibial preparation and bone cuts. This tends to happen while cutting the anterolateral portion of the tibial plateau. It can however also be due to vascular issues, for example following a lateral release in close proximity to the lateral edge of the patella for a maltracking patella with disruption to the lateral patella tendon blood supply.

Patella fractures: these are more common in resurfaced patellae, so the advice here when resurfacing patellae is to avoid over-resection. The resection landmarks should be the osteochondral junction medially to osteochondral junction laterally. It should be a flat surface superior to inferior. When doing so, you will notice a good quality cortical rim circumferentially inferring a lot of strength. Always ensure that this rim is kept intact by not cutting obliquely during patella resection. Expose the osteochondral margins by removing the surrounding soft tissue before placing the cutting guide. Another technical tip is to upsize the patella button to ensure coverage of the cortical rim. Finally, joint line restoration and its impact on patello-femoral joint mechanics, particularly avoiding overstuffing in posterior-based hinges as previously discussed in Chap. 10.

Quads failure: again, we see attrition failure akin to what we see in quads failure in native knees. The other TKA-specific potential cause is over-resecting the patella superiorly adjacent to the quads tendon insertion or the use of proximally based extensile approaches such as a quadriceps turndown.

Top Tip: Minimise surgical risks to the extensor mechanism intraoperatively, avoid over-tensioning during tibial exposure, ensure central tracking and avoid overstuffing the patellofemoral joint.

15.3   Management Options

Different strategies can be used for acute and chronic presentations. For acute cases, primary repair or fixation is needed with adjunctive secondary fixation or protection. We tend to over-tension the repair acknowledging that all repairs will stretch out. This is followed by a strict rehabilitation and mobilisation programme with the knee locked in full extension for 4–6 weeks followed by graduated flexion and range of motion rehabilitation.

(a) **Patella tendon failure:** if *acute*, it is eminently fixable applying first principles in opposing the tendon ends if it is a mid-substance failure or reattaching to the bone in cases of avulsions using anchors. Tendon length should be restored and the repair protected. A variety of techniques can be deployed, but we prefer the technique described by *Cadambi and Engh* [3] as an augmentation to the primary repair using an autograft. We harvest *semitendinosus* and *gracilis* leaving the hamstrings attached to the proximal tibia at the *pes anserinus*. We then prepare the graft with a whip stitch, feed the graft through drill holes medial to lateral in the patella forming a sling around it and fix the graft into the proximal tibia using anchors or staples. Alternatively, if the patella is thin or already resurfaced, the graft can be weaved through the extensor mechanism and quads tendon more proximally. We ensure that we also have an allograft hamstrings tendon on standby to supplement the repair if needed.

Other techniques include the use of Bard polypropylene mesh (Bard hernia mesh, BD, Franklin Lakes, NJ), which involves creating a window of bone in the proximal tibia and cementing the mesh in to be used as a scaffold which can then be weaved into the extensors more proximally.

(b) **Patella fracture:** if displaced these require fixation. It is a difficult fixation particularly with a resurfaced patella. We keep the button if it is well-fixed, but if it is loose we remove it, fix the fracture and consider cementing a new button. Tension band wiring techniques remain the mainstay option using wires or other alternatives.

(c) **Quads failure:** the hardest to treat with the least favourable outcome is quads failure. The main issue here is that we cannot easily protect the repair. We have used direct repair techniques with adjunctive fixation such as a free harvest of semitendinosus which with a native patella can be used as a sling through the patella and weaved through the quads proximally using the *'Pulvertaft weave'* principle to get a secondary fix. Similarly, this technique can also be used with a mesh or allograft.

15.4 Managing Failed Acute Repairs or Chronic Salvage Failures

Over the years, we have had more success with extensor mechanism allograft reconstruction than mesh or synthetic grafts techniques. We currently use bone-tendon-patella-quads (full extensor mechanism allograft). Tissue banks offer a variety of lengths, choosing an appropriately measured allograft is crucial. We use fresh-frozen irradiated allografts.

This could be used in isolation for chronic extensor mechanism reconstruction in an otherwise well-balanced and previously well-functioning knee. It can also be performed as part of a major reconstruction with combined knee revision and extensor mechanism allograft reconstruction. In the latter, most of these patients are elderly and at the end of their reconstructive salvage options. We therefore opt for a fixed-hinge implant for a number of reasons; if the allograft fails, patients can still have some function albeit limited, and the risk of dissociation and hinge dislocation is eliminated in cases of allograft failure with a fixed-hinge. Other options in terms of longevity of a fixed-hinge implant in younger patients have to be considered.

15.4.1   Surgical Technique

Incision: use the old midline skin incision.

Approach: direct midline approach through the existing native extensor mechanism. The patella and patella tendon are excised. The quads tendon is split in the midline shelling out the patella leaving a flap of native quads/retinaculum medially and laterally which can be later used as a soft tissue envelope to fold over the extensor allograft; otherwise there is little protection of the allograft under the skin.

Allograft preparation: at this point, once the trial components are in situ we offer up the allograft and decide where the patella position would be in relation to the joint line and to create a tibial box to attach the allograft. A box is fashioned in the proximal tibia. The allograft comes with a distal bone block which can be modified and fashioned based on the individual case and the space we have in the anterior aspect of the proximal tibia. The patella tendon length, on the other hand, is fixed and it is important to choose the appropriate length patella tendon allograft as

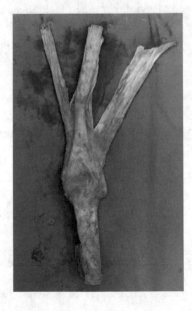

Fig. 15.1 Extensor mechanism allograft with quadriceps, patella and patella tendon allograft. The bone block is fashioned to fit he proximal tibial window. The quadriceps allograft tendon is fashioned into three strips; central rectus, vastus medialis and lateralis

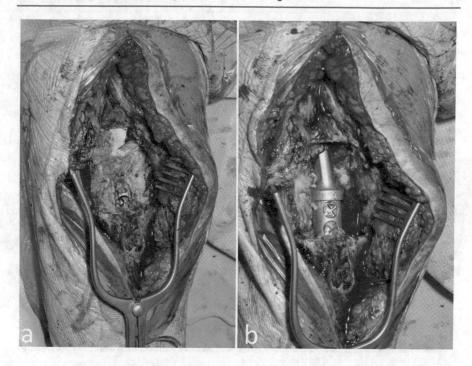

Fig. 15.2 Case demonstration of allograft extensor mechanism reconstruction at time of 2nd stage revision with **a**) temporary modular fusion nail in situ following midline approach through the remining quadriceps; **b**) cement is removed with exposure of the proximal tibial and distal femur

per preoperative planning and liaison with your soft tissue bank. The allograft patella is aneural and does not cause pain, the consideration is mechanical for extension power and impingement during range of motion.

Feel for the native tibial tubercle and use it as a site for the tibial box. The box should be minimum 3–4 cm long to be able to secure the block with at least two wires. We then mark the box on the tibia with a diathermy, use a 2.5 mm drill around the box and complete it with an osteotome lifting off the cortical window off the anterior aspect of the proximal tibia. We attempt to taper the box inferiorly, chamfering it in keeping with the shape of the proximal tibia as it tapers proximal to distal.

Once the block is thawed it is fashioned to the required shape to match the box on a trial-and-error basis until we get a perfect match and a tight press-fit at the end.

Distal Allograft fixation: we then drill for cerclage wires medial to lateral in the proximal tibia deep to where the block would sit. We then punch the allograft block in the box gently using a wide punch. The cancellous bone on the posterior aspect of the block is usually malleable and will disperse facilitating a flush fit on the anterior aspect of the proximal tibia. In cases of combined revision and extensor reconstruction we only tighten the wires once the definitive components are implanted.

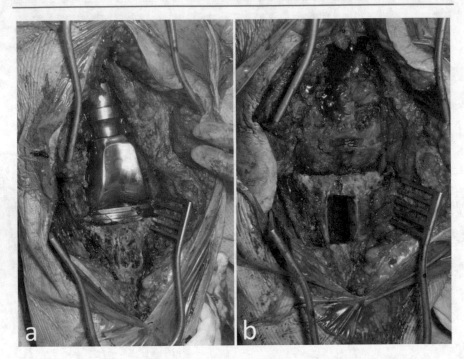

Fig. 15.3 a) trial distal femoral replacement components are in situ; **b)** preparation for the allograft bed by creating a box in the proximal tibia

Proximal allograft fixation: the allograft usually has the main central slip of rectus tendon which is a robust structure and its adjacent expansions *(vastus medialis and lateralis)* which can be split into three strands; lateral, central rectus and medial strands. With the knee in extension, we use a stay suture in the allograft rectus tendon and the remaining native tendon which we had divided midline, using a *Pulvertaft weave* technique, we weave the allograft rectus slip into the remaining native extensor tendon both medially and laterally extending as far proximally as the tendinous material allows. This offers a better pull-out strength than side-to-side repair. Then we bring the two lateral slips and sutures to the native vastus medialis and lateralis using a *Pulvertaft weave* technique.

We use non-absorbable sutures *(5 Ethibond)* for the *Pulvertaft weave* and supplemented by absorbable 1 *Vicryl*. The principle for these weaves is to get different anchor points of the allograft to enhance repair. We then close the knee in layers suturing the subcutaneous tissues onto the allograft.

Postoperatively: we mobilise the patients in full extension for 4 weeks with isometric exercises closely monitored by a physiotherapist followed by graduated range of motion exercises (Figs. 15.7 and 15.8).

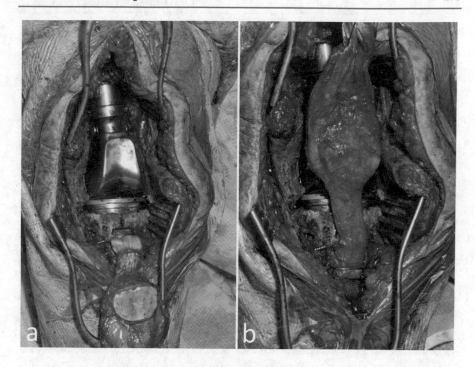

Fig. 15.4 a) the allograft bone block is secured and punched flat over two cerclage wires; **b)** patella height is checked as per preoperative plan ensuring no impingement to during range of motion

15.5 Outcomes of Allograft Reconstructions

The failures are almost always proximal; the distal bony fixation heals with reasonable outcomes reported in the literature when used for chronic patella tendon ruptures [4–8]. The allograft technique has a number of advantages including the absence of donor site morbidity and the abundance of tissue available for fixation to the native quadriceps. On the other hand, some drawbacks include possible host immune reaction, disease transmission, and the mechanical properties of the allograft, although the latter is minimised by using fresh frozen allografts [9]. Significant extensor lag remains the most common complication and has been reported in up to 45% of cases, followed by re-rupture and infection [1].

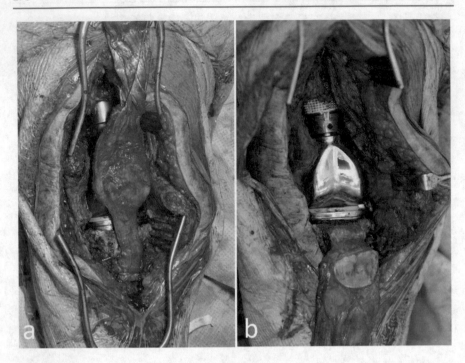

Fig. 15.5 a) final trials and check completed; **b**) definitive implants are cemented in place, the wires can now be tightened over the bone block in the proximal tibia

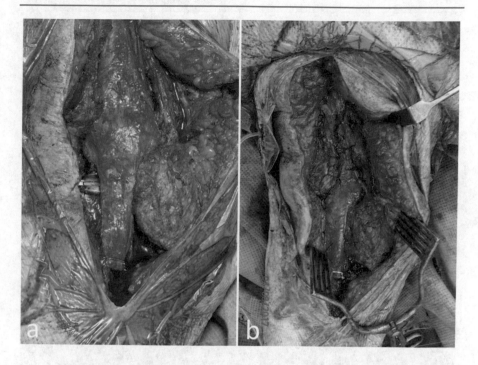

Fig. 15.6 a) allograft is secured proximally through a 3-slip technique and Pulvertaft weave to the native quadriceps; **b**) retinaculum and native vastus medialis and lateralis are sutured over the allograft before closing the subcutaneous tissues in layers

(i)

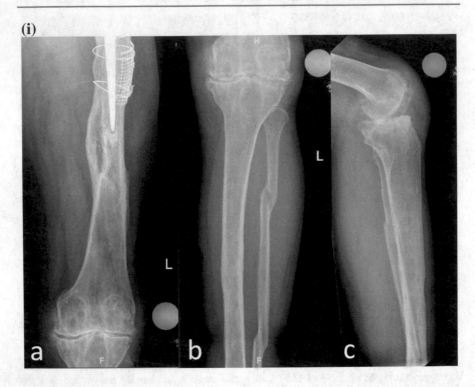

Fig. 15.7 i) Example of a complex primary case in a 54 years old man with previous patellectomy from major trauma and a failed extensor mechanism, he underwent attempted reconstruction using carbon fibre at the age of 19 and had declined knee arthrodesis at that time. He had coped throughout his life with a back-stepping gait. Now he presents with a painful arthritic knee. Further, he has an ipsilateral femoral shaft and tibial/fibular malunited fractures and an ipsilateral revision hip arthroplasty 15 years ago. The main indication for surgery was a debilitating pain. Clinically, he had no leg extension with well-healed scars but otherwise motivated patient with healthy skin. Operative options, in our view, were arthrodesis or major reconstruction with allograft and a hinge implant accepting that if the allograft fail he would be able to mobilise with a fixed hinge that will not dislocate and with better control of his pain; (a-c) anteroposterior and lateral radiographs of the left knee. **ii)** Full length alignment views; as noted the femoral fixation would be limited by the malunited fracture with only 140 mm remaining distal femur which is not enough to support a standard off-shelf hinge implant. Further, on the tibial side the canal is narrow with tibial deformity. **iii)** Magnetic resonance imaging further confirmed the extent of proximal quadriceps deficiency and revealed significant bony cysts. **iv)** Anteroposterior and lateral radiograph at 1 year follow up following major reconstruction with a custom-made fixed hinge implant (Stanmore) and allograft extensor mechanism reconstruction with satisfactory clinical outcome. **v)** Anteroposterior, lateral and skyline views at 3 years follow up with satisfactory clinical outcome and active extension lagging only by 10°

(ii)

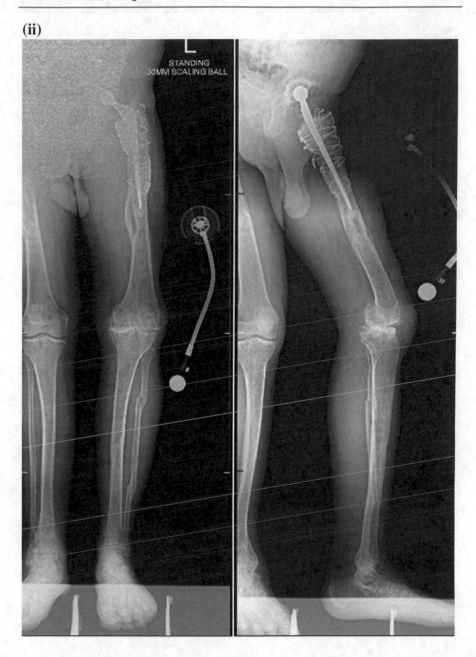

Fig. 15.7 (continued)

(iii)

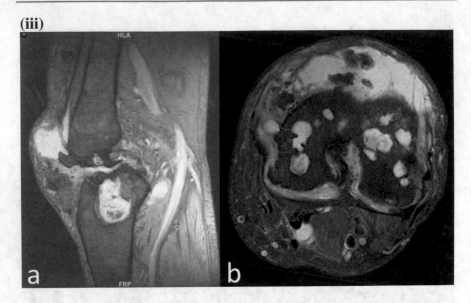

Fig. 15.7 (continued)

(iv)

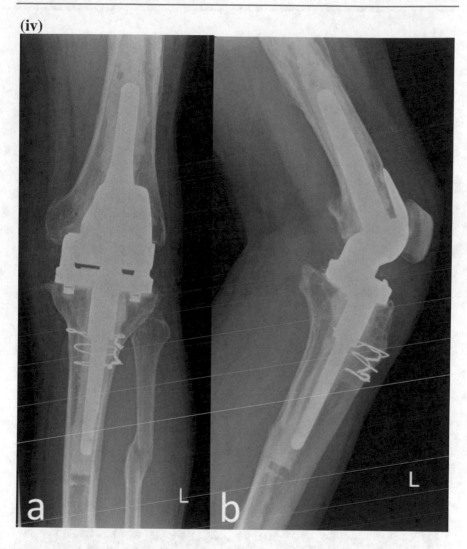

Fig. 15.7 (continued)

(v)

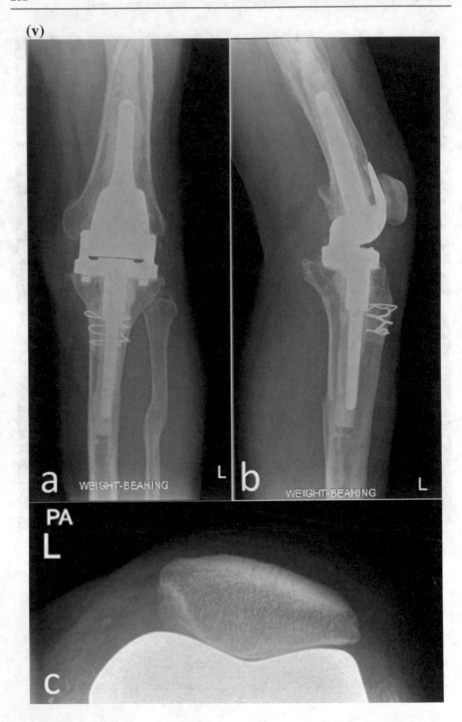

Fig. 15.7 (continued)

(i)

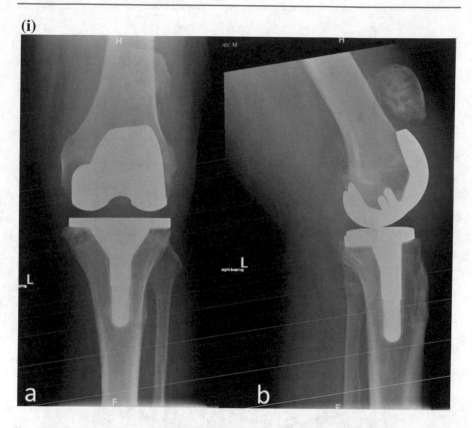

Fig. 15.8 i) Anteroposterior and lateral radiographs of a left knee in a 61 years old man with infected TKA (mixed growth Enterococcus and Coagulate Negative Staphylococcus infection) and a chronically failed extensor mechanism. **ii**) Anteroposterior radiograph following 1st stage revision with a temporary static spacer. **iii**) Anteroposterior and lateral radiographs at 3 years follow up following combined 2nd stage reconstruction with a rotating-hinge implant and satisfactory clinical outcome

(ii)

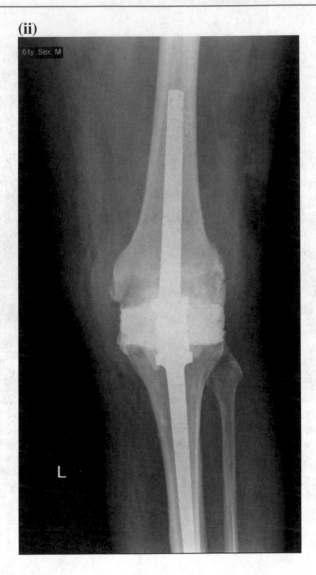

Fig. 15.8 (continued)

(iii)

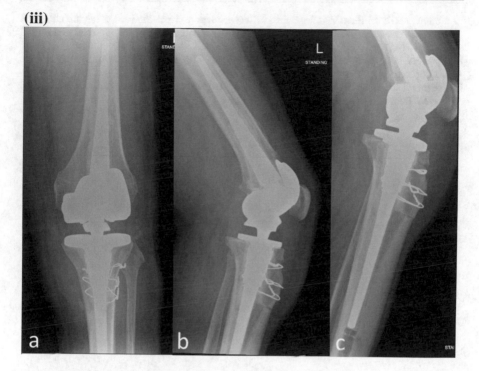

Fig. 15.8 (continued)

References

1. Vajapey SP, et al. Treatment of extensor tendon disruption after total knee arthroplasty: a systematic review. J Arthroplasty. 2019;34(6):1279–86.
2. Maffulli N, et al. The management of extensor mechanism disruption after total knee arthroplasty: a systematic review. Sports Med Arthrosc Rev. 2017;25(1):41–50.
3. Cadambi A, Engh GA. Use of a semitendinosus tendon autogenous graft for rupture of the patellar ligament after total knee arthroplasty. A report of seven cases. J Bone Joint Surg Am. 1992; 74(7):974–9.
4. Barrack RL, Stanley T, Allen Butler R. Treating extensor mechanism disruption after total knee arthroplasty. Clin Orthop Relat Res. 2003(416):98–104.
5. Burnett RS et al. Extensor mechanism allograft reconstruction after total knee arthroplasty. A comparison of two techniques. J Bone Joint Surg Am. 2004; 86(12):2694–9.
6. Burnett RS, Butler RA, Barrack RL. Extensor mechanism allograft reconstruction in TKA at a mean of 56 months. Clin Orthop Relat Res. 2006;452:159–65.

7. Emerson RH, Jr, Head WC, Malinin TI. Reconstruction of patellar tendon rupture after total knee arthroplasty with an extensor mechanism allograft. Clin Orthop Relat Res. 1990 (260):154–61.
8. Springer BD, Della Valle CJ. Extensor mechanism allograft reconstruction after total knee arthroplasty. J Arthroplasty. 2008; 23(7 Suppl):35–8.
9. Eastlund T. Bacterial infection transmitted by human tissue allograft transplantation. Cell Tissue Bank. 2006;7(3):147–66.

Periprosthetic Knee Fractures: An Arthroplasty Perspective

16

> *You look closely enough, you'll find that everything has a weak spot where it can break, sooner or later.*
>
> Anthony Hopkins

16.1 Introduction

Periprosthetic fractures following TKA are defined as fractures of the femur or tibia occurring within 15 cm of the joint line or 5 cm from an intramedullary stem when present [1]. The rate of these fractures ranges from 0.3 to 5.5% in the published literature and is projected to rise with increasing demand for TKA [2], with the distal femur being most commonly affected [3, 4]. The mechanism of injury is commonly a low energy trauma in elderly patients [5]. Osteoporosis with advanced age is considered one of the main risk factors with a high stress mismatch zone between the osteoporotic metaphyseal bone and the implant [3, 4, 6]. Other surgical risk factors include component malalignment, anterior femoral notching particularly with distal fractures and with increased time since primary TKA [7–9].

In this chapter, we will discuss the management of periprosthetic fractures around knee implants from a revision arthroplasty point of view and present our experience using distal femoral replacements for managing acute comminuted distal femoral fractures.

© The Author(s), under exclusive license to Springer Nature Switzerland AG 2021
H. E. Matar et al., *Revision Total Knee Arthroplasty*,
https://doi.org/10.1007/978-3-030-81285-0_16

16.2 Principles of Management

The mortality rate of periprosthetic knee fractures is similar or higher than that of hip fracture patients [10]. Conservative management of displaced periprosthetic fractures is limited only to moribund patients. The aim of surgical management is to restore function to, or near, pre-injury level of activity, to minimise complications, and allow pain-free full weight-bearing status with adequate alignment.

(a) Proximal Tibial Fractures

Intraoperative fractures: can occur during tibial preparation or use of the keel punch, usually at the joint line. These fractures often require reduction and fixation with screws with the aim of keeping the proximal tibial ring intact. Occasionally, a buttress plate is needed if the fracture involves a large fragment or extending more distally. In those cases, a cemented stem extension is needed for further protection.

Acute Periprosthetic fractures: these are fortunately rare and most are below or at the level of the keel or stem, there have been few cases reported of fractures associated with pins from navigation or robotic systems [11]. If the tibial component is well-fixed, these can be plated in the usual fashion with lateral locking plates. Proximal tibial replacements play little role in managing these fractures compared to distal femoral fractures.

(b) Distal Femoral Fractures

Surgical treatments for distal femoral periprosthetic fractures include open reduction and internal fixation with lateral locking plates, retrograde intramedullary nailing, or revision arthroplasty with distal femoral replacement (DFR) [5, 8, 12, 13]. Rorabeck et al. [14] devised a commonly used classification system to describe these fractures; type-1 (non-displaced, well-fixed component), type-2 (displaced, well-fixed component) and type-3 (fractures around a loose component). However, this system does not take into account the location of the fracture which is a key determinant of the choice of treatment [7]. Other important factors that dictate surgical treatment include the remaining bone stock, bone quality, fracture morphology and degree of comminution, the patient's functional level, cognitive function and medical comorbidities.

Fracture fixation techniques generally require a period of restricted weight-bearing until the fracture heals with high rates of delayed- or non-union, whilst revision arthroplasty with endoprostheses allows immediate weight-bearing and a quicker recovery. This is especially true in cases where internal fixation is likely to fail due to mechanical factors, loose implants, or patients' factors [3, 15, 16].

Intraoperative distal femoral fractures: more common with PS implants if the box cut is not accurate causing condylar fractures during impaction at a wrong angle. These are treated when recognised with a buttress plate. If it happens during trialling then a short-cemented stem on a revision femoral component can be used instead.

Acute Periprosthetic Distal Femoral Fractures: these are the biggest group of periprosthetic fractures, usually at the level of the anterior flange, supracondylar into the intercondylar region, and often associated with significant comminution in frail elderly patients with osteoporosis.

The question of whether to fix or replace depends on patient factors, fracture factors and surgeon factors. Our approach, in younger fitter patients with good quality bone, with a well-fixed and well-functioning implant is to fix them. The options are either a supracondylar nail through the centre of the implant or more commonly a lateral locking plate with a medial buttress plate as an adjunctive fixation for stability in selected cases with medial comminution. Alternatively, a combined lateral plate and anterior strut allograft can be used. In a multicentre study of 36 periprosthetic fractures around *primary* knees (18 plating vs. 18 combined plating and cortical strut), significantly better union rates (77.8% vs. 100%) and patient-reported outcomes were obtained with the combined use of a plate and struts [17].

In older patients with comminuted fractures, almost all fixation techniques necessitate protected weight-bearing which is difficult for elderly patients. This has an impact on their recovery and increases their risk of medical complications. Our strategy is therefore to use distal femoral replacements with immediate stability and early mobilisation. Most fractures are low and most revision systems have a distal femoral replacement with a cemented stem option.

Surgical technique: utilising the old midline incision and extending as far proximally as needed to expose the distal femur, knees were approached through a standard medial parapatellar arthrotomy. Then by distracting the leg, the joint line would be apparent. Here, we provisionally offer up the shortest trial DFR to determine the level of distal femoral resection. We mark the resection level with diathermy but under-resect by approximately 1 cm on the principle that we can always resect more bone if needed. Then, using bone holding forceps above the resection level, we dissect out the distal femur, protecting the posterior structures, shelling out the distal femur, fracture fragments and component. We release the tourniquet at this point to ensure haemostasis. The femoral canal is then prepared with reamers to accept an appropriate diameter cemented stem.

Attention is then turned to the tibia which is prepared in the standard fashion, removing the component with minimal bone loss. The canal is reamed to accept an appropriate diameter cemented stem. A trial is then assembled and articulated with the tibial component. On the femoral trial, use a larger stem trial of a similar size to the last reamer to give some stability during trialling. The joint line level is restored and checked using a combination of anatomical markers and length measurements including the patellofemoral articulation. Achieving correct rotation of the components is crucial to ensure patellofemoral tracking, and this can be challenging with the loss of traditional landmarks such as the trans-epicondylar axis. Once satisfactory trial positioning is obtained, a mark is placed on the femur and the tibia using diathermy to identify the position of the definitive implants which are assembled to match the trials and cemented in place. We fully cement the stems, using cement restrictors, cement guns and pressurisation. Routine closure is then performed in layers over a drain which is removed in 24 h. Full weight-bearing is commenced as tolerated with routine physiotherapy.

Top Tip: Do not distalise the joint line, ensure adequate component rotation and tension in the PFJ at 90° flexion similar to a primary.

Periprosthetic distal femoral fractures around stemmed or revision implants: most of these fractures are around or at the tip of the stem. Therefore, these are diaphyseal fractures and require fixation if the implants are well-fixed. A combined technique of lateral locking plates and anterior strut allograft provide better mechanical stability and union rate compared to plating alone [18].

16.3 Our Experience in DFRs for Acute Comminuted Periprosthetic Fractures

In a retrospective consecutive study, we reported our series of 30 patients who underwent a DFR for periprosthetic distal femoral fractures with minimum 2-year follow up between 2010–2018 [19]. Patients were identified using a prospective database. Demographic, clinical, and surgical data were collected from patients' electronic health records. All patients underwent routine preoperative anaesthetic assessment and received a spinal anaesthetic with upper thigh tourniquet and perioperative prophylactic antibiotics.

Implants: we used the METS® SMILES Total Knee Replacement (Stanmore Implants Worldwide Ltd) which is a modular system consisting of a SMILES distal femoral component, a range of shafts in 15 mm increments to suit differing lengths of resections, options of hydroxyapatite coated or uncoated collars, and a range of cemented stems to fit the intramedullary canal. We routinely use the SMILES knee rotating hinge metal casing tibia with cemented stems (140 or 180 mm). We also used the LPS™ Limb Preservation System (DePuy, Warsaw, IN) with cemented stems, cemented metaphyseal sleeves and a mobile bearing hinge. The minimum distal femoral resection for LPS™ is 70 mm when using the extra-small DFR component. Choice of implant was dictated by the degree of bone loss and adjunctive fixation required as well as patient factors, the soft tissue envelope, and some consideration to the overall cost of the construct with the SMILES system being considerably cheaper and therefore preferentially used for older patients.

Outcome Measures: clinical outcomes, surgical complications, hospital length of stay, revision for any cause, loosening and mortality data were collected. Knee Society Score (KSS) [20] at final follow up was used as patient' reported outcome measure; if KSS score was not collected at final follow up, we contacted the patients/caregivers for the purposes of the study to undertake clinical assessment.

Results: average age was 81 years (range 65–90); 6 males and 24 females. Mechanism of injury was a simple mechanical fall in 24 patients, and a fall due to medical compilations (dizziness, loss of balance and collapse) in the remaining 6 patients. Only 5 patients had been mobilising independently prior to their falls and 25 with walking aids. All patients had multiple comorbidities (ASA-II 1/30, ASA-III 26/30, ASA-IV 3/30). All had comminuted fractures (*Rorabeck* type-2/3) and were thought to have a high risk of failure using fracture fixation techniques. All patients had cemented distal femoral replacements; 21 patients (70%) had SMILES and 9 patients had LPS™ DFRs. Three patients (10%) with multiple comorbidities died postoperatively; 2 patients within the same acute admission (hospital acquired pneumonia, myocardial infarction), and a third died in a nursing home facility 9 weeks postoperatively. Average time from admission to being fit for discharge was 9 days (range 3–14). Clinical outcomes and follow up was available for 27 patients with median follow up of 4 years (2–13 years).

Two patients (2/27; 7.4%) developed complications; One patient, required reoperation at 7 years for change of polyethylene which had dislocated following a fall. Her implant remains in situ at a total of 13 years follow-up. Another patient dislocated her patella but was able to continue mobilising and opted for conservative management due to her low demands and medical comorbidities. Both of these patients had poor functional scores. There were no cases of infection and none of the patients have been revised to date. The average KSS score at final follow up was 78 (range 57–92) with median arc of motion flexion–extension 100° (range 60–125) (Tables 16.1).

Survivorship analysis: 3/30 patients died postoperatively and further 4 patients later died at 1.2, 2, 3.5 and 5 years for unrelated causes. At median 4 year follow up, patients' survivorship for the entire data set was 74.6%.

Our indications to use a DFR in favour of fixation techniques is when the distal segment does not offer enough support for the retained prosthesis. Further with the use of cemented stemmed DFR implants, immediate weight bearing is encouraged and non-union as a surgical complication of fixation techniques is eliminated. Further, similar to hip fracture patients, this cohort of patients is elderly with multiple comorbidities and early mobilisation is crucial to minimise perioperative medical complications associated with these fractures [10, 21, 22] (Figs. 16.1, 16.2, 16.3, 16.4, 16.5 and 16.6).

Table 16.1   Clinical outcomes at final follow up

Outcome	Number of patients Median (range)	
Operative time (n = 30)	128 min (105–153)	
Blood loss (n = 30)	523 mls (419–838)	
Follow up (years)	4 (2–13)	
Arc Flexion–Extension	100° (60–125)	
Knee Society Score (n = 27)	78 (57–92)	Poor 4 (14.8%) Fair 4 (14.8%) Good 3 (11.1%) Excellent 16 (59.3%)
Complications	2/27	1 reoperation for insert dislocation 1 patella dislocation

*(combined- intra-operative and drain output)

Table 16.2 Outcomes of DFR for periprosthetic fractures in the literature

Study [number]	Average follow up (months)	Number of patients	Revision rate	Early Postoperative Mortality rate
Mortazavi 2010 [25]	58.6	20	10%	10%
Jassim 2014 [26]	33	11	0	9.1%
Rao 2014 [27]	20	12	0	0
Rahamn 2016 [15]	33.9	17	11.8%	5.8%
Darrith 2020 [28]	58.2	22	13.6%	31.8%
Our series [19]	48	30	0	10%

(i)

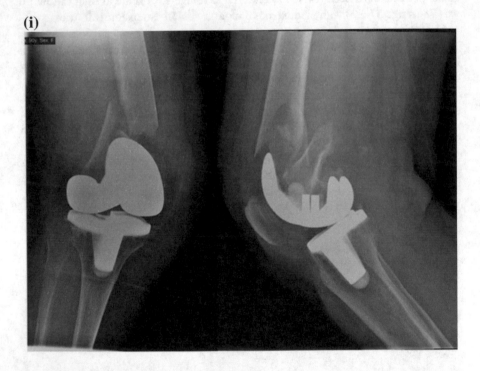

Fig. 16.1 i) Preoperative anteroposterior and lateral radiograph of the right knee with a comminuted periprosthetic fracture in a 90 years old female. **ii)** Anteroposterior and lateral postoperative radiographs at 2 years follow up

(ii)

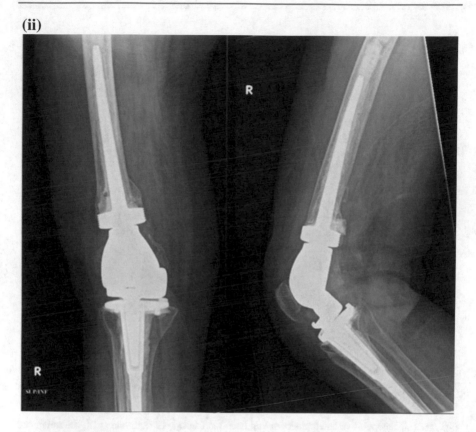

Fig. 16.1 (continued)

Literature Overview (Table 16.2): In a multicentre retrospective study of 55 patients (3 level-I trauma centres) with distal femoral periprosthetic fractures treated with a precontoured locking plate, overall complication rates of 24% and non-union rates of 18% were reported [23]. Similarly, another report of 36 periprosthetic distal femoral fractures (35 patients from 2 trauma centres) managed with locking plate fixation had an overall non-union rate of 30.6% [7]. In a systematic review comparing the outcomes of locking compression plating and retrograde intramedullary nailing for periprosthetic supracondylar femoral fractures, six studies reported non-union rates between the two treatment modalities, which were 24/221 (10.9%) in the locking plate group versus 19/136 (14.0%) in the nailing group. Of those, four studies reported on further revision surgery required for non-union cases: 24/109 (22.0%) versus 26/98 (26.5%) [24]. Finally, in a systematic review of 41 studies of distal femur periprosthetic fracture fixation by fracture type, locking plates used to treat *Rorabeck type II* fractures had a complication rate of 35% and those treated with intramedullary nailing had a higher complication rate of 53% [12].

(i)

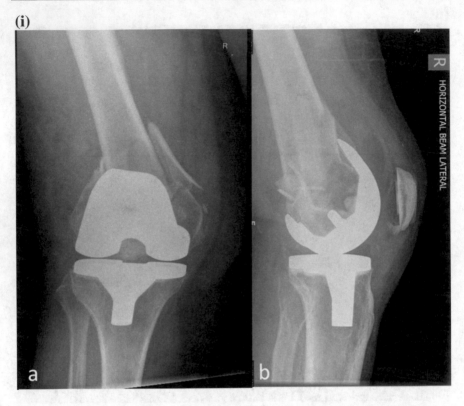

Fig. 16.2 **i)** Preoperative anteroposterior and lateral radiograph of right knee with a comminuted periprosthetic fracture in 70 years old female. **ii)** Anteroposterior and lateral postoperative radiographs at 2 years follow up

In our series, patients were all *Rorabeck type II/III* and our overall complication rate was 7.4%. The early postoperative mortality rate was 10%. However, mortality rates as high as 30% at 1 year after periprosthetic distal femoral fractures have been reported for this complex cohort of patients [10]. The functional scores achieved at various points of follow up using the KSS indicate that almost two thirds of our patients had good/excellent outcomes.

The use of DFR for managing periprosthetic fractures in distal femur is gaining popularity. Several small case-series have reported similar clinical outcomes at short- to medium-term follow up [15, 25–28]. A recent report from the Mayo Clinic on their experience using DFRs in 144 cases (11 native fractures, 55 periprosthetic femoral fractures, 40 2-stage reconstruction for infection, 28 aseptic loosening, and 10 other indications) [29], reported 10-year cumulative incidences of revision for aseptic loosening, all-cause revision, and any reoperation of 17, 27.5, and 46.3%, respectively [29].

(ii)

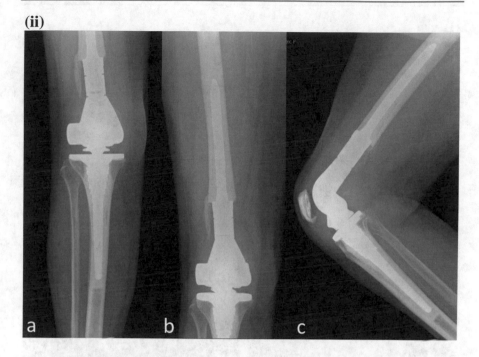

Fig. 16.2 (continued)

In a consecutive series of 60 periprosthetic distal femoral fractures at mean follow up 3.8 years (1–10.4), DFRs were compared with lateral locking plate fixation. (LLP-ORIF) or distal femoral arthroplasty (DFA). Reoperations were more common following fixation 7/33 versus 0/27 (P = 0.008). Five-year survival for reoperation was significantly better following DFRs; 100% compared to 70.8% (95% CI; 51.8% to 89.8%, P = 0.006). There was no significant difference for the endpoint mechanical failure (including radiological loosening); fixation 74.5% versus DFR 78.2% (P = 0.182). Reoperation following fixation was independently associated with medial comminution and anatomical reduction was protective against reoperation [30].

Top Tip: Periprosthetic knee fractures should be treated expeditiously, similar to neck of femur fractures, and with early discussion between trauma and revision arthroplasty surgeons to decide the best option for individual cases; fixation versus DFR.

In conclusion, periprosthetic distal femoral fractures are the most common around the knee and expected to increase with the high demand for TKA. For acute comminuted fractures, we found that the use of DFRs lead to satisfactory clinical outcomes with acceptable complication rate for this challenging group of patients. Meticulous preoperative planning is crucial with appropriate surgical skills in using endoprostheses. Further, avoiding excessive tension/load on the extensor

(i)

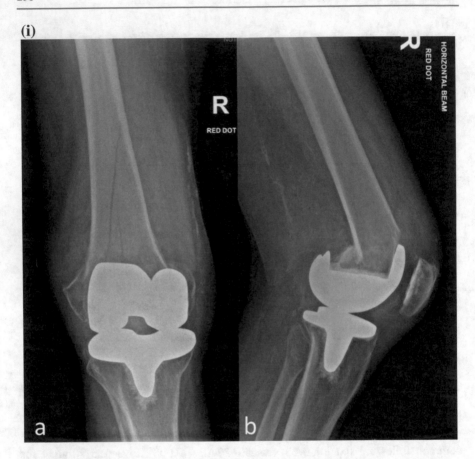

Fig. 16.3 i) Preoperative anteroposterior and lateral radiograph of right knee in a 78 years old male with comminuted periprosthetic fracture of the distal femur propagating proximally around a posterior-stabilised knee. **ii)** Postoperative radiographs at 5 years follow up demonstrating the use of a cable around the distal femur ensuring anatomical reduction and "reconstituting the tube"; then cementing a distal femoral replacement component and allowing the patient to mobilise fully weight bearing in the immediate postoperative period

mechanism and subsequent "overstuffing of the patellofemoral joint", particularly with the use of hinged implants to minimise risk of extensor mechanism' complications. Adequate restoration of the joint line also helps to restore normal mechanics of the patellofemoral joint. Immediate mobilisation with the ability to fully weight-bear helps to reduce perioperative medical complications.

(ii)

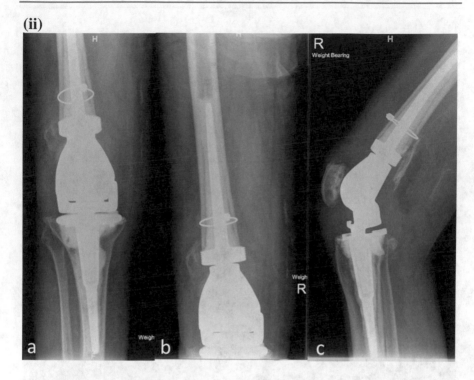

Fig. 16.3 (continued)

(i)

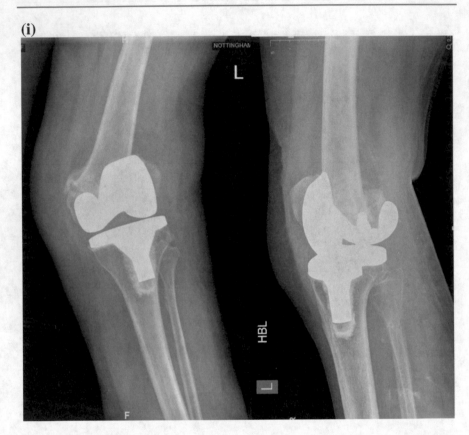

Fig. 16.4 i) Preoperative anteroposterior and lateral radiograph of the left knee in an 81 years old female with a distal femoral fracture and a loose CR knee. **ii)** Postoperative radiographs at 3 years follow up following a SMILES cemented DFR with a fixed hinge due to the narrow tibial intramedullary canal

(ii)

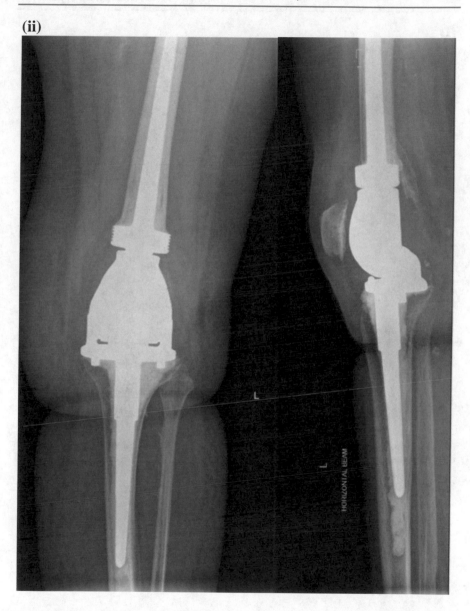

Fig. 16.4 (continued)

(i)

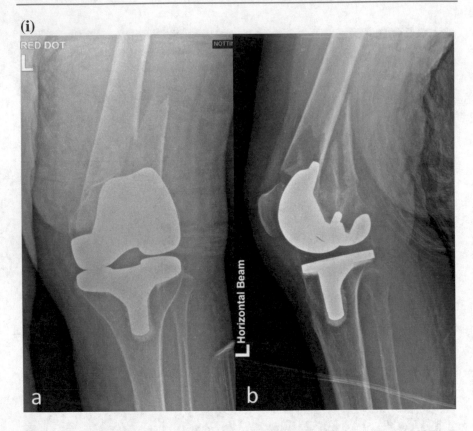

Fig. 16.5 i) Anteroposterior and lateral radiographs of the right knee in an 82 years old female with a comminuted distal femoral fracture. **ii)** Postoperative radiographs following DFR reconstruction with an adjunctive HA coated collar as a body extension to the DFR with high level resection due to the fracture configuration

(ii)

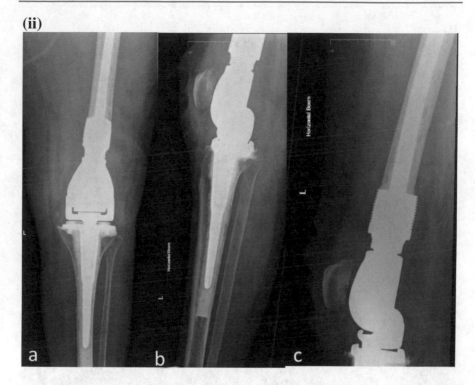

Fig. 16.5 (continued)

(i)

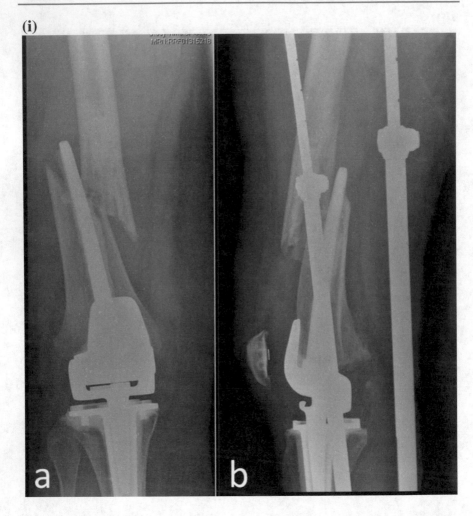

Fig. 16.6 i) Anteroposterior and lateral radiographs of right knee with a cemented rotating hinge implant with a periprosthetic fracture in the distal femur. **ii) a, b** Postoperative radiographs following open reduction and internal fixation using a combination of lateral long locking plate and anterior strut allograft; **c, d** 1-year radiographs with a healed fracture and integrated allograft

(ii)

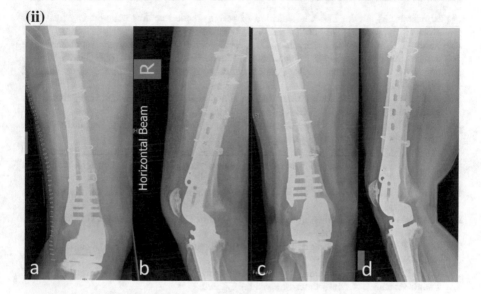

Fig. 16.6 (continued)

References

1. Dennis DA. Periprosthetic fractures following total knee arthroplasty. Instr Course Lect. 2001;50:379–89.
2. Della Rocca GJ, Leung KS, Pape HC. Periprosthetic fractures: epidemiology and future projections. J Orthop Trauma. 2011:S66–70.
3. Ricci WM. Periprosthetic femur fractures. J Orthop Trauma. 2015;29(3):130–7.
4. Kim KI, et al. Periprosthetic fractures after total knee arthroplasties. Clin Orthop Relat Res. 2006;446:167–75.
5. Herrera DA, et al. Treatment of acute distal femur fractures above a total knee arthroplasty: systematic review of 415 cases (1981–2006). Acta Orthop. 2008;79(1):22–7.
6. Singh JA, Jensen M, Lewallen D. Predictors of periprosthetic fracture after total knee replacement: an analysis of 21,723 cases. Acta Orthop. 2013;84(2):170–7.
7. Hoffmann MF, et al. Outcome of periprosthetic distal femoral fractures following knee arthroplasty. Injury. 2012;43(7):1084–9.
8. Yoo JD, Kim NK. Periprosthetic fractures following total knee arthroplasty. Knee Surg Relat Res. 2015;27(1):1–9.
9. Meek RM, et al. The risk of peri-prosthetic fracture after primary and revision total hip and knee replacement. J Bone Joint Surg Br. 2011;93(1):96–101.
10. Streubel PN. Mortality after periprosthetic femur fractures. J Knee Surg. 2013;26(1):27–30.
11. Smith TJ et al. Periprosthetic fractures through tracking pin sites following computer navigated and robotic total and unicompartmental knee arthroplasty: a systematic review. JBJS Rev. 2021; 9(1):e20.00091.
12. Ebraheim NA, et al. Periprosthetic distal femur fracture after total Knee arthroplasty: a systematic review. Orthop Surg. 2015;7(4):297–305.
13. Konan S et al. Periprosthetic fractures associated with total knee arthroplasty: an update. Bone Joint J. 2016; **98-b**(11):1489–96.

14. Rorabeck CH, Taylor JW. Classification of periprosthetic fractures complicating total knee arthroplasty. Orthop Clin North Am. 1999;30(2):209–14.
15. Rahman WA, Vial TA, Backstein DJ. Distal femoral arthroplasty for management of periprosthetic supracondylar fractures of the femur. J Arthroplasty. 2016;31(3):676–9.
16. Parvizi J, Jain N, Schmidt AH. Periprosthetic knee fractures. J Orthop Trauma. 2008;22 (9):663–71.
17. Rollo G et al. Standard plating vs. cortical strut and plating for periprosthetic knee fractures: a multicentre experience. Med Glas (Zenica). 2020; 17(1):170–7.
18. Matar HE, et al. Cortical strut allografts in salvage revision arthroplasty: Surgical technique and clinical outcomes. J Clin Orthop Trauma. 2021;17:37–43.
19. Matar HE, Bloch BV, James PJ. Distal femoral replacements for acute comminuted periprosthetic knee fractures: satisfactory clinical outcomes at medium-term follow-up. Arthroplast Today. 2021;7:37–42.
20. Insall JN, et al. Rationale of the Knee Society clinical rating system. Clin Orthop Relat Res. 1989;248:13–4.
21. Streubel PN, et al. Mortality after distal femur fractures in elderly patients. Clin Orthop Relat Res. 2011;469(4):1188–96.
22. Myers P, et al. Patient mortality in geriatric distal femur fractures. J Orthop Trauma. 2018;32 (3):111–5.
23. Campbell ST et al. Complication Rates after Lateral Plate Fixation of Periprosthetic Distal Femur Fractures: A Multicenter Study. Injury, 2020.
24. Shin YS, Kim HJ, Lee DH. Similar outcomes of locking compression plating and retrograde intramedullary nailing for periprosthetic supracondylar femoral fractures following total knee arthroplasty: a meta-analysis. Knee Surg Sports Traumatol Arthrosc. 2017;25(9):2921–8.
25. Mortazavi SM, et al. Distal femoral arthroplasty for the treatment of periprosthetic fractures after total knee arthroplasty. J Arthroplasty. 2010;25(5):775–80.
26. Jassim SS, McNamara I, Hopgood P. Distal femoral replacement in periprosthetic fracture around total knee arthroplasty. Injury. 2014;45(3):550–3.
27. Rao B, et al. Distal femoral replacement for selective periprosthetic fractures above a total knee arthroplasty. Eur J Trauma Emerg Surg. 2014;40(2):191–9.
28. Darrith B, et al. Periprosthetic fractures of the distal femur: is open reduction and internal fixation or distal femoral replacement superior? J Arthroplasty. 2020;35(5):1402–6.
29. Wyles CC, et al. Long-term results of total knee arthroplasty with contemporary distal femoral replacement. J Bone Joint Surg Am. 2020;102(1):45–51.
30. Ross LA et al. Management of low periprosthetic distal femoral fractures. Bone Joint J. 2021; 103-b(4):635–43.

Mortality in Revision Knee Arthroplasty

17

You can die of the cure before you die of the illness.
Michael Landon.

17.1 Introduction

Mortality after primary hip and knee arthroplasty is thought to be lower than the general population in the first decade after surgery but gradually increases to higher than expected after 12 years [1]. It is thought that this initial decrease in mortality is due to the fact that patients undergoing TKA are more likely to be in good physical health. However, in rTKA populations, the overall risk of failure and complications is much higher particularly with septic revisions [2, 3]. The demand for primary TKA continues to rise worldwide with a corresponding projected increase in rTKA [4, 5].

Periprosthetic joint infection (PJI) is a devastating complication with significant implications on patient-reported outcomes [6] and increased costs to healthcare systems with a significant economic burden [7–10]. Early 90-day complications and mortality rates are also higher following septic- compared to aseptic- rTKA [11]. Five-year mortality following septic rTKA has been reported in numerous studies as high as 21% [12] and up to 34% at 7-year [13]. These are significantly high mortality rates and reflect the complexity of this cohort of patients.

In this chapter, we will present our tertiary series comparing long-term mortality rates between septic and aseptic rTKA and the important implications on patients' selection and informed consent [14].

© The Author(s), under exclusive license to Springer Nature Switzerland AG 2021
H. E. Matar et al., *Revision Total Knee Arthroplasty*,
https://doi.org/10.1007/978-3-030-81285-0_17

17.2   The Scale of the Problem

The demand for TKA is rising worldwide. In this context of increasing demand, particularly with more younger patients offered TKAs [15], understanding mortality trends in rTKA is crucial in counselling patients at time of primary TKA. This is particularly important for high-risk patients of developing PJI. Most published mortality studies in rTKA are of short- to medium- term follow up with the main focus on perioperative mortality [16–18]. Little is known about the long-term mortality trends of rTKA patients. Therefore, we aimed to examine the differences in long-term mortality rates between septic and aseptic rTKA in a single specialist centre over 17-year period.

17.3   Our Series on Mortality in Septic Versus Aseptic rTKA

Methods: we undertook a retrospective study of all consecutive patients who underwent rTKA at our tertiary centre between 1st April 2003 and 31st Dec 2019. We identified our cohort through local prospective electronic databases and linkable data obtained from the UK National Joint Registry (NJR) for rTKA. Revisions were classified as single-stage, stage-1, or stage-2 of two-stage revision; a two-stage procedure was considered as a single revision episode. For calculation of mortality statistics in two-stage revisions, the date of the first procedure was recorded as the date of index procedure. Patients who underwent a two-stage revision would have at least two NJR-linked procedures. For patients who had bilateral revisions, the date of the first revision was also recorded as the index procedure.

We identified patients' age, gender, American Society of Anesthesiologists (ASA) score [19], body mass index (BMI kg/m^2) and indication for revision surgery which was grouped into "septic" or "aseptic". The latter included aseptic loosening, instability, polyethylene wear, malalignment, periprosthetic fracture, implant failure, stiffness, and pain.

Outcome measures: The primary outcome measure was all-cause mortality at 5-years, 10-years and over the whole study period (17-years). Death was identified through both local hospital electronic databases and linked data from the NJR which uses data from the NHS Personal Demographic Service; a national database that holds demographic details of all users of health and care services in England.

Operative strategies: Our standard practice in treating PJIs is to consider debridement, antibiotics, and implant retention (DAIR) in selected cases of early postoperative infection (<4–6 weeks duration) or late haematogenous infection with acute onset of symptoms in previously well-functioning TKA [20, 21]. We also consider a single-stage approach in selected patients with a single infecting organism of low virulence and known sensitivities, in immunocompetent patients without soft tissue compromise and in the absence of a draining sinus [22]. Our two-stage approach involves a thorough debridement, removal of the infected prosthesis, and implantation of either an articulating spacer using a standard TKA prosthesis with an all-poly tibia component (PFC Sigma, DePuy Synthes, Warsaw, Indiana), or a static spacer using a temporary fusion nail (Waldemar LINK GmbH & Co, Hamburg, Germany). These spacers are implanted with antibiotic-loaded cement, and additional antibiotics can be added, tailored to the infecting organism. Following a period of antibiotic therapy, the definitive rTKA is then implanted in a second stage procedure [24]. Aseptic revisions are performed, and coded, as single-stage revisions using either cemented or cementless components with varying degrees of constraint based on the individual factors such as bone loss, joint line restoration and ligamentous insufficiency.

Statistical Analysis: Differences in patient characteristics were assessed using the *chi-square test* for categorical variables and the *t-test* for continuous variables; differences were considered significant for P-value < 0.05. *Kaplan–Meier survival* curves were used to estimate time to death. The *log-rank test* was used to test statistical significance. The 10-year risk of death for septic versus aseptic revisions was estimated using generalised linear models. A priori confounders included age, gender, ASA, and BMI. Modification of the risk ratios were examined. Statistical analyses were performed using SPSS 16.0 software (SPSS Inc., Chicago, IL).

Results: During the study period, 1,298 consecutive knee revisions were performed on 1,254 patients. Forty-four patients had bilateral revisions. There were 985 aseptic revisions in 945 patients (75.4%) and 313 septic revisions in 309 patients (24.6%). PJI was diagnosed based on the Musculoskelctal Infection Society (MSIS) classification which was applied retrospectively prior to 2011. The infecting organisms were identified in 84.3% of revisions (15.7% were culture negative PJI). The average age was 70.6 years (range 27–95) with 720 females (57.4%). The BMI data was available for 879 (68%) patients with mean 31.2 (range 16–53). There were no statistically significant differences in baseline characteristics between the two groups in age, gender, or BMI (Table 17.1). However, there were statistically significant differences in ASA grades between the two groups with higher grades for the septic group, which is suggestive of an increased prevalence of comorbidities in the septic population (Table 17.1).

In the septic group, there were 17 successful DAIRs (5.4%), 111 (35.6%) single-stage revisions, and the remaining 186 (59%) were two-stage revisions of which 7 required further salvage procedures (6 arthrodesis and 1 above-knee amputation). The total number of surgical episodes for the septic group was 496 NJR-linked procedures. In the aseptic group, there were 985 revisions with a total number of 1,159 NJR-linked procedures.

Patients' survivorship and Mortality Rates: Kaplan–Meier survivorship curves demonstrate that septic revisions had a higher mortality rates at 5 years, 10 years, and throughout the 17 year study period (Figs. 17.1 and 17.2). Patients' survivorship for septic versus aseptic revisions was 77.6% vs. 89.5% at 5 years, 68.7% vs. 80.2% at 10 years and 66.1% vs. 75.0% at 17 years; these differences were all statistically significant $P < 0.0001$ (Table 17.2).

Table 17.1 Demographic and surgical data

Demographics	TOTAL	Septic	Aseptic	P-value
Number of patients	N = 1,254	N = 309	N = 945	
Number of revisions	N = 1,298	N = 313	N = 985	
Demographics:				
Patient Age (y) [Median (IQR)]	71 (64–78)	72 (65–79)	71 (64–78)	0.928
Female [N (%)]	720 (57.4%)	179 (57.9%)	539 (57%)	0.781
BMI [Median (IQR)] Mean ± SD (range) (number of patients)	31 (27–35) 31.2 ± 5.9(16–53) (n = 879)	30 (27–34) 31.0 ± 6.1 (20–53) (n = 187)	31 (27–35) 31.3 ± 5.8 (16–51) (n = 692)	0.699
ASA: N (%) I	108 (8.3)	14 (4.5)	94 (9.5)	0.0056
II	768 (59.2)	156 (49.8)	612 (62.2)	0.0001
III	389 (30)	128 (40.9)	261 (26.5)	0.0001
IV	33 (2.5)	15 (4.8)	18 (1.8)	0.0036

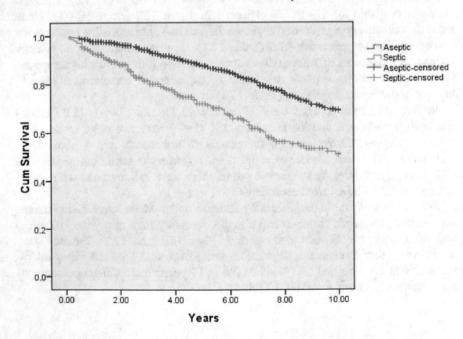

Fig. 17.1 Patients' Kaplan–Meier survivorship curve at 10-years

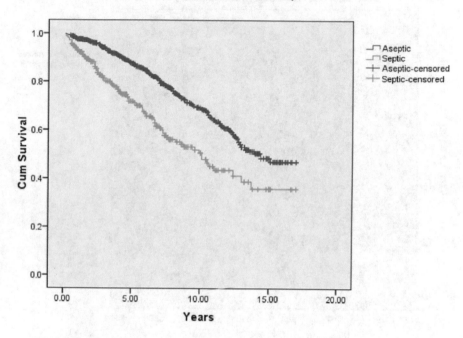

Fig. 17.2 Patients' Kaplan–Meier survivorship curve over the study period (17-years)

Table 17.2 Patients' survivorship in septic versus aseptic revisions at 5-, 10- and 17-years

Survivorship (years)	Septic		Aseptic		P-value
	%	Mean survivorship (95% CI)	%	Mean Survivorship (95% CI)	
5 yrs	77.6	4.26 (4.09 to 4.42)	89.5	4.73 (4.68 to 4.79	<0.0001
10 yrs	68.7	7.26 (6.82 to 7.69)	80.2	8.65 (8.48 to 8.83)	<0.0001
17 yrs	66.1	10.04 (9.10 to 10.98)	75.0	12.48 (12.04 to 12.92)	<0.0001

Finally, to account for the early excess deaths seen in the first 5 years, we compared mortality rates beyond 5 years. There were 713 patients with a minimum 5-year follow up (125 septic vs. 588 aseptic) with a higher mortality rate in the septic group (Fig. 17.3).

In the regression models, the unadjusted 10-year risk ratio of death after septic revision was 1.59 (95% CI; 1.29 to 1.96) compared to aseptic revisions. When adjusting for age, gender, BMI and ASA grade the risk ratio was 1.68 (95% CI; 1.37 to 1.98) (Table 17.3).

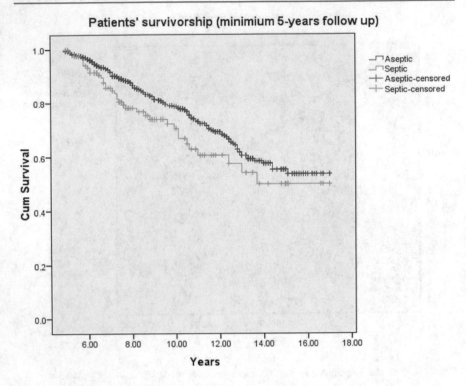

Fig. 17.3 Patients' Kaplan–Meier survivorship curve with minimum 5 years follow up

Table 17.3 Crude and Adjusted 10-year Risk Ratio of Death in Septic compared to Aseptic revisions

Exposure	Alive N = 968	Dead N = 286	Total N = 1,254	Unadjusted RR (95% CI)	Adjusted[a] RR (95% CI)
Septic	211 (21.8%)	98 (34.3%)	309 (24.6%)	1.59 (1.29 to 1.96)	1.68 (1.37 to 1.98)
Aseptic	757 (78.2%)	188 (65.7%)	945 (75.4%)		

[a]Adjusted for age, gender, BMI and ASA

Limitations: the use of administrative data has its inherent limitations as we could not fully account for unmeasured confounders. Secondly, we lacked data on background mortality and associated comorbidities and instead we used the ASA grade as a *surrogate* measure. However, patients' characteristics were similar in both groups except for ASA grade which reflects the morbidity of infection and host risk factors [23]. Finally, although the practice of rTKA in different healthcare systems is variable, this study has a large sample size and high internal validity as our data was collected uniformly for all patients and mortality data was collected nationally making these findings generalisable. Further, our unit is a specialist tertiary centre with a dedicated microbiology support in a multidisciplinary team approach which ensures standardisation of care.

17.4   rTKA Mortality in the Literature

Our findings indicate that patients who underwent septic revisions had persistently higher mortality rates at 5- *(22.4 vs.10.5)*, 10- *(31.3 vs. 19.8)* and 17-year *(33.1 vs. 25%)* compared to aseptic revisions.

In their meta-analysis of 14 studies of mortality rate following rTKA in PJI, with a total of 20,719 patients, Lum et al.reported an aggregated 1-year mortality of 4.33% and 5-year mortality rate of 21.64% [12]. Further, in their matched cohort of 88 patients with septic/aseptic rTKA, Choi et al., reported mortality rate of 18% vs. 3% at median 4 years follow up [24]. In their series from the Mayo clinic, Yao et al.reported on their cohort of 4,907 patients between 1985 and 2015. Their 10-year mortality rate was 47% for septic revisions, 46% in revisions for periprosthetic fractures, 34% in revisions for aseptic loosening and 31% in revisions for instability [25].

17.5   Practical Implications

In our cohort, the 10-year survivorship of septic revisions was 68.7% and 80.2% for aseptic revisions. These findings have important practical implications as these outcomes are comparable to what we see in some cancer patients with risk of mortality following septic rTKA being higher than some of the most common cancers [26]. For example, in the UK, the most common types of cancer are breast, prostate, lung and bowel respectively with 10-year survivorship rates of 78% for breast, 77.6% for prostate, 9.5% for lung and 60% for bowel cancer [27]. This reality should be highlighted in candid discussions when counselling patients not only at time of revision surgery, when patients have little choice where infection has already developed, but more importantly at time of primary TKA particularly for those patients who are at higher risk for developing PJI [28, 29].

In conclusion, revision total knee arthroplasty performed for infection is associated with significantly higher post-operative mortality at all time points compared with aseptic revision surgery.

References

1. Harris IA, et al. How does mortality risk change over time after hip and knee arthroplasty? Clin Orthop Relat Res. 2019;477(6):1414–21.
2. Hamilton DF, et al. Dealing with the predicted increase in demand for revision total knee arthroplasty: challenges, risks and opportunities. Bone Joint J. 2015;97-b(6):723–8.

3. Geary MB, et al. Why do revision total knee arthroplasties fail? A single-center review of 1632 revision total knees comparing historic and modern cohorts. J Arthroplasty. 2020.
4. Singh JA, et al. Rates of total joint replacement in the United States: Future projections to 2020–2040 using the national inpatient sample. J Rheumatol. 2019;46(9):1134–40.
5. 17th Annual Report of the National Joint Registry for England, Wales, Northern Ireland, the Isle of Man and the States of Guernsey. https://reports.njrcentre.org.uk/Portals/0/PDFdownloads/NJR%2017th%20Annual%20Report%202020.pdf. Accessed 23 Oct 2020.
6. Greidanus NV, et al. Quality of life outcomes in revision versus primary total knee arthroplasty. J Arthroplasty. 2011;26(4):615–20.
7. Blom AW, et al. Infection after total knee arthroplasty. J Bone Joint Surg Br. 2004;86(5):688–91.
8. Huotari K, Peltola M, Jämsen E. The incidence of late prosthetic joint infections: a registry-based study of 112,708 primary hip and knee replacements. Acta Orthop. 2015;86 (3):321–5.
9. Kurtz SM, et al. Economic burden of periprosthetic joint infection in the United States. J Arthroplasty. 2012;27(8 Suppl):61-5.e1.
10. Meyer E, et al. Impact of department volume on surgical site infections following arthroscopy, knee replacement or hip replacement. BMJ Qual Saf. 2011;20(12):1069–74.
11. Boddapati V, et al. Revision total knee arthroplasty for periprosthetic joint infection is associated with increased postoperative morbidity and mortality relative to noninfectious revisions. J Arthroplasty. 2018;33(2):521–6.
12. Lum ZC, et al. Mortality during total knee periprosthetic joint infection. J Arthroplasty. 2018;33(12):3783–8.
13. Haleem AA, Berry DJ, Hanssen AD. Mid-term to long-term followup of two-stage reimplantation for infected total knee arthroplasty. Clin Orthop Relat Res. 2004;428:35–9.
14. Matar HE, et al. Septic revision total knee arthroplasty is associated with significantly higher mortality than aseptic revisions: Long-term single-center study (1254 Patients). J Arthroplasty. 2021.
15. Bayliss LE, et al. The effect of patient age at intervention on risk of implant revision after total replacement of the hip or knee: a population-based cohort study. Lancet. 2017;389 (10077):1424–30.
16. Jones MD, et al. Early death following revision total knee arthroplasty. J Orthop. 2020;19:114–7.
17. Memtsoudis SG, et al. Risk factors for perioperative mortality after lower extremity arthroplasty: A population-based study of 6,901,324 patient discharges. J Arthroplasty. 2010;25(1):19–26.
18. Traven SA, et al. Frailty predicts medical complications, length of stay, readmission, and mortality in revision hip and knee arthroplasty. J Arthroplasty. 2019;34(7):1412–6.
19. Saklad M. Grading of patients for surgical procedures. Anesthesiology. 1941;2:281–4.
20. Leone JM, Hanssen AD. Management of infection at the site of a total knee arthroplasty. Instr Course Lect. 2006;55:449–61.
21. Parvizi J, et al. The 2018 definition of periprosthetic hip and knee infection: An evidence-based and validated criteria. J Arthroplasty. 2018;33(5):1309-1314.e2.
22. Freeman MA, et al. The management of infected total knee replacements. J Bone Joint Surg Br. 1985;67(5):764–8.
23. Mayhew D, Mendonca V, Murthy BVS. A review of ASA physical status-historical perspectives and modern developments. Anaesthesia. 2019;74(3):373–9.
24. Choi HR, Bedair H. Mortality following revision total knee arthroplasty: A matched cohort study of septic versus aseptic revisions. J Arthroplasty. 2014;29(6):1216–8.
25. Yao JJ, et al. Long-term mortality trends after revision total knee arthroplasty. J Arthroplasty. 2019;34(3):542–8.
26. Zmistowski B, et al. Periprosthetic joint infection increases the risk of one-year mortality. J Bone Joint Surg Am. 2013;95(24):2177–84.

27. Cancer Statistics for the UK. https://www.cancerresearchuk.org/health-professional/cancer-statistics-for-the-uk. Accessed 2 Aug 2020.
28. Alamanda VK, Springer BD. The prevention of infection: 12 modifiable risk factors. Bone Joint J. 2019;101-b(1_Supple_A):3–9.
29. Lenguerrand E, et al. Risk factors associated with revision for prosthetic joint infection following knee replacement: An observational cohort study from England and Wales. Lancet Infect Dis. 2019;19(6):589–600.

Starting Out in Revision Knee Arthroplasty

18

Benjamin V. Bloch

No Man is an Island. John Donne

18.1 Training, Mentoring and Support

I have been very fortunate to have developed a high-volume revision TKA practice relatively early in my career, but for the new surgeon it can be a daunting prospect to start offering this surgery. It can be complex and technically difficult to perform, and while it can be very gratifying and life-changing surgery with excellent outcomes [1, 2], it can also carry a high complication rate [3] and mortality rate, particularly for infection [4]. It is therefore essential to have appropriate training, mentoring and support when starting out in revision TKA—this is not a procedure that should be adopted by the occasional knee surgeon.

Most revision TKA surgeons will now have completed one or two specialist rTKA fellowships prior to starting out in their consultant career. As well as providing you with excellent training and exposure to rTKA surgery, this also gives you lifelong contacts for advice, case discussions and an informal second opinion! It is always a pleasure to hear from former fellows who have been through our unit and one should not be afraid of seeking a range of opinions, particularly for a complicated or complex case. There is rarely only one correct answer to the problem!

As you start out in your consultant career, it is important to develop local and regional links for mentoring and support. There is new guidance from the British Association for Surgery of the Knee that suggests individual surgeons should be performing at least 15 rTKAs per year, and 30 at the unit level [5]. This is because there is evidence of a volume effect on outcomes [6]. It is accepted that this is going to be tricky for a new consultant, so the concept of dual-consultant operating is supported by specialist societies to help maintain surgeon numbers, and it is hugely valuable for ongoing support in the first few years following your appointment. It can help to develop confidence in the young revision TKA surgeon, and by performing the rarer and more complex techniques such as proximal tibial replacement or extensor mechanism allograft reconstruction together it means that all surgeons in your unit maintain their skills.

A joint complex knee clinic can be a very useful learning experience too that also allows for assessment and discussion of difficult cases, and can only enhance surgical decision making. One should never be afraid to ask for a second opinion in a difficult case, and don't let yourself be persuaded to operate on an unhappy knee if you cannot find a specific cause for the failure that you can correct with surgery [5]. These cases certainly benefit from a senior colleague's opinion and a multidisciplinary assessment.

It is not just orthopaedic support that you will need. As a revision TKA surgeon, you will want the support of a specialist orthopaedic microbiologist, with access to outpatient parenteral antibiotic therapy (OPAT) teams, as well as experienced musculoskeletal radiologists and plastic surgeons. There will be those patients who will not benefit from surgery, and here having access to a good pain management service is invaluable.

You will unfortunately have complications—any surgeon who has no complications is not performing any operations! Infections and early failures are sadly a fact of life with these complex operations, and can have a significant effect on your confidence and your own self-esteem [7]. An experienced colleague and mentor is invaluable to debrief with in the event of an adverse outcome.

18.2   Clinical Networks

In order to support the development of rTKA service provision in the U.K., a hub-and-spoke model of clinical networks is being set up [8, 9]. This provides regional support for units performing rTKA with a specialist hub hospital available for advice and guidance, as well as a referral stream for the most complex cases. This is in keeping with the principles of the *Getting it Right First Time (GIRFT)* initiative [10].

The *East Midlands Specialist Orthopaedic Network (EMSON)* [11] was set up in 2015 as a pilot and has acted as the blueprint for further rTKA networks within the United Kingdom. It covers much of the East Midlands—a geographical area with a population of 4 million—and currently has a hub tertiary hospital in our unit and four spoke hospitals.

All rTKA cases to be performed at these hospitals are discussed at a weekly meeting over a virtual videoconferencing platform. The meeting is chaired by a senior revision knee surgeon, and other specialties such as plastics, radiology and microbiology are all available to provide input if required. The surgeon presenting the case shares his computer screen and controls the imaging on display. Following discussion, a summary of the recommendations is typed and returned to the originating surgeon as a record for the medical notes.

Our early analysis of this network's effect was that a significant number of patients had a change to their proposed surgical plan as a result of discussion—either advice on exposure or technique, changes to kit required or further investigations suggested. Few patients were transferred to the hub for surgery after discussion but we did notice an increase in tertiary referrals, perhaps reflecting a natural move towards centralisation of more complex work [12].

In summary, an early career in rTKA surgery will have many high and low points; having an excellent team around you will make it all the more rewarding!

References

1. Bloch BV, et al. Metaphyseal sleeves in revision total knee arthroplasty provide reliable fixation and excellent medium to long-term implant survivorship. J Arthroplasty. 2020;35 (2):495–9.
2. Stirling P, et al. Revision total knee arthroplasty versus primary total knee arthroplasty. Bone Joint Open. 2020;1(3):29–34.
3. Mortazavi SMJ, et al. Failure following revision total knee arthroplasty: infection is the major cause. Int Orthop. 2011;35(8):1157–64.
4. Matar HE, et al. Septic revision total knee arthroplasty is associated with significantly higher mortality than aseptic revisions: long-term single-center study (1254 Patients). J Arthroplasty. 2021;36(6):2131–6.
5. Kalson NS, et al. Revision knee replacement surgery in the NHS: A BASK surgical practice guideline. Knee. 2021;29:353–64.
6. Yapp LZ, et al. The effect of hospital case volume on re-revision following revision total knee arthroplasty. Bone Joint J. 2021;103-B(4):602–09
7. Svensson K et al. Reflecting on and managing the emotional impact of prosthetic joint infections on orthopaedic surgeons—a qualitative study. Bone Joint J. 2020;102-B(6):736–43.
8. Bloch BV, James PJ, Phillips JRA. Clinical networking in revision knee replacement. Knee. 2020;27(5):1690–2.
9. Kalson NS, et al. Provision of revision knee surgery and calculation of the effect of a network service reconfiguration: An analysis from the National Joint Registry for England, Wales, Northern Ireland and the Isle of Man. Knee. 2020;27(5):1593–600.
10. Briggs T. A national review of adult elective orthopaedic services in England; Getting It Right First Time;2015.
11. Bloch BV, et al. The East Midlands specialist orthopaedic network: The future of revision arthroplasty? Bull R Coll Surg Engl . 2017;99(2):66–70.
12. Bloch BV et al. Two-year experience of a 'hub and spoke' revision arthroplasty network: 1000 cases and counting. Orthopaedic Proc. 2018;100-B(SUPP_11):18–18.

A Lifetime of Revision Knee Arthroplasty

19

Hugh U Cameron

Festina lente, hasten slowly.

19.1 Revision–Why?

Why is a revision being contemplated? There are six main reasons: wear, stiffness, loosening, infection, instability, and pain.

19.2 Wear

In the eighties and nineties, this was a significant problem. It was due to the use of too thin and too constrained plastic components and poor-quality polyethylene. We did not know then that polyethylene oxidises in air. Inert gas packaging and better-quality polyethylene seem to have solved those problems.

It was the medial tibia plateau which wore, leading to a posteromedial pivot, with pain and instability [2]. So far with the Profix knee (Smith and Nephew), which I began to insert about 25 years ago, I have seen no cases which have shown significant wear. As I was never shy about doing young patients, as I always believed that technology would catch up with their problem, it looks like this is not going to be a major issue in the future.

Wear of a replaced patella is a problem. Curiously it is a minor problem in an isolated patellofemoral replacement. As these fail if the tracking is not correct, this suggests that wear of the patellar component in TKR is actually a tracking problem, rather than a wear problem. Fortunately as I described in 1987 [3], the patellar component rapidly becomes covered by an aneural avascular meniscus which protects it. Revision of a thin brittle hollowed out cortical shell is so difficult that after a few tries even the most ardent patellar resurfacer should have second thoughts.

There are three solutions to this problem of the hollow patella, none of which are good. In younger patients the Gull-wing osteotomy as described by Kelly Vince can be done [4]. What is left of the patella is split vertically and wired together like the wings of a gull. I have minimal experience with this, so what I did in these cases was to just to leave it, expecting AVN to occur, and I could worry about that later. In the elderly I placed transverse screws across the gap in the centre of the patella like rebars and cemented the plastic component to the screws. As there never was any integration of the cement and bone, the X-rays always looked terrible, but surprisingly I never had to revise one of these cases, but they were all elderly. Fortunately, in Canada not that many surgeons were seduced into replacing patellae.

The only modern tibial component likely to show significant wear is the central post of a high central post knee. The usual cause for this surprisingly is not medio lateral instability but tibial torsion. A high central post knee can easily handle up to 30° of tibial torsion. But attempting more produces such intolerable stress on the central post that it will likely deform and break. When you revise these cases derotation of the proximal tibia is required, which should have been done either prior to the initial surgery as an interval procedure, or for the brave, at the time of the initial knee replacement. Simply changing the plastic will result in another fracture a few years later.

19.3   Loosening

For most of my life I preferred to use cruciate-retaining knees, although this is a misnomer as I usually sacrificed the cruciates, and I usually used uncemented ingrowth components. The loosening rates for such components was almost zero. I never, with 40 years follow-up, saw an aseptic loosening of an uncemented Tricon knee. This was an opening wedge component so any loosening would simply jam it on tighter. Parallel-sided femoral components should not be used. Cruciate substituting knees were always cemented, as none of the designers of these knees, such as John Insall or Chit Ranawat were interested in uncemented components.

There is a certain loosening rate with cemented knees, especially on the tibial side, where stubby stems have been used. This is obvious on x-ray, and a revision to a longer stemmed component is all that is necessary. If a long stem is used there is no need to resect the tibia to produce a flat bony surface. Minimal contact is required as it is only resisting vertical load. The stem must resist the other loads. In other words, the implant is stem-dependent for fixation. If a cementless stem is used it should be fluted for rotational stability, canal filling and split like clothes peg in the sagittal plane to reduce the tendency to end of stem pain. End of stem pain with a non-flexible stem is a problem with the tibia, but not so much in the femur.

I initially had several cases of significant tibial end of stem pain, as the tibia is much more flexible than the femur. All bones flex under load, which is why they are bent like a leaf spring. The femur obviously flexes into the bow. Years ago, by strain gauging a tibia. I could show that a loaded tibia flexes mediolaterally, rather than anteroposteriorly. To get around the problem when a screw on stem as opposed to a unidirectional taper lock stem was used, the distal few centimetres of the stem can be split in a cruciate fashion.

In a couple of cases I strut allografted the tibia at the pain site to try to stiffen the bone, as we did in hip replacement. I was unconvinced about the result. In several cases it was necessary to revise to a shorter cemented stem. I never had any end of stem pain with a split stem, like an SROM hip stem. On the femur a cementless canal filling stem has to be long, about 200 mm to get up to where the femoral canal is a circular tube. To do so, it has to be bowed. It should also be fluted and split in the coronal plane.

19.4 Stiffness

The first question is why did the joint become stiff, or rather why did the patient fail to regain movement? There are, I am sure, some cases of fibrosis, like the stiff man syndrome. These are very unusual and usually multiple joints are involved, often with periarticular calcification. I had one such case and discussed perioperative radiation with an oncologist. Canada unfortunately was going through one of its numerous austerity binges and he was unwilling to radiate someone for a non-lethal condition, as the waiting list for cancer treatment was so long.

I did treat the few other cases I was worried about with prednisolone 20 mg daily for a week. As there were so few cases I don't know if that helped, or simply the fact that I and my fellows were dancing around these cases so they got much more attention than normal.

Patients who have been stiff for years prior to surgery are going to have a difficult time regaining movement as the quadriceps will have shortened. They may need a tibial tubercle osteotomy and a patellar proximalisation at time of the initial surgery. They must be warned not to expect too much.

If the patient fails to regain movement post-surgery, then manipulation under anaesthesia within the first two weeks, with a femoral nerve block and Continuous Passive Motion (CPM), may be employed. Tibial tubercle osteotomy patients must not be manipulated.

Manipulation after a month post-surgery seldom is useful and risks an avulsion of the patellar tendon, or a fracture of the patella or a supracondylar fracture. If they are stiff at six to eight weeks then a scope, breaking down the adhesions, may help, along with a femoral nerve block and CPM.

If seen after three months, none of that helps, so what to do? When we began knee replacement seventies an excellent was 90° of flexion. Nowadays we expect essentially full flexion, but 75° is all a patient needs to go upstairs, and to come downstairs backwards. At least 90° or more likely 105° is necessary to come downstairs normally.

If the patient is frail and elderly and lives in an apartment with an elevator, then there is not a great concern. A raised toilet solves that problem and portable ejector seats, which help them stand up from an easy chair, are now very reasonably priced. So, I would not hurry too much to do anything to these cases, as many will graciously accept what they have, as their main goal was pain relief. The elderly are often far more realistic than the young.

After one-year post surgery range of movement will not change, so if the patient finds the result intolerable, then revision may be attempted. It however should only be done if the patient is realistic and prepared to work at it.

If there is a fixed flexion deformity, the extension gap must be increased to get the knee out straight. To get more flexion the flexion gap must be increased to such an extent that the knee is unstable AP. A CR knee therefore cannot be used, and I would recommend a high central post knee. If a small post is used the femoral component may jump the post resulting in dislocation. While intraoperatively these cases may seem frighteningly unstable, within six weeks they all scar down, and I have never seen late AP instability as a problem.

If the cause of stiffness is severe patella baja, this must be corrected. A minor degree of baja is helped by hollowing out the lower pole of the patella, so that there is no contact with the tibial component. This should be done at the time of the initial surgery. During a revision, a tibial tubercle osteotomy at least 7 or 8 cms long and 1.5 to 2cms wide is necessary. A lateral parapatellar approach is required. If a medial approach is used the proximalised patella will sublux laterally. A compensatory lateral release may result in patellar avascular necrosis.

If patellar AVN occurs then do nothing for one year. It will disintegrate and about half to one third will dislocate laterally. At one year, remove all bone lateral to the trochlea. Do not attempt to reposition.

The patella can be proximalised 2cms maximum. More than that will result in a permanent quadriceps lag. I prefer to reattach the osteotomy with two or three angled countersunk screws. If they become a nuisance, they may have to be removed later. If wires are used to reattach the tubercle they must be angled otherwise some escape will likely occur. The medial retinaculum is left untouched. The lateral retinaculum is sewn up with the knee in 90° of flexion. Most of the vastus lateralis can be reattached but a fair amount of the retinaculum cannot be closed. If the retinaculum is closed with the knee in extension, the patella will dislocate.

As a general rule, if you are doing anything fancy with the patella, do not resurface it. The risks of AVN far outweigh any benefits. Revision of an infected or loose patella is a thankless procedure. There is no reason to replace the patella -it does not improve the result of a properly done knee replacement.

19.5 Infection

This is a whole separate subject and is far too complex for this chapter. All I would say is not to put any trust in any test for infection. Negative cultures and negative blood work mean nothing. I was so disappointed with aspirations and cultures preop, I stopped doing it decades ago. A bone scan is useful, but I never found any other test of value.

Diagnosing sepsis is a bit like the diagnosis of schizophrenia. If you think about it, that is probably what it is. Listen to the patient. The pain of infection has been present since the operation. it is constant, often worse at night. If the components are not loose, it is non-mechanical. Unlike RSD it is helped by morphine.

The best test is a straightforward X-ray. The loosening rates of knee replacement now are so low, or if properly done in the first case should be so low, that loosening means infection. Early loosening of any component is a sign of infection and loosening of both components is definitely infected. And don't let the Infectious Disease doctors tell you otherwise. If I was clinically convinced of infection I kept all patients on antibiotics for a year.

If the infection is not overt at the time of revision, then an immediate exchange can be tried. If it is overt, I preferred a temporary prosthesis. Only primary TKA components should be used, cemented in place with antibiotic laden cement. I used to fill all bone defects with antibiotic-laden resorbable artificial bone graft. And then wait. If the patient is coping, there is no hurry about doing a definitive exchange. The longer the temporary prosthesis remains in place the more host bone regenerates, which makes revision easier. I had some patients pass on years later with their temporary prosthesis still in place.

One cost saving trick, if your hospital will let you, is to reuse the implant you are taking out. Remove all stems, bells and whistles, autoclave it and cement back in the femoral component and the plastic tibia only. The plastic is damaged, but so what? It is going to be replaced again anyway.

19.6 Instability

The patellofemoral joint and the tibiofemoral joint have to be considered separately.

A dislocated patella is not something I have seen for 30 years as now most surgeons are reasonably competent. But patellar maltracking leading to pain is not that uncommon. Unless the condition is congenital patellar dislocation, of which I have only seen two cases, the problem is never the patella maltracking, it is internal rotation of the femoral component.

The usual cause for this is a valgus knee with an underdeveloped posterior lateral femoral condyle. If the surgeon is unaware of this condition and uses posterior referencing guides, he will always internally rotate the femoral component. If they notice this during the operation they may try to compensate with a lateral release.

Two wrongs do not make a right. They simply make a mess which someone else will have to clean up.

If you find intraoperatively that you are thinking about a lateral release, remember that it is almost always the patella which is tracking properly. So externally rotate the femoral component to match the patella. And remember, if you are doing that, build up anteromedial, and resect posteromedial. Do not resect anterolateral as that results in significant notching.

Tibiofemoral instability can be in all planes. AP, mediolateral and rotation. Lateral Rotatory instability was the hardest to understand [5]. It never happened medially. Initially I had all sorts of theories but eventually realised that it was due to external tibial torsion. I never saw a problem from internal tibial torsion, a fact which I constantly have to share with the anxious parents of little children who in-toe when they walk.

A cruciate retaining knee must not be used in these cases. Up to 30° of tibial torsion can be handled by a high central post knee. If it is more than that, I preferred to do a proximal tibial derotation osteotomy as an interim procedure, and I waited for a year or two to make sure that I had not devascularised the tibial metaphysis. One of my partners, John Cameron, frequently used to do it during total knee replacement. But thinking of the potential problems of non-union of the osteotomy and avascular necrosis, I never had the courage to do that.

Mediolateral instability is usually due to rupture of the MCL or loosening and sinking of the knee. One does see it in patients with Marfan's syndrome, who fortunately are very uncommon. They are very difficult to treat, as they run into knee problems at an early age. At two or three years, a perfectly done knee will be showing instability. You will have to revise it once otherwise the patient will simply not believe you, that stretching of the ligaments is inevitable, as it is with a Charcot joint. Start off with as thin a plastic as possible. At two years an 8 mm poly will show instability. When you revise, it will be necessary to go to 14 mm and in two years the knee will again be unstable. Do not use a rotating hinge as inevitably there will be major problems and these patients are far too young for a fixed axis non-rotating hinge. After his first revision the patient will have to realise that he must use a hinged knee brace for the rest of his life. Hopefully you will never see a case.

If mediolateral instability is due to component wear or sinkage, revision is straightforward. If it is due to rupture or stretching of the MCL, then in general thickening the plastic alone is seldom satisfactory. It is much better to go with a high central post knee. Just remember, if you thicken the poly only, you are producing a patella baja, so be mindful of that.

I have never found attempts to tighten the MCL or LCL of value. It is theoretically possible if it is done by advancing the bony attachment such as the whole medial or lateral epicondyle, and fixing it with a screw, in the same way I have described releasing the lateral epicondyle in a severe fixed valgus knee [6], but it is very difficult to find the isometric point.

Ken Krakow did describe how to tighten the LCL by doing a shortening osteotomy of the fibula, but as the shortening takes place through the bed of the lateral popliteal nerve, I never had the courage to try.

Correcting AP instability is difficult. Simply thickening the poly is usually a very short-term solution as the knee will rapidly stretch out. If you feel you have to try that, make the poly thick enough to give a 5 to 10° fixed flexion deformity. It is much better to go with a high central post knee. Even that may not be enough. If the flexion space is greater than 2cms the femoral component may be able to jump the post, so brace these patients in full extension for several weeks, hoping that they never get good flexion.

It is preferable however to narrow the flexion gap by building up the femoral component posteriorly. If the company does not make a posterior spacer, then put a couple of screws in the posterior femoral condyles leaving them protruding to hold the component out to length until the cement hardens. These patients also should be left with a fixed flexion deformity of 5° at the close of the operation. They will almost certainly work it out.

If the flexion gap is 3 or 4 cm there is no alternative to a fixed axis hinge. Preferably not one that rotates, as these can produce severe patellofemoral problems, which are almost impossible to correct.

19.7 Pain

This is an interesting and puzzling field, mostly because of our complete inability to measure it. As Lord Kelvin said, "if you can't measure it, you know nothing about it." My research nurse, Yvonne Ramlall and I have found that all current measurements, such as an analogue scale, are useless [7]. We have adopted a scale which relies on what the patient does, not says.

Grade 1—no medication.

Grade 2—A- occasional OTC analgesics.

    B—regular OTC.

Grade 3—A- occasional opioids.

    B—regular opioids.

Grade 4—neurogenic/ RSD.

Everyone feels pain at the same temperature, but the emotional reaction to pain is quite different. When you touch a hot stove, your reflexes pull your hand away immediately without you thinking about it. Someone said that the reason you feel pain is to remind you not to do that action again.

The simplest division of pain is mechanical, which means that when you move it hurts, such as the pain of a broken bone, and nonmechanical, which is unrelated to activity. Mechanical pain is helped or controlled by opiates.

Excluding the patellofemoral joint, which is a separate issue, mechanical knee pain is usually from loosening. The history is quite characteristic. The knee goes from painless to painful. The sensation of wear is different. The worn knee is not necessarily painful, but the patient knows something has changed. This is seldom seen in knees nowadays, but is still seen in hips.

The hallmark of loosening is a new pain which is 'start up'. 'Start-up 'means that when the patient first bears weight, they have to stand for a minute or so before they can walk. What is happening is that at rest fluid enters the gap between the implant and bone. This will not tolerate weight, as it is an unstable loading platform. When loaded, the fluid is forced out, and when the implant rests on bone the patient can walk. Patients don't know this and therefore it is usually organic. It doesn't matter what the X-rays look like, the implant is loose, and if the patient lives long enough, it will have to be revised.

It must be clearly understood that minor loosening and some pain does not necessarily mean that a revision is required. An elderly, low demand patient may be reasonably content knowing what the problem is and that revision can be carried out if necessary.

Nonmechanical pain is an extremely difficult, even when divided into neurogenic and non-neurogenic.

Causalgia, or a nerve injury is now called Complex Regional Pain Syndrome, Type 2. It is fortunately exceedingly rare in TKR surgery. Division or injury to the infrapatellar branch of the saphenous nerve occurs in about 25% of cases. Patients will notice numbness, and some have local tenderness over the neuroma. This is best handled with a simple explanation, which satisfies most patients. Repetitive finger tapping on the neuroma often dulls the symptoms.

Damage to the fibular nerve can occur, but fortunately seldom produces causalgia. There may be many causes of this, but after I stopped using a laterally placed Hohmann retractor I never saw another case.

Complex Regional Pain Syndrome, Type 1, or Reflex Sympathetic Dystrophy is not that common, and in consequence, most surgeons miss the diagnosis as they may never see a case. As in the early days, I did many revisions, at one time I collected 40 cases. My favourite pain expert in Toronto always told me that I was over-diagnosing these cases, and she may have been correct.

The diagnosis is non-mechanical pain, usually worse at night, not relieved by opiates, and unaffected by a knee revision. In some cases, the pain may have predated the knee replacement. There is always allodynia, or skin sensitivity, which usually extends above and below the knee. There are very seldom the classic skin changes seen in RSD of the hand or foot. Bone scan changes may be equivocal. Given the subjective nature of this diagnosis, one can readily understand why many surgeons question its authenticity, especially if compensation is at issue.

The best treatment I found was a lumbar sympathetic block, which was effective in about 40% of cases [8]. But in the last couple of decades I could not find anyone who was capable of doing these. You can tell if the block is in the correct place by placing a thermocouple on the big toe. The toe temperature must go up by 2 °C. If the patient does not respond with two blocks it is ineffective and further blocks will not help.

Nowadays I use Lyrica, or if that is ineffective or the patient cannot tolerate the dose required, which occurs in 40% of cases, then the antidepressant Cymbalta may be of value. I found no other drugs of any use. If the patient can tolerate it, aerobic exercise helps. Aerobic means you sweat. If you do so, you release endorphins in the brain, the so-called runner's high, which seems to help RSD. The only possible way they can get aerobic is an exercise bicycle or better, an elliptical trainer. Obviously, this is simply not possible for elderly patients. The Lyrica must start with a very low dose and be built up gradually. If there is no effect by six weeks there will not be an effect so it should be stopped. If it works then the patient should stay on it for six months to a year and very gradually decrease the dose.

In general, a revision does not help these cases, but I did it twice as the patients were very stiff, changing the knee from a PS-Knee to a high central post knee. These patients did get better, so we have a long way to go in our understanding of this condition.

Perceived pain is an interesting topic, and probably comprises the largest group seen by an experienced knee surgeon for a second opinion. These cases require careful consideration as the cause is often a deep-rooted unhappiness with life, and this is difficult, as there may be no good answer. I will describe a few groups, but doubtless there are many others. It is very important that the young surgeon knows of at least some of these conditions, otherwise a great deal of unnecessary and unhelpful revision surgery will occur.

19.8 Workman's Compensation Knee

A change in legislation made this less of a problem than it used to be. In the late 70 s my colleagues and I looked at knee revisions in Toronto, we found that the only cases which ended in amputation were all WCB. The reason was that as long as the patient complained of pain he would be paid and the more operations the more money they got. This was therefore a huge incentive, not only to continue to complain but also to submit oneself to further surgery.

There were other cultural reasons. In the 70 s Toronto was bursting with immigrants bent on fame and fortune. Those who were not working were not regarded with favour by family or friends, unless they had some sort of medical excuse. Times have changed and this is no longer an issue, so the necessity to seem to be disabled has decreased. It is still there, especially with new immigrants who don't quite understand how the system works. The old joke about Jesus going around laying on hands healing the sick still applies. "Don't touch me," says one cripple, "I'm on compensation."

In the seventies and eighties, it was so bad that our recommendations were that compensation knees were not to be revised for pain complaints. Repeated unnecessary revisions were ending in infection and amputation. The low back has been the target organ for compensation complaints since compensation was introduced and a young joint replacement surgeon would do well running a back clinic for a few months to develop a healthy scepticism. A personal injuries medico-legal practice, under the supervision of an experienced lawyer, is also quite helpful.

For inexperienced surgeons who might be inclined to ignore the effects of compensation I should point out a study I did on return to work in the car plants [9], where the men are on their feet on the assembly line for 8 to 12 h shifts. My patients returned to work usually at around six months. The patients of Adolph Lombardi in Columbus, Ohio, returned to similar work in three months. I know Adolph is a good surgeon, but I did not think he was that much better than I was. Eventually we found that Canadian car workers had benefits for 6 months, while in the US it was for three months.

19.9   Perceived Pain

This is possibly the biggest group of post-surgery knee pain. In Europe it is called The Princess And The Pea Syndrome. A classic European princess can feel a pea on her bed under 7 mattresses. Why it should be seven I don't know, it just is.

These patients complain of pain after surgery and usually there is nothing to find. The history is frequently of long-standing pain complaints, with multiple injections of this and that, multiple knee scopes when arthroscopy was popular, and finally a knee replacement which did not change the pain. These patients do not have allodynia, and many seem to have 'belle indifference' and really are not taking much in the way of analgesics in spite of their agony.

It is relatively easy to separate these people from drug seekers. If they are on opiates, the dose has not been increasing. If one can get the preoperative X-rays, usually the degree of arthritic change was pretty minimal. So, it is quite understandable why the TKA didn't help. There is always some pain or at least some awareness of a knee post-surgery. Patients can forget which hip was replaced, but no patient ever has to think which knee was done. If the pain prior to knee replacement was not much, then the pain after will be no better.

It was for this reason that I would only operate if the standing X-ray showed bone on bone. I was totally uninterested in what the MRI reported, as it is far too sensitive. Perhaps I was too slow to operate. In an unpublished study, I once compared my results of hip replacement with Wayne Paprosky in Chicago and Chit Ranawat in New York. This was when my waiting list in Toronto was over two years. Canada has a state medicare and private practice is illegal. At year one, the American patients, who don't wait for anything, scored better in the Harris rating system, which I sort of expected. What was of interest was that at year five, a certain percentage of Canadian patients still lagged behind. We never got around to publishing that, but a later study, eventually showed that if the patient pre op was below 60 or 70 in the rating, they never got back up to 100 [10]. I don't know of any comparable knee studies, but I suspect that that is true there also.

These Princess and the Pea cases should not have revision surgery as it will not help. Eventually, after a few years, most accept the situation, and the complaints tail off. To gain a better understanding of these cases, I would recommend that young surgeons read Dr Ian Macnab's book 'Backache'. He was an experienced spine surgeon who developed many of the validity tests we routinely use in examining the back, such as pseudorotation, dissociated straight leg raising, bent leg raising and hip rotation, to differentiate true sciatica from pain complaints.

He describes many categories of back pain, but some of these translate well into knee pain. There is the Racehorse syndrome, the Razor's Edge, the Worried Sick, the Last Straw, and Concealed Emotional Breakdown. Above all things, remember that surgery on the soma does not help the psyche.

19.10 The Flat on Flat Knee

This is the one exception to the rule to avoid revision if you are not absolutely sure what the problem is. If a patient with a 'flat on flat' knee *(older designs with a flat polyethylene and a flat femoral component in the coronal plane)* complains of pain, even if there is nothing obvious, I would recommend revising it. Quite why a 'flat on flat' knee should be so sensitive to presumably the most minor error which would not bother a 'round on round' knee I do not know. I would simply revise it to a high central post knee.

19.11 Drug Seekers

Surgeons have always been deeply concerned about those who are on opiates prior to knee replacement. Our impression has always been that they do not do well. However, in a study conducted by my research nurse, Yvonne Ramlall [7], to our surprise we found that this was not the case, and many did indeed get off opiates post-surgery. Our numbers however were so small that I hesitate to draw any definitive conclusion, and I would suggest that this question still needs study.

I did and do have some patients on chronic opiates, but as long as their intake remains level, I simply accept it. I do not increase the dose and do not accept that 'the dog ate the prescription'. Eventually drug seekers go away to find some softer touch.

19.12   Conclusion

For the young surgeon, unless it is an infected case, do not rush into a revision. If you are uncertain, have the patient seen by senior colleagues and other surgeons across the town. Spread the grief around. If it is unclear what the problem is today, maybe tomorrow or next month or next year will make it obvious.

Top Tip: *Festina lente*, hasten slowly. Apart from infection, fractures and tendon ruptures, don't do anything today you can put off until tomorrow.

References

1. Cameron HU. *Have Knife Will Travel. 2019; 1–152. Xlibris US. ISBN: 9781796053418.* 2019: Xlibris US. 1–152.
2. Kilgus DJ, et al. Catastrophic wear of tibial polyethylene inserts. Clin Orthop Relat Res. 1991;273:223–31.
3. Cameron HU, Cameron GM. The patellar meniscus in total knee replacement. Orthop Rev. 1987;16(3):170–2.
4. Vince K. et al. *'Gull-wing' osteotomy of the patella in total knee arthroplasty.* American Association of Hip and Knee Surgeons Nonth Annual Meeting. Dallas, TX. J Arthroplasty. 1999:254.
5. Hughes JD, et al. Diagnosis and treatment of rotatory knee instability. J Exp Orthop. 2019;6 (1):48.
6. Cameron HU, Botsford DJ, Park YS. Prognostic factors in the outcome of supracondylar femoral osteotomy for lateral compartment osteoarthritis of the knee. Can J Surg. 1997;40 (2):114–8.
7. Ramlall Y, et al. Examining pain before and after primary total knee replacement (TKR): A retrospective chart review. Int J Orthop Trauma Nurs. 2019;34:43–7.
8. Cameron HU, Park YS, Krestow M. Reflex sympathetic dystrophy following total knee replacement. Contemp Orthop. 1994;29(4):279–81.
9. Cameron HU, Wadey VMR, Silverman F. The post-operative painful knee—Clinical and societal causation. Seminars in Arthroplasty. 2015;26(4):251–4.
10. Fortin PR, et al. Timing of total joint replacement affects clinical outcomes among patients with osteoarthritis of the hip or knee. Arthritis Rheum. 2002;46(12):3327–30.

A Lifetime of Revision Knee Arthroplasty

20

Peter J James

> *Let our advance worrying become advance thinking and planning Winston Churchill.*

20.1 Introduction

Your career is often defined by those who teach you in your formative years. It was my time spent under the guidance of *Professor David Beverland* that formed the basis of my understanding and philosophy of TKA surgery. I have taken these principles, built on them and applied them to my revision TKA practice with some success. I am indebted to David for his mentorship, advice and guidance which continues to this day.

20.2 It is All About Planning

In providing a set of messages and lessons to arthroplasty surgeons throughout this book, the one word that I would emphasise is *planning*. A successful outcome of revision surgery will only come to fruition by identifying and understanding the problem in the primary knee. Never be forced to operate on an unhappy knee unless you fully understand the mechanism of failure; only then can you plan your solution.

Once you plan the solution, the most important next step is getting adequate *exposure*. I do believe that this is the most important step in revision surgery. If you can see what you are doing, protect the important structures i.e. extensor

© The Author(s), under exclusive license to Springer Nature Switzerland AG 2021
H. E. Matar et al., *Revision Total Knee Arthroplasty*,
https://doi.org/10.1007/978-3-030-81285-0_20

mechanism, collateral ligaments (when present), and posterior capsule, then it becomes a predictable technical exercise in positioning the joint line, balancing the gaps and getting fixation. Always be patient, clear the gutters, clear the posterior space, and consider early extensile exposure through a tibial crest osteotomy. What I have learnt over years of practice is that if you do not clear the posterior space, you will have an apparently slack flexion gap when in fact what you actually have is a tight extension gap due to scarring and granulation tissues in the posterior space.

Plan your surgical reconstruction, the alphabet has 26 letters, always have alternative plans in a stepwise fashion particularly when you are starting out in revision practice or have a low-volume practice. Plan your joint line, plan your constraint, and plan your fixation. You should know beforehand whether the collateral ligaments are intact or not, whether the joint line is raised or not i.e. do you need to distalise with augments, what type of fixation you are aiming for i.e. metaphyseal fixation, press-fit diaphyseal fixation, cemented or hybrid fixation.

Having all those plans in mind before you start the operation makes the whole process more fluent and efficient which leads to familiarity and getting to a consistent endpoint.

Implant removal for a primary cemented knee is relatively straightforward gently working on the implant–cement interface. Find out as much as you can about the implants you are planning to take out particularly in re-revision cases focusing on areas of fixation, modular junctions, special instruments and compatibility for single component revisions in some cases.

20.3 Frame Principle

Here, I would reiterate the point which has been made repeatedly throughout this book. What is the difference between a primary TKA and a condylar revision? Someone has been there before, but we can deal with that through adequate exposure. There is missing bone, but we can deal with that using revision components. Providing we have intact collaterals, all that we are trying to achieve is having stable tibial and femoral components within the collateral frame that are balanced in flexion and extension throughout the range of motion. The logical way of achieving that is by getting a stable tibial platform against which gap balancing can be done within the frame. I always start with the flexion space, balancing it with appropriately sized trials in terms of anteroposterior and mediolateral dimensions as well as rotation. Here, the routine use of tibial metaphyseal sleeves offers great advantages in balancing the frame in an efficient and reproducible manner. A tibial metaphyseal trial sleeve gives me a stable platform to work with akin to that of a primary knee after the tibial bony cut. One might ask if there any alternatives? The problem I have had with using press-fit stems is that it is very difficult to get an absolutely stable tibial platform to gap balance off when the trial stem and component is rocking mediolaterally; even with a larger diameter stem which requires extensive reaming with the potential problems that can ensue. On the femoral side, however, it is different. Metaphyseal sleeves are only indicated when you have significant metaphyseal or condylar bone loss. All that is needed here is some stability to the trial components to balance with before making any bony cuts. This is achieved through a system that delivers that ability during preparation such as cut through trials or cutting guides attached to stable intramedullary trial stems. In many series, including my own, metaphyseal sleeves have proven to provide excellent long-term fixation and durability in addition to their role in reconstructing the joint within the frame principle.

20.4 Choice of Constraint

The emerging evidence and survivorship data from joint registries and large series supports my view that some degree of rotational freedom in the reconstruction is beneficial. This is not surprising; the difference in outcomes between a fixed- and a rotating-hinge is only too obvious. Using a fixed-bearing VVC-type constraint in the construct does have an impact in terms of torque transmission to the fixation interfaces. The divergence in survivorship data between a rotating-platform (RP) VVC implant with metaphyseal sleeves versus fixed-bearing VVC implants is becoming obvious in longitudinal survivorship data. In my view, an RP-VVC type construct gives the stability and reassurance of a VVC without any detrimental effect on fixation as the torque is dissipated with the presence of an RP insert. This has long been my practice and it is evident in my series that this approach has been successful with the RP-VVC having no negative impact on durability of fixation. If I do not have an intact MCL, then I believe a hinge implant is the only alternative. A VVC implant can cope with LCL deficiency, up to a point, as the IT band gives some dynamic stability laterally, but certainly not with MCL deficiency.

20.5 Fixation

In my practice, the use of metaphyseal tibial sleeves is mandatory to simplify the process and establish a stable tibial platform with durable fixation near the joint line. On the femoral side, in most simple revisions there is usually a relatively stable distal femur to work with and femoral sleeves are unnecessary adjuncts in simple revision surgery. However, I do maintain the benefits of having fixation close to the joint line. Short cemented stems are therefore the logical alternative when there is good bone stock and when only using smaller augments; no more than 8 mm.

20.6   Infection

It is evident that managing periprosthetic joint infection in modern practice has to be within a multidisciplinary team approach with involvement of microbiology specialists and meticulous surgical technique. Increasingly, single stage revisions are becoming more widespread with the usual caveats of patients' selection, status of soft tissues and the infecting organism.

20.7   Megaprostheses

Unfortunately, periprosthetic fractures are becoming more common and likely to increase over time. For comminuted fractures, the use of distal femoral replacements gives reliable outcomes with early mobilisation and are being used more frequently. Similarly, a lot of patients are coming to their third or fourth revisions with depleted bone stock with salvage options relying on distal femoral replacements or proximal tibial replacements. This is an area where further development in implants is needed over time, particularly in terms of fixation, as their use becomes more prevalent in arthroplasty patients. Remember, most of these implants were originally developed for tumour patients, often young with good periosteum that allows for a secondary fixation interface.

20.8   Learning Never Stops

Self-discipline in planning revision cases is incredibly important. Even with extensive experience in the field, once can still face unexpected scenarios and you have to be prepared for it. For example, a tertiary case was referred to me—an elderly lady with longstanding rheumatoid arthritis and recent inability to mobilise. Plain radiographs clearly show an old periprosthetic fracture around the stem of a revision femoral component with significant bone loss and an ipsilateral hip replacement (Fig. 1a). Seemingly, the complexity here is all around the femoral component and how to salvage this situation using a distal femoral replacement. Do I have enough bone proximally to cement a DFR? What to do with the junction between the hip stem and the DFR?

However, planning what to do with the tibia is equally important. This is an old design with grit-blasted roughened surface along the length of its cemented stem (*Biomet Rotating Hinge*). It may well be the case that when you deal with old unfamiliar implants, this information can be easily overlooked. Although in this case, tibial extraction may look relatively straightforward, but for a grit blasted cemented stem nothing could be further from the truth. The initial plan is therefore to work on the implant cement interface, remove the component leaving the cement behind and consider cement-in-cement revision. Plan *B* would be to do a crest

(i)

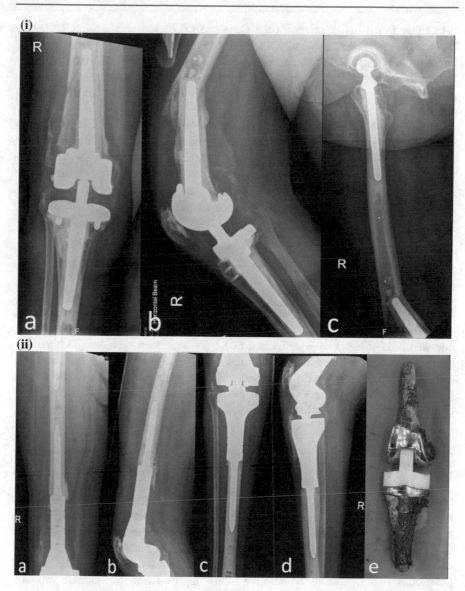

(ii)

Fig. 1 **i** Preoperative anteroposterior and lateral radiograph of right knee and femur with an old periprosthetic fracture around the tip of revision femoral component with significant bone loss and an ipsilateral total hip replacement. **ii** Postoperative radiographs following distal femoral replacement and proximal tibial replacements

osteotomy to get better access to the stem and work around it. Failing that, in a rheumatoid osteopaenic bone with a well-fixed implant, our plan C was to negate an uncontrolled complication and consider osteotomising the proximal tibia and plan for a proximal tibial replacement. On the femoral side the plan was for a DFR, protecting the junction between the hip and the DFR stem with intramedullary cement.

Intraoperatively, extraction attempts of the tibial component with varying manoeuvres were unsuccessful. A proximal tibial replacement was the only alternative for this case (Fig. 1b). The lesson here is that you have to predict the potential problems and difficulty and have the resources to deal with it before you start surgery. A multidisciplinary approach, and discussions with like-minded colleagues, is very important to bring one's attention to certain aspects that may have been overlooked.

20.9 Personal Series

Over the years, I have been fortunate in achieving satisfactory outcomes applying the principles outlined in this book. Using the UK *National Joint Registry* data, between 2005–2018, I have performed 604 unique revision episodes (36 bilateral), excluding secondary patella resurfacings. Multiple operations for infection, for example, including a DAIR, 1st stage and 2nd stage in the same knee are all counted as one revision episode. My re-revision rate for any cause was 4.5%, this is externally validated nationally collected mandated data ensuring high validity.

20.10 Future of Revision Knee Arthroplasty

Great advances have been made in revision surgery with ever increasing portfolios of revision systems and versatility to deal with difficult scenarios. Although digital technology and navigation techniques are being used in primary knees which are fairly consistent and repeatable procedures, revision cases are unique with often the need for intraoperative surgical decision making and judgment calls. The surgical process, however, remains an area for future improvement to minimise variation and standardise care. With the projected increased burden of revision surgery, working within a specialist network with a collaborative structure has proven beneficial in driving up standards and improving outcomes.

20.11 Conclusion

This book represents most of what I have learnt as I have developed my revision knee practice. As with all surgeons, early setbacks occur which can test your resolve particularly in this area of work. Taking advice, working closely with colleagues and for difficult cases dual consultant operating are all important attributes for a successful outcome even with experience.

I hope this book helps surgeons by delivering a simplified approach to the management of patients requiring revision TKA. It has been a pleasure to work with my co-authors on this book to produce what I believe to be a practical guide to this complex subject. I hope you gain as much from reading it as I have from contributing to it.

Finally, as Winston Churchill put it, success is not final, failure is not fatal, it is the courage to continue that counts.

Index

A

Allograft reconstruction, 40, 170, 208, 269, 271, 272, 275, 316

Amputation, 195, 196, 202, 208, 209, 213, 219, 236, 238, 307, 327

Anterior knee pain, 14, 61, 62

Arthrotomy, 94, 97, 180, 215, 227, 253, 289

Aseptic loosening, 59, 67, 68, 72, 75, 77, 81, 151, 154, 155, 163, 166, 169, 178, 181, 191, 192, 195, 219, 220, 230, 294, 306, 311, 320

Aseptic revision knee arthroplasty, 305

B

Balanced approach, 5, 6, 11–13, 26, 34, 62, 84, 123–127, 129, 137, 143

Bone scan, 64, 323, 326

C

Cam-post mechanism, 165

Cemented components, 320

Cementless components, 122, 307

Clinical assessment, 230, 290

Clinical outcomes, 1, 12, 40, 74, 103, 163, 169, 181, 189, 204, 219, 283, 287, 290, 291, 294, 295

Complex primary knee arthroplasty, 17, 45–47, 170, 209

Condylar revision, 72, 77, 79, 123, 124, 127, 130, 139, 142, 163, 166, 234, 235, 332

Constraint, 34, 42, 63, 77, 83, 129, 140, 148, 163–166, 168, 169, 176, 197, 227, 307, 332, 333

Cruciate-substituting, 13, 320

Culture negative infections, 226, 238, 307

D

DAIR, 119, 150, 226–229, 241, 306, 307, 336

Distal femoral replacement, 44, 148, 169, 170, 180, 196, 274, 287–289, 291, 296, 334, 335

E

Examination under anaesthetic, 63, 83

Extensor mechanism failure, 170–172, 174, 191, 208, 269

Extensor mechanism reconstruction, 209, 269, 271, 273

F

Fixation, 2, 10, 12, 13, 17–19, 26–28, 30, 35, 40, 42, 46, 62, 72, 74, 77, 79, 81, 82, 99, 103, 107, 108, 110–112, 114, 116, 118–120, 123, 124, 126, 128, 129, 139–143, 145, 147, 148, 151, 154, 156, 157, 163–166, 168, 169, 175, 177, 179, 180, 185, 196–198, 202, 204, 206, 210, 215, 217, 231, 235, 270, 271, 273–275, 288 291, 293, 295, 320, 332–334

Fixed-hinge implants, 164, 172, 188, 208, 272

Frame principle, 4, 5, 14, 26, 42, 45, 123, 125, 130, 132, 139, 156, 332, 333

G

Gap balancing, 3, 13, 332

H

Hinge implants, 17, 44, 84, 169, 174, 197, 333

Hinge kinematics, 174

Hybrid fixation, 74, 77, 79, 135, 136, 139, 142, 156, 198, 216, 332

I

Implant-arthrodesis, 195, 209–212, 236
Implant removal, 94, 107, 332
Infection, 2, 27, 42, 59, 60, 62, 67, 68, 81, 82,
        120, 142, 150, 151, 163, 169, 181, 188,
        191, 192, 195, 196, 207, 209–213, 219,
        220, 223–232, 235–237, 241, 245–250,
        269, 275, 283, 291, 294, 305–307, 310,
        311, 315, 316, 319, 323, 327, 330, 334,
        336
Infrapatellar defects, 247, 248
Instability, 2–5, 10, 12, 17, 40–43, 59–63, 68,
        70, 74, 82–84, 86, 88, 125, 128, 129,
        150, 163, 169, 172, 174, 176, 177, 181,
        183, 186, 189, 191, 192, 195, 203, 209,
        231, 233, 251, 252, 262, 306, 311, 319,
        320, 322–325

J

Joint line, 10, 11, 42, 43, 70, 79, 86–88, 96, 98,
        99, 103, 123–130, 139–143, 145, 148,
        149, 165, 166, 168, 172, 174, 180, 185,
        200, 202, 216, 217, 231, 270, 272,
        287–290, 296, 307, 332, 333

L

Local flaps, 233, 249
Long-term outcomes, 17, 19, 139

M

Massive endoprosthesis, 195–198, 208, 287
Matar procedure, 251
Measured resection, 5, 12, 13
Medial gastrocnemius flap, 245, 248
Metal augments, 143
Metaphyseal cones, 142
Metaphyseal sleeves, 19, 35, 72, 84, 107, 118,
        120, 128, 130, 139–143, 148, 149, 151,
        152, 154–156, 170, 179, 180, 214, 216,
        231, 235, 290, 332, 333
Mid-flexion instability, 62, 63, 83, 84, 163
Mobile-bearing, 2, 12, 136, 141, 142, 148, 163,
        166, 180, 214, 290
Mortality, 219, 223, 236, 288, 290, 292, 294,
        305–307, 309–311, 315
Multidisciplinary team approach, 65, 220, 245,
        246, 250, 311, 334

O

Open reduction and internal fixation, 288, 302

P

Painful total knee arthroplasty, 60, 62, 63, 65,
        225
Patella dislocation, 41, 219, 251, 264, 265, 291
Patella resurfacing, 2, 14, 61, 64, 68, 81, 255,
        270, 336
Patellectomy, 17, 40–42, 183
Patellofemoral complications, 183
Patellofemoral joint, 35, 40, 42, 61, 128, 130,
        166, 270, 296, 323, 325
Patient-specific instrumentations, 17
Periarticular fracture, 26, 28, 30
Periprosthetic joint infection, 59, 68, 223, 229,
        305, 334
Periprosthetic knee fractures, 287, 288, 295
Polyethylene wear, 34, 67, 68, 71, 74, 306
Posterior space, 11, 69, 84, 85, 90, 94, 95,
        124–126, 130, 227, 229, 235, 332
Press-fit stems, 72, 126, 128, 139–141, 332
Primary total knee arthroplasty, 1, 70
Proximal tibial replacement, 79, 178, 196, 214,
        219, 288, 316, 334–336

R

Removal of metaphyseal sleeves, 120
Revising unicompartmental knee arthroplasty,
        17, 34
Rotating-hinge implants, 23, 164, 169, 170,
        179, 181, 184, 191, 197, 283, 302
Rotational constraint, 129, 165, 166, 176, 197

S

Salvage endoprosthesis, 79, 195, 198, 202,
        208, 213, 235
Salvage surgery, 195
Septic revision knee arthroplasty, 305
Single-stage revision, 223, 235, 236, 241, 307,
        334
Soft tissue defects, 229, 234, 236, 241, 245
Stiffness, 5, 42, 68, 88, 89, 95, 142, 191, 192,
        306, 319, 321, 322
Surgical approach, 1, 2, 18, 22
Synovectomy, 89, 94, 97, 111, 180, 215, 227,
        229, 231

T

Tibial crest osteotomy, 19, 42, 89, 93, 95, 97,
        103, 107, 109, 119, 198, 332
Two-stage revision, 223, 229, 236, 306, 307

V

Varus-valgus constraint, 129, 166, 197
Vastus medialis advancement, 253, 255, 262

Printed in the United States
by Baker & Taylor Publisher Services